Management of Limb-Length Discrepancies

EDITED BY

Reggie C. Hamdy, MB, ChB, MSc, FRCSC
Chief of Staff, Shriners Hospital for Children, Canada
Associate Professor of Surgery, Montreal Children's Hospital
Director of Pediatric Orthopaedics, McGill University
Montreal, Quebec, Canada

James J. McCarthy, MD
Director of Pediatric Orthopaedic Surgery
Alvin Crawford Chair in Pediatric Orthopaedics
Professor, Department of Orthopaedic Surgery
University of Cincinnati College of Medicine
Cincinnati Children's Hospital Medical Center
Cincinnati, Ohio

SERIES EDITOR

Henry D. Clarke, MD
Consultant, Department of Orthopedic Surgery
Associate Professor of Orthopedic Surgery, College of Medicine
Mayo Clinic
Phoenix, Arizona

AAOS
AMERICAN ACADEMY OF ORTHOPAEDIC SURGEONS

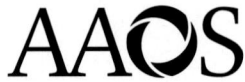

AAOS
AMERICAN ACADEMY OF ORTHOPAEDIC SURGEONS

Management of Limb-Length Discrepancies

Published 2011 by the
American Academy of Orthopaedic Surgeons
6300 North River Road
Rosemont, IL 60018

The material presented in *Management of Limb-Length Discrepancies* has been made available by the American Academy of Orthopaedic Surgeons for educational purposes only. This material is not intended to present the only, or necessarily best, methods or procedures for the medical situations discussed, but rather is intended to represent an approach, view, statement, or opinion of the author(s) or producer(s), which may be helpful to others who face similar situations.

Some drugs or medical devices demonstrated in Academy courses or described in Academy print or electronic publications have not been cleared by the Food and Drug Administration (FDA) or have been cleared for specific uses only. The FDA has stated that it is the responsibility of the physician to determine the FDA clearance status of each drug or device he or she wishes to use in clinical practice.

Furthermore, any statements about commercial products are solely the opinion(s) of the author(s) and do not represent an Academy endorsement or evaluation of these products. These statements may not be used in advertising or for any commercial purpose.

ISBN: 978-0-89203-746-9
Printed in the USA

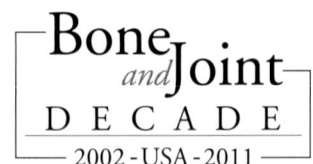

Bone *and* Joint
DECADE
2002 - USA - 2011

CONTRIBUTORS

John G. Birch, MD
Assistant Chief of Staff
Texas Scottish Rite Hospital for Children
Dallas, Texas

Timothy P. Carey, MD
Associate Professor
Department of Orthopedic Surgery
University of Western Ontario
London, Ontario, Canada

Sonia Chaudhry, MD
Resident Physician
Department of Orthopaedic Surgery
NYU Hospital for Joint Diseases
New York, New York

George Cierny III, MD
Senior Consultant
REO Orthopaedics
San Diego, California

Janet D. Conway, MD
Head of Bone and Joint Infection
International Center for Limb Lengthening
Rubin Institute for Advanced Orthopedics
Baltimore, Maryland

Maria Julia Cornes, MD
Research Fellow
Department of Orthopaedics
Alfred I. duPont Hospital for Children
Wilmington, Delaware

Doreen DiPasquale, MD
Senior Consultant
REOrthopaedics
San Diego, California

David S. Feldman, MD
Chief of Pediatric Orthopaedic Surgery
Associate Professor of Orthopaedic Surgery
Department of Orthopaedic Surgery
New York University
Hospital for Joint Diseases
New York, New York

Stuart A. Green, MD
Clinical Professor of Orthopaedic Surgery
Department of Orthopaedic Surgery
University of California, Irvine
Orange, California

Reggie C. Hamdy, MB, ChB, MSc, FRCSC
Chief of Staff, Shriners Hospital for Children,
  Canada
Associate Professor of Surgery,
  Montreal Children's Hospital
Director of Pediatric Orthopaedics,
  McGill University
Montreal, Quebec, Canada

John E. Herzenberg, MD, FRCSC
Director
International Center for Limb Lengthening
Head of Pediatric Orthopedics
Rubin Institute for Advanced Orthopedics
Sinai Hospital of Baltimore
Baltimore, Maryland

Joseph Ivan Krajbich, MD, FRCSC
Adjunct Associate Professor
Department of Orthopaedics and Rehabilitation
Oregon Health Sciences University
Staff Surgeon
Shriners Hospital for Children
Portland, Oregon

David W. Lowenberg, MD
Chairman of the Department of Orthopaedic
  Surgery
Co-Director of the Buncke Microsurgical
Research Lab
California Pacific Medical Center
San Francisco, California

William G. Mackenzie, MD, FRCSC, FACS
Chairman
Department of Orthopaedics
Alfred I. duPont Hospital for Children
Wilmington, Delaware

CONTRIBUTORS (CONT.)

James J. McCarthy, MD
Director of Peidatric Orthopaedic Surgery
Alvin Crawford Chair in Pediatric
Orthopaedics
Professor, Department of Orthopaedic Surgery
University of Cincinnati College of Medicine
Cincinnati Children's Hospital Medical Center
Cincinnati, Ohio

Norman Y. Otsuka, MD
Clinical Professor
Department of Orthopaedic Surgery
Shriners Hospitals for Children
Los Angeles, California

Dror Paley, MD, FRCSC
Paley Advanced Limb Lengthening Institute
Joint Preservation and Bone Reconstruction
Center
Saint Mary's Medical Center
West Palm Beach, Flordia

Karl E. Rathjen, MD
Associate Professor
Department of Orthopaedic Surgery
UT Southwestern Medical Center
Texas Scottish Rite Hospital
Dallas, Texas

S. Robert Rozbruch, MD
Chief of Limb Lengthening and Deformity Service
Hospital for Special Surgery
Associate Professor of Clinical Orthopaedic Surgery
Weill Medical College of Cornell University
New York, New York

Sanjeev Sabharwal, MD
Professor, Department of Orthopaedics and
Pediatrics
Chief, Division of Pediatric Orthopaedics
University of Medicine and Dentistry of
New Jersey
Newark, New Jersey

Neil Saran, MD, FRCSC
Department of Pediatric Orthopaedics
McGill University Health Center
Shriners Hospital for Children, Canada
Montreal, Quebec, Canada

Anthony Scaduto, MD
Lowman Professor and Chief of Pediatric
Orthopaedics
Los Angeles Orthopaedic Hospital
University of California, Los Angeles
Los Angeles, California

Alec C. Stall, MD, MPH
Orthopaedic Resident
Department of Orthopaedics
University of Maryland
Baltimore, Maryland

Shawn C. Standard, MD
Pediatric Orthopedic Surgeon
Department of Pediatric Orthopedics
Rubin Institute for Advanced Orthopedics
Sinai Hospital of Baltimore
Baltimore, Maryland

Mihir M. Thacker, MD
Assistant Professor of Orthopedic Surgery and
Pediatrics
Thomas Jefferson University
Philadelphia, Pennsylvania
Attending Orthopedic Surgeon
Alfred I. duPont Hospital for Children
Wilmington, Delaware

Hiroyuki Tsuchiya, MD, PhD
Professor
Department of Orthopaedic Surgery
Graduate School of Medical Science
Kanazawa University
Kanazawa, Japan

Harold J.P. van Bosse, MD
Pediatric Orthopaedic Surgeon
Shriners Hospital for Children
Philadelphia, Pennsylvania

CONTENTS

PREFACE

Limb-length discrepancy (LLD) is a complex and challenging problem encountered not only by orthopaedic surgeons but also by many other medical specialties and allied health care professionals. To properly manage this condition, the treating physician must have in-depth knowledge of all aspects of LLD, including its etiology, its effects on function and gait, its clinical and radiologic assessment, and the many medical and surgical treatment options that are available. Very few books, if any, cover all these aspects of LLD in a single source of information.

This monograph, *Management of Limb-Length Discrepancies,* is an attempt to provide such a comprehensive source of current information. It contains a wealth of information for orthopaedic surgeons, residents, fellows, pediatricians, family medicine and primary care physicians, and allied health care professionals who manage such conditions in both the pediatric and adult populations.

The 22 chapters of this monograph provide cutting-edge information on the etiology, functional effects and disability, and clinical and radiologic assessment of LLD, as well as techniques for predicting LLD at skeletal maturity. Chapters on various treatment options for LLD also are included. Gradual lengthening by distraction osteogenesis, including the newest surgical techniques using both external and internal fixation, is discussed extensively. Lengthening in specific conditions such as congenital deficiencies, upper limb deficiencies, short stature, and soft-tissue contractures and lengthening in adults are addressed. Chapters dealing with bone transport in cases of segmental bone loss secondary to trauma, infection, and tumor provide the most recent information in these fields.

We would like to thank the contributing authors, all recognized leaders in the field, for their valuable time and effort they have dedicated to this monograph. We also would like to acknowledge the efforts of Marilyn Fox, PhD, Director of the Department of Publications; Laurie Braun, Managing Editor; Steven Kellert, Senior Editor; and Michelle Bruno, Publications Assistant, who have guided this project through to its completion. Finally, we would like to acknowledge all of our colleagues for their ongoing efforts to improve the care of patients with LLDs.

Reggie C. Hamdy, MB, ChB, MSc, FRCSC
James J. McCarthy, MD
Editors

CHAPTER 1

PREVALENCE, SIGNIFICANCE, AND ETIOLOGY OF LIMB-LENGTH DISCREPANCIES

NEIL SARAN, MD, FRCSC

PREVALENCE

Limb-length discrepancies (LLDs) are more common than might be expected. Not only are they common in children with congenital or acquired musculoskeletal conditions, but relatively high rates also are seen in healthy individuals, although great variance in the prevalence of LLD is seen in the literature, depending partly on the magnitude of LLD used as a cutoff. Hellsing[1] studied 600 healthy military recruits and found an LLD of 0.5 to 1.5 cm in 32% and an LLD of greater than 1.5 cm in 4%. Rush and Steiner[2] reported an LLD greater than 11 mm in 15% of 1,000 US Army recruits with low back pain. Soukka et al[3] reported an LLD of 1.0 cm or greater in 13% of 247 patients that were evaluated as part of a comprehensive clinical survey of civil servants of the Helsinki City Council. The prevalence of LLD appears to be inversely correlated to the threshold level used to define it.

CLINICAL SIGNIFICANCE

Large LLDs can cause functional scoliosis,[4,5] gait abnormalities,[6] and cosmetic concerns, and some studies suggest that smaller discrepancies (LLDs of 5 to 15 mm) may be associated with low back pain,[5,7] osteoarthritis of the hip,[8] and an increased propensity for knee injuries.[9,10] Friberg[11] reported a higher-than-normal incidence of stress fractures in Finnish Army conscripts with LLDs greater than 1.0 cm. Gurney et al[6] created artificial LLDs in healthy individuals using shoe lifts and showed that an artificial LLD as small as 2 cm could increase oxygen consumption and perceived exertion in older adults as compared with no LLD. Gofton and Trueman[8] reported that 29 of 36 idiopathic cases of hip osteoarthritis were in the longer leg and speculated that increased joint forces predisposed the longer side to osteoarthritis, whereas decreased forces across the shorter side protected it.

Results of many studies suggest that small discrepancies can become symptomatic, whereas others demonstrate that small discrepancies appear to be well tolerated and asymptomatic. Soukka et al[3] examined 247 patients for an association between low back pain and mild LLDs and found that an LLD of up to 10 mm was similar in distribution in the symptom-free group as in the groups with recent or past low back pain. Similarly, a 10- to 20-mm LLD was not associated with low back pain.[3] Hoikka et al[12] examined scoliosis in 100 patients with chronic low back pain and reported poor correlation between scoliosis and LLD ($r = 0.338$). Gross[13] administered a four-question survey to 74 skeletally mature patients with an LLD of 1.5 cm or greater and concluded that little evidence existed to support treating LLDs smaller than 2 cm. Brand and Yack[14] showed that an LLD of up to 2 cm does not significantly alter hip mechanics. Song et al[15] evaluated the gait of 35 children with an LLD of 0.6 to 11.1 cm and found no correlation between the actual discrepancy or percentage of discrepancy and any of the dependent kinematic or kinetic

---

Dr. Saran or an immediate family member has received research or institutional support from Stryker.

TABLE 1 Commonly Seen Causes of LLD

Congenital
  Hemihypertrophy or hemiatrophy
    Idiopathic
    Klippel-Trenaunay-Weber syndrome
    Beckwith-Wiedemann syndrome
  Femoral and tibial dysplasia
    Proximal femoral focal deficiency
    Congenital short femur
    Fibular hemimelia
    Tibial hemimelia
    Posterior medial bowing of the tibia
  Skeletal dysplasia
    Ollier disease
    Multiple hereditary exostosis
    Congenital pseudarthrosis of the tibia
    Neurofibromatosis
    Fibrous dysplasia

Acquired
  Trauma
    Physeal disruption
    Fracture malunion
    Femoral fracture overgrowth
  Infection
    Osteomyelitis
    Septic arthritis
    Fulminant meningococcemia
  Inflammatory arthropathy
  Neuropathic
    Poliomyelitis
    Cerebral palsy
    Myelodysplasia
    Sacral agenesis
  Miscellaneous
    Radiation therapy
    Slipped capital femoral epiphysis
    Legg-Calvé-Perthes disease
    Joint dislocation or contracture
    Suprapelvic obliquity

variables, including pelvic obliquity. They found no compensatory strategies in children with discrepancies less than 3%, whereas increased mechanical work was performed by the long leg and there was a greater displacement of the center of body mass when the discrepancy was 5.5% or more.[15]

Asymptomatic LLD is relatively prevalent in the healthy population, and little evidence exists to support treatment of discrepancies smaller than 2 to 3 cm. Although some studies claim that a small LLD may become symptomatic, no evidence exists to suggest that treatment of a small, asymptomatic LLD will prevent these problems. If artificial equalization of these small LLDs by means of shoe inserts or shoe lifts decreases symptoms in a symptomatic patient with an LLD, then surgical treatment strategies to equalize the LLD can be considered.

The functional and physiologic impairments associated with LLDs greater than 2 to 3 cm are difficult to quantify; however, they are generally associated with an underlying etiology or diagnosis such as those listed in **Table 1**. The direct effect of the LLD in these situations is difficult to discern because separating the effects of the LLD from the associated effects of the underlying diagnosis is difficult. The effects of LLD on pelvic obliquity, scoliosis, and low back pain are highly controversial. Unfortunately, little data exist on such effects in patients with larger LLDs (greater than 2 to 3 cm); however, they have been associated with decreased psychosocial scores. Moraal et al[16] reviewed 37 patients who underwent limb lengthening and found that patients with persistent discrepancies greater than 2 cm had lower "perceived competence" scores and health-related quality-of-life scores compared with those with persistent discrepancies smaller than 2 cm. Vitale et al[17] reported on 76 patients with surgically untreated LLDs and showed that LLD was inversely correlated to psychosocial function. Also, Bhave et al[18] showed that gait parameters are significantly improved after treatment of large LLDs. Multiple studies[18-21] have shown asymmetric gait patterns in patients with LLDs greater than 2 to 3 cm, but the implications of these patterns are not fully understood.

Although evidence is lacking, LLDs may plausibly affect pelvic obliquity, scoliosis, hip arthritis, and low back pain significantly as the magnitude of the discrepancy increases. These anticipated effects and the psychosocial effects of LLDs can warrant surgical treatment of discrepancies greater than 3 to 5 cm.

ETIOLOGY
Classification
The etiologies of LLD often are categorized as congenital or acquired. Etiology is a major factor that influences

both the progression and the treatment strategies of the LLD. **Table 1** lists the most common causes of LLDs.

In 1982, Shapiro[22] reported on lower extremity LLD data in 803 patients, looking specifically at the rate of change in the limb length in skeletally immature patients. **Figure 1** outlines the five major developmental discrepancy patterns described by Shapiro. Although it is not commonly used, the classification provides insight into the different discrepancy patterns and their effects on LLD predictions. Type I is a constant upward slope, indicating that the LLD continues to progress at a constant rate. Complete physeal arrest and congenital LLD are examples of this type of discrepancy pattern. The Paley multiplier method,[23] Menelaus method,[24] Moseley straight-line graph,[25,26] as well as the Anderson, Messner, and Green lengths of normal femur and tibia charts,[27,28] all rely on this type of developmental discrepancy pattern to predict the final LLD at skeletal maturity. Type II starts with an upward slope and is followed by deceleration. This can be a difficult pattern to deal with. If the patient is followed during the first stage and a prediction is made assuming that a type I pattern is occurring, the predicted discrepancy will be larger than the final discrepancy, and early treatment may result in overcorrection. Type III starts with an upward slope and is followed by a plateau. Subtype IIIA starts with a downward slope and then plateaus; subtype IIIB is detected after the initial discrepancy has developed and then remains unchanged. In Shapiro's study, 93% of the femoral diaphyseal fractures followed the type III pattern. Type IV is an upward sloping pattern interrupted by a period of a plateau. This pattern is seen mainly when the etiology involves the proximal femur such as in some cases of septic arthritis and Legg-Calvé-Perthes (LCP) disease. Type V is an upward slope followed by a plateau, then a downward slope. This is a less common pattern except in the setting of LCP disease; 49 of 140 patients with LCP disease followed this pattern. Type I was the usual pattern seen in proximal femoral focal deficiency (proximal longitudinal deficiency of the femur), congenital short femur (CSF) measuring greater than 6 cm, Ollier disease, and physeal destruction or premature fusion. Diaphyseal femoral fractures demonstrated a type III pattern. Patients with hemihypertrophy and hemiatrophy demonstrated predominantly the type I pattern with

FIGURE 1

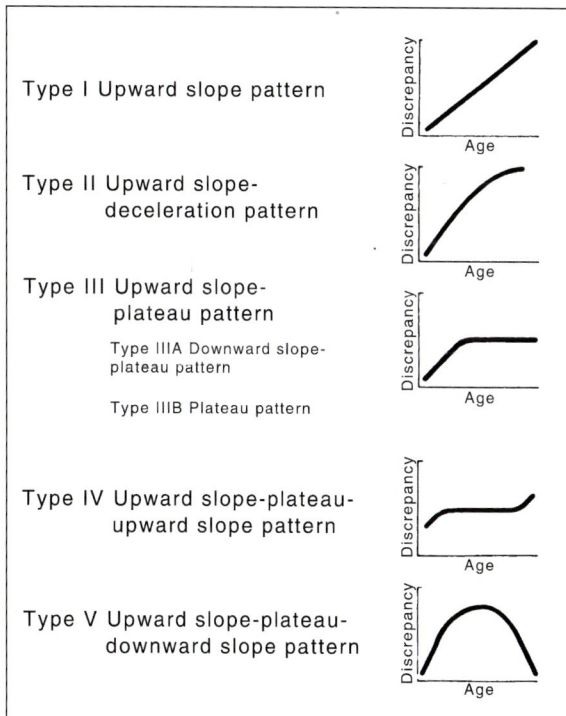

LLD patterns described by Shapiro.[17] (Adapted with permission from Shapiro F: Developmental patterns in lower-extremity length discrepancies. *J Bone Joint Surg Am* 1982;64:639-651.)

some type II and III patterns. Patients with neurofibromatosis demonstrated mainly type I patterns with some type II, III, and V patterns. Patients with juvenile idiopathic arthritis demonstrated type I, III, and V patterns, and patients with poliomyelitis demonstrated a predominantly type I pattern with some type II, III, and IV patterns. Patients with LCP disease demonstrated all five patterns; however, types III and V predominated, occurring in 101 of 140 patients. Although Shapiro did not include fibular hemimelias (longitudinal fibular deficiencies) in his study, these also appear to follow the type I pattern.[25] It is clearly evident from Shapiro's study that not all LLDs follow a linear pattern (type I); therefore, the etiology of the LLD must be considered and care must be taken when determining a predicted LLD because all available predictive models rely on a linear discrepancy pattern.

Effect of Etiology on the Treatment of LLDs

LLD etiology influences the pattern of the discrepancy and it can have important implications for treatment strategies. Whereas lengthening of idiopathic LLDs or posttraumatic physeal arrests can be relatively straightforward, congenital deficiencies can be fraught with complications. It is imperative to recognize that an increased number of problems, obstacles, and complications may be faced when treating certain nonidiopathic causes of LLDs that include but are not limited to CSF, congenital pseudarthrosis of the tibia, skeletal dysplasia, and purpura fulminans.

The absence of cruciate ligaments or the presence of acetabular abnormalities in CSF can result in joint subluxation during lengthening. Bowen et al[29] suggested that the combination of coxa vara and varus femoral bowing seen in CSF contributes to hip subluxation and dislocation during lengthening, and they recommended correction of the varus bow of the femur and the neckshaft angle to 120° and the acetabular index to less than 25° before lengthening. Suzuki et al[30] reviewed 26 femora of 18 patients with varying diagnoses undergoing femoral lengthening. Of 14 hips with a centeredge angle (CEA) greater than 20°, none deteriorated, during or after the lengthening procedure, whereas 5 of 12 hips with a CEA of 20° or less did deteriorate, and one hip completely dislocated. Suzuki et al[30] suggested that a CEA of 20° or less requires a surgical procedure such as an innominate osteotomy before proceeding with a femoral lengthening procedure. Noonan and Price[31] noted that it may be necessary to release the iliotibial band, intramuscular septum, rectus femoris, hamstrings, and hip adductors to decrease the risk of joint subluxation in patients with CSF undergoing femoral lengthening.

Lengthening for short stature in skeletal dysplasias is a controversial topic, with many researchers suggesting that it may be performed safely with close follow-up and careful monitoring.[32-36] Nogueira et al[36] reported a high rate of peripheral nerve lesions (48%; 55 of 115 procedures) in patients with skeletal dysplasia who underwent limb lengthening. The authors recommended a high level of vigilance in monitoring for nerve lesions in these patients and stated that they routinely perform biweekly testing with a pressure-specified sensory device to detect early signs of a nerve lesion.

Congenital pseudarthrosis of the tibia (CPT) is a challenging orthopaedic problem. Multiple efforts to heal the pseudarthrosis can result in significant shortening of the affected limb.[37] Distraction osteogenesis has been used to treat CPT as well as to gain limb length. Paley et al[38] have reported good results with this technique, with a 94% union rate after one treatment and a 100% union rate after two; however, healing indices for the regeneration can be extremely high. Cho et al[39] reported that 17 of 27 patients had a healing index greater than 65 d/cm (mean, 117 d/cm). Some of these patients required autologous bone grafting, bone marrow injections, or demineralized bone matrix insertion. Cho et al also stated that patients with proximal tibial dysplasia or undergoing a repeat lengthening were at higher risk of having a higher healing index.

Purpura fulminans is a devastating infectious condition that primarily affects children and results in diffuse vasculitis and disseminated intravascular coagulation. The acute phase is associated with a high mortality rate[40,41] and a high rate of amputations secondary to gangrene.[41,42] In the last few decades, a handful of studies have reported on the late orthopaedic manifestations and sequelae of purpura fulminans, including physeal abnormalities such as premature, asymmetric, and incomplete arrest.[40,43-45] These physeal growth disturbances can result in angular deformities and/or LLDs. The individual physis may exhibit a Shapiro type IV pattern of growth compared with a normal physis.[42] The initial insult may result in an upward-sloping LLD that then plateaus and, later in skeletal maturity, begins to slope upward again secondary to early closure of the physis. This is very similar to the pattern seen in septic arthritis of the hip. In addition to this nonlinear pattern of discrepancy, variability due to asymmetric bilateral involvement of multiple physes can make the eventual LLD extremely unpredictable. The physician treating such a problem must understand this before embarking on possible treatment of future predicted discrepancies.

REFERENCES

1. Hellsing AL: Leg length inequality: A prospective study of young men during their military service. *Ups J Med Sci* 1988;93(3):245-253.

2. Rush WA, Steiner HA: A study of lower extremity length inequality. *Am J Roentgen* 1946;56:616-623.

3. Soukka A, Alaranta H, Tallroth K, Heliövaara M: Leg-length inequality in people of working age: The association between mild inequality and low-back pain is questionable. *Spine (Phila Pa 1976)* 1991;16(4):429-431.

4. Papaioannou T, Stokes I, Kenwright J: Scoliosis associated with limb-length inequality. *J Bone Joint Surg Am* 1982;64(1):59-62.

5. Giles LG, Taylor JR: Low-back pain associated with leg length inequality. *Spine (Phila Pa 1976)* 1981;6(5):510-521.

6. Gurney B, Mermier C, Robergs R, Gibson A, Rivero D: Effects of limb-length discrepancy on gait economy and lower-extremity muscle activity in older adults. *J Bone Joint Surg Am* 2001;83-A(6):907-915.

7. Friberg O: Clinical symptoms and biomechanics of lumbar spine and hip joint in leg length inequality. *Spine (Phila Pa 1976)* 1983;8(6):643-651.

8. Gofton JP, Trueman GE: Studies in osteoarthritis of the hip: II. Osteoarthritis of the hip and leg-length disparity. *Can Med Assoc J* 1971;104(9):791-799.

9. McCaw ST: Leg length inequality: Implications for running injury prevention. *Sports Med* 1992;14(6):422-429.

10. Kujala UM, Kvist M, Osterman K, Friberg O, Aalto T: Factors predisposing Army conscripts to knee exertion injuries incurred in a physical training program. *Clin Orthop Relat Res* 1986(210):203-212.

11. Friberg O: Leg length asymmetry in stress fractures: A clinical and radiological study. *J Sports Med Phys Fitness* 1982;22(4):485-488.

12. Hoikka V, Ylikoski M, Tallroth K: Leg-length inequality has poor correlation with lumbar scoliosis: A radiological study of 100 patients with chronic low-back pain. *Arch Orthop Trauma Surg* 1989;108(3):173-175.

13. Gross RH: Leg length discrepancy: How much is too much? *Orthopedics* 1978;1(4):307-310.

14. Brand RA, Yack HJ: Effects of leg length discrepancies on the forces at the hip joint. *Clin Orthop Relat Res* 1996(333):172-180.

15. Song KM, Halliday SE, Little DG: The effect of limb-length discrepancy on gait. *J Bone Joint Surg Am* 1997;79(11):1690-1698.

16. Moraal JM, Elzinga-Plomp A, Jongmans MJ, et al: Long-term psychosocial functioning after Ilizarov limb lengthening during childhood. *Acta Orthop* 2009;80(6):704-710.

17. Vitale MA, Choe JC, Sesko AM, et al: The effect of limb length discrepancy on health-related quality of life: Is the '2 cm rule' appropriate? *J Pediatr Orthop B* 2006;15(1):1-5.

18. Bhave A, Paley D, Herzenberg JE: Improvement in gait parameters after lengthening for the treatment of limb-length discrepancy. *J Bone Joint Surg Am* 1999;81(4):529-534.

19. White SC, Gilchrist LA, Wilk BE: Asymmetric limb loading with true or simulated leg-length differences. *Clin Orthop Relat Res* 2004(421):287-292.

20. Perttunen JR, Anttila E, Sodergard J, Merikanto J, Komi PV: Gait asymmetry in patients with limb length discrepancy. *Scand J Med Sci Sports* 2004;14(1):49-56.

21. Kaufman KR, Miller LS, Sutherland DH: Gait asymmetry in patients with limb-length inequality. *J Pediatr Orthop* 1996;16(2):144-150.

22. Shapiro F: Developmental patterns in lower-extremity length discrepancies. *J Bone Joint Surg Am* 1982;64(5):639-651.

23. Paley D, Bhave A, Herzenberg JE, Bowen JR: Multiplier method for predicting limb-length discrepancy. *J Bone Joint Surg Am* 2000;82-A(10):1432-1446.

24. Menelaus MB: Correction of leg length discrepancy by epiphysial arrest. *J Bone Joint Surg Br* 1966;48(2):336-339.

25. Moseley CF: A straight-line graph for leg-length discrepancies. *J Bone Joint Surg Am* 1977;59(2):174-179.

26. Moseley CF: A straight line graph for leg length discrepancies. *Clin Orthop Relat Res* 1978(136):33-40.

27. Anderson M, Messner MB, Green WT: Distribution of lengths of the normal femur and tibia in children from one to eighteen years of age. *J Bone Joint Surg Am* 1964;46(6):1197-1202.

28. Anderson M, Green WT, Messner MB: Growth and predictions of growth in the lower extremities. *J Bone Joint Surg Am* 1963;45-A:1-14.

29. Bowen JR, Kumar SJ, Orellana CA, Andreacchio A, Cardona JI: Factors leading to hip subluxation and dislocation in femoral lengthening of unilateral congenital short femur. *J Pediatr Orthop* 2001;21(3):354-359.

30. Suzuki S, Kasahara Y, Seto Y, Futami T, Furukawa K, Nishino Y: Dislocation and subluxation during femoral lengthening. *J Pediatr Orthop* 1994;14(3):343-346.

31. Noonan KJ, Price CT: Pearls and pitfalls of deformity correction and limb lengthening via monolateral external fixation. *Iowa Orthop J* 1996;16:58-69.

32. Ganel A, Horoszowski H: Limb lengthening in children with achondroplasia: Differences based on gender. *Clin Orthop Relat Res* 1996(332):179-183.

33. Myers GJ, Bache CE, Bradish CF: Use of distraction osteogenesis techniques in skeletal dysplasias. *J Pediatr Orthop* 2003;23(1):41-45.

34. Bell DF, Boyer MI, Armstrong PF: The use of the Ilizarov technique in the correction of limb deformities associated with skeletal dysplasia. *J Pediatr Orthop* 1992;12(3):283-290.

35. Aldegheri R: Distraction osteogenesis for lengthening of the tibia in patients who have limb-length discrepancy or short stature. *J Bone Joint Surg Am* 1999;81(5):624-634.

36. Nogueira MP, Paley D, Bhave A, Herbert A, Nocente C, Herzenberg JE: Nerve lesions associated with limb-lengthening. *J Bone Joint Surg Am* 2003;85-A(8):1502-1510.

37. Dobbs MB, Rich MM, Gordon JE, Szymanski DA, Schoenecker PL: Use of an intramedullary rod for treatment of congenital pseudarthrosis of the tibia: A long-term follow-up study. *J Bone Joint Surg Am* 2004;86-A(6):1186-1197.

38. Paley D, Catagni M, Argnani F, Prevot J, Bell D, Armstrong P: Treatment of congenital pseudoarthrosis of the tibia using the Ilizarov technique. *Clin Orthop Relat Res* 1992(280):81-93.

39. Cho TJ, Choi IH, Lee KS, et al: Proximal tibial lengthening by distraction osteogenesis in congenital pseudarthrosis of the tibia. *J Pediatr Orthop* 2007;27(8):915-920.

40. Bache CE, Torode IP: Orthopaedic sequelae of meningococcal septicemia. *J Pediatr Orthop* 2006;26(1):135-139.

41. Davies MS, Nadel S, Habibi P, Levin M, Hunt DM: The orthopaedic management of peripheral ischaemia in meningococcal septicaemia in children. *J Bone Joint Surg Br* 2000;82(3):383-386.

42. Farrar MJ, Bennet GC, Wilson NI, Azmy A: The orthopaedic implications of peripheral limb ischaemia in infants and children. *J Bone Joint Surg Br* 1996;78(6):930-933.

43. Grogan DP, Love SM, Ogden JA, Millar EA, Johnson LO: Chondro-osseous growth abnormalities after meningococcemia: A clinical and histopathological study. *J Bone Joint Surg Am* 1989;71(6):920-928.

44. Watson CH, Ashworth MA: Growth disturbance and meningococcal septicemia: Report of two cases. *J Bone Joint Surg Am* 1983;65(8):1181-1183.

45. Patriquin HB, Trias A, Jecquier S, Marton D: Late sequelae of infantile meningococcemia in growing bones of children. *Radiology* 1981;141(1):77-82.

CHAPTER 2

CLINICAL ASSESSMENT OF LIMB-LENGTH DISCREPANCIES

REGGIE C. HAMDY, MB, CHB, MSC, FRCSC

INTRODUCTION

A thorough clinical assessment is of paramount importance in a patient with a suspected limb-length discrepancy (LLD). This assessment will help determine the etiology, site, and amount of the LLD, and if it is real or apparent.

HISTORY AND PHYSICAL EXAMINATION

Clinical assessment of a patient with LLD includes a full history, followed by a general physical examination and assessment of the LLD.[1,2] The history includes a family history of similar or other musculoskeletal abnormalities, any specific problems during the mother's pregnancy, the birth history, any previous trauma or infection, when the discrepancy first was noticed (at or after birth), and whether it is progressive. A history of any symptoms related to the LLD such as leg, back, or hip pain, and the presence of functional disability related to the LLD should be documented, as well as any previous treatment related to the LLD.

For a complete physical examination, the patient is asked to undress appropriately. First, the gait is examined. Generally, children can compensate for an LLD better than adults.[3] Young children may compensate for an LLD by flexing the knee or walking on their toes, whereas adolescents and adults rarely walk on their toes

and usually display a vaulting gait. The patient also is asked to run, as this will magnify any mild gait abnormality.

Examination of the spine should be performed with the patient in both standing and sitting positions. The patient is examined while standing for the presence of any pelvic obliquity. The range of motion of the spine also is assessed while standing and the presence of any spinal deformity is noted. The spine is examined for any overlying abnormalities such as skin dimples, a sinus, or a hairy patch. The spine is also examined with the patient sitting on the side of the examination table to eliminate the effect of the LLD on the spine. If any spinal curvature is still apparent while the patient is sitting, its etiology is suprapelvic and not compensatory to the LLD.

With the patient standing, the alignment of the lower limbs is examined in both the frontal and sagittal planes. Any angular deformities such as genu varum or genu valgum and any contractures in the hip or knee joints should be noted, as these may cause an apparent LLD, as shown in **Figure 1**.

The skin should be examined for café au lait spots, vascular malformations, or other abnormalities. The lower limbs also are examined for signs of hemihypertrophy syndromes that could be associated with an LLD. The range of motion of the joints of the lower limb is

---

Neither Dr. Hamdy nor any member of his immediate family has received anything of value from or owns stock in a commercial company or institution related directly or indirectly to the subject of this chapter.

FIGURE 1

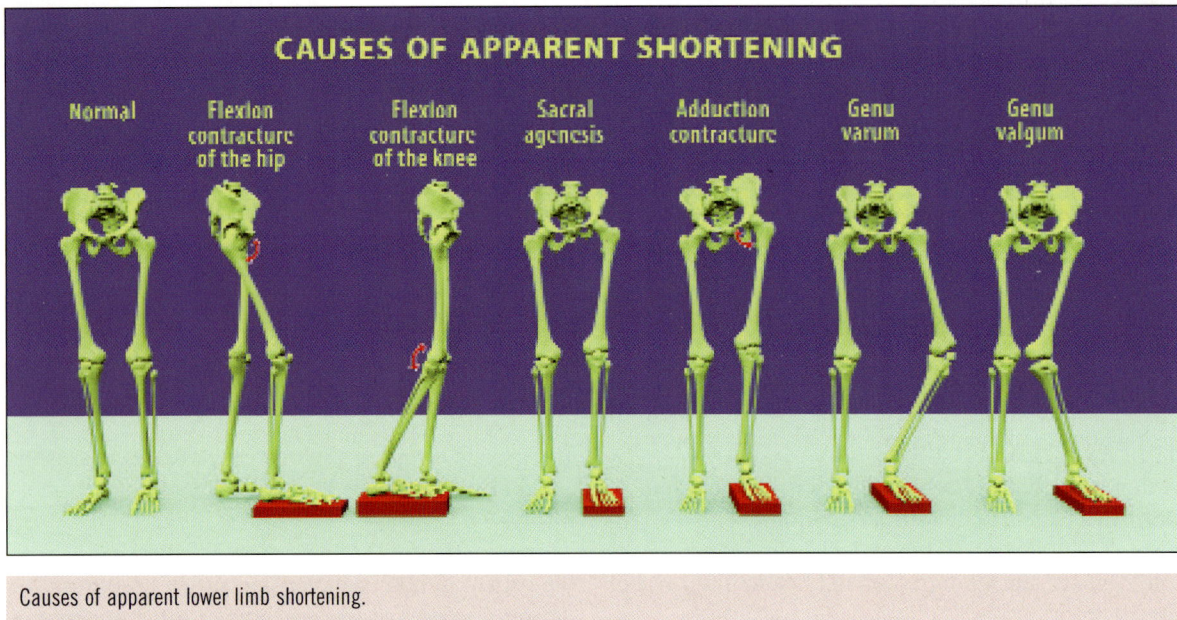

Causes of apparent lower limb shortening.

FIGURE 2

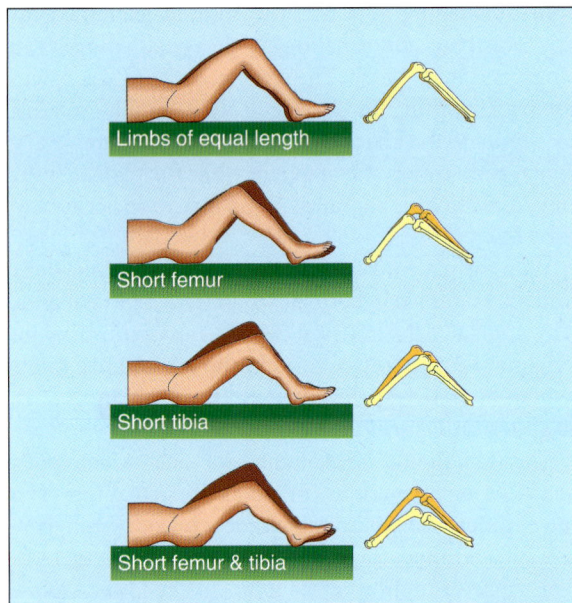

The Galeazzi test is used to determine the site of lower limb shortening (femur, tibia, or both).

assessed for any contractures that may cause an apparent LLD (**Figure 1**). The presence of joint instability also should be looked for, as this may affect surgical treatment, especially lengthening procedures. A complete neurovascular examination is performed to assess for neuromuscular disorders.

ASSESSING LLD IN THE LOWER LIMB

Several methods are used to assess LLD clinically.

Visual Estimation

First, the site of the LLD should be determined. Have the patient lie supine with the hips and knees flexed as shown in **Figure 2**. This method roughly estimates which bones are affected: the femur, the tibia, or both.

Tape Measurement

Have the patient lie supine on the examination table with all clothes removed below the waist except for underwear. Use a tape measure to obtain direct measurement of the LLD between two constant bony landmarks: the anterior superior iliac spine and the medial

FIGURE 3

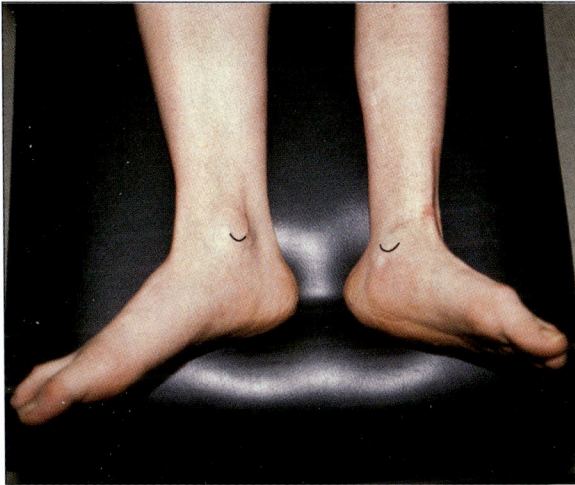

Clinical photograph demonstrates heel height discrepancy measured from the medial malleolus (black lines) to the plantar aspect of the heel.

FIGURE 4

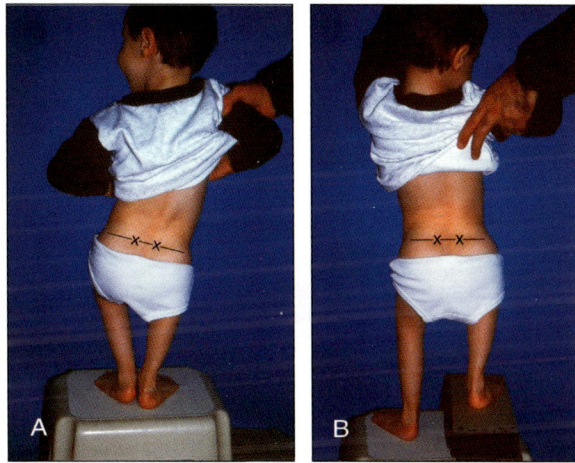

In the blocks method of measuring limb-length discrepancies, blocks are placed underneath the short leg to level the pelvis. In these photographs, the dimples over the posterior superior iliac spine (x) are used as landmarks to determine the alignment of the pelvis before (**A**) and after (**B**) the blocks are placed.

or lateral malleolus. This method provides only a gross assessment of lengths of the lower limbs. It does not take into account any discrepancy that may be present in the foot and ankle (**Figure 3**), any apparent discrepancy secondary to contractures of the hip and knee, or angular deformities in the knee.

Blocks Method

With the patient standing, blocks are placed under the short leg, adding blocks until the pelvis is level. A level pelvis is determined by palpating the iliac crest or by comparing the level of the dimples overlying the posterior superior iliac spine (**Figure 4**). This is the most accurate clinical method because it takes heel height into account. It does not take into account, however, any angular deformities or contractures around the hip or knee or an equinus contracture.

ASSESSING LLD IN THE UPPER LIMB

Accurate measurement of LLD in the upper limb is rarely necessary, but a rough estimate may be useful. To determine if any length discrepancy exists between the

FIGURE 5

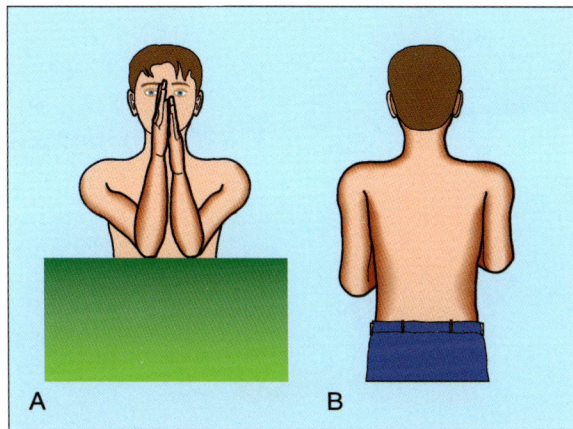

Drawings illustrate methods of measuring length discrepancy in the forearm (**A**) and the upper arm (**B**).

upper limbs, the patient is asked to undress appropriately above the waist. The patient is asked to stand and then fully extend the elbows and wrists, placing the hands beside the thighs. Any difference between the level of the fingertips is noted. If a difference is observed, the next step is to determine if the difference is in the arm or in the forearm. To assess whether a discrepancy exists in the forearms, the patient is asked to place the elbows on the table with the forearms side by side and place the hands together, as shown in **Figure 5,** *A*. To assess whether a discrepancy exists in lengths of the humeri, the patient is asked to flex the elbows and keep the arms beside the chest and is examined from the back, as shown in **Figure 5,** *B*.

REFERENCES

1. Stanitski DF: Limb-length inequality: Assessment and treatment options. *J Am Acad Orthop Surg* 1999;7(3):143-153.

2. Carey RPL: Clinical examination and measurement of limb length inequality, in Menelaus MB, ed: *The Management of Limb Inequality.* Edinburgh, Scotland, Churchill Livingstone, 1991, pp 50-52.

3. Wenger DR, Rang M, eds: Leg length discrepancy, in Wenger DR, Rang M: *The Art and Practice of Children's Orthopaedics.* New York, NY, Raven Press, 1993, pp 524-528.

CHAPTER 3

IMAGING ASSESSMENT OF LIMB-LENGTH DISCREPANCY

SANJEEV SABHARWAL, MD

INTRODUCTION

Radiographs are considered more accurate and reliable than clinical examination for analysis of limb-length discrepancy (LLD).[1-3] Accuracy is defined in terms of the variation between the measurements obtained using the imaging method and the actual length, whereas reliability is the variation in measurements between observers (interobserver reliability) and within a single observer (intraobserver reliability) in obtaining measurements. Over the last 6 decades, several imaging modalities have been used to assess patients with LLD. In addition to a variety of plain radiographic techniques, computed radiography (CR), microdose digital radiography, ultrasonography, CT, and MRI also have been advocated. When choosing an imaging technique to help assess LLD, in addition to accuracy and reliability, one needs to consider the magnification, radiation dose, cost, need for special equipment, convenience, and ability to image the entire extremity[4] (Table 1).

PLAIN RADIOGRAPHY

The three types of images obtained for assessing LLD using standard radiography include an orthoradiograph, a scanogram, and a teleoradiograph. The patient is supine for the orthoradiograph and scanogram and stands erect for the teleoradiograph. With supine radiographs, measurement error secondary to magnification is minimized by using three exposures centered over the hip, knee, and ankle, using either a single 35 × 110–cm long cassette for an orthoradiograph (**Figure 1,** *A*) or a standard 35 × 43–cm cassette for a scanogram (**Figure 1,** *B*). Both imaging methods, however, are prone to errors related to patient movement between radiographic exposures; moreover, the radiation exposure to the patient for a scanogram or orthoradiograph is greater than that associated with a full-length weight-bearing radiograph or a CT scanogram[5-7] (**Table 1**). Patients with unequal leg lengths often have associated angular deformities of the lower limb. Because the entire lower extremity is imaged on a single full-length radiograph with the patient in the erect position (**Figure 1,** *C*), a comprehensive analysis of limb deformities can be performed along with the assessment of LLD.[6-8] Furthermore, the difference in height of the feet is incorporated in the measurement of LLD when obtaining the full-length weight-bearing radiograph, unlike a scanogram. Despite a magnification of approximately 5%, the measurement of LLD using full-length weight-bearing AP radiographs is similar in accuracy to that of the scanogram, especially in the absence of significant mechanical axis deviation.[7] The potential drawbacks of full-length weight-bearing AP radiographs include the need for special radiographic equipment, such as grids, filters, and processors, as well as the need for long

Dr. Sabharwal or an immediate family member serves as a board member, owner, officer, or committee member of the Limb Lengthening and Reconstruction Society and has received research or institutional support from Smith & Nephew.

TABLE 1 Comparison of Imaging Modalities for Assessing Limb-Length Discrepancy

Imaging Modality/Technique	Reliability[a]	Accuracy[a]	Magnification	Approximate Radiation Exposure (mrad)[b,c]
Teleoradiography	+ + + +	+ + +	~5%	42
Orthoradiography	+ + +	+ + +	Minimal	200
Scanogram	+ + + +	+ + +	Minimal	200
Computed radiography	+ + + +	+ + +	Varies with technique (scanogram vs teleoradiograph)	Varies with technique, less exposure than standard radiography
Microdose digital radiography	+ + +	+ + + +	None	2
Ultrasonography	+ + +	+ +	None	None
CT (digital localization image)	+ + + +	+ + + +	Minimal	60
MRI	+ + + +	+ + +	Minimal	None

[a] An increasing number of "+" signs indicates a greater degree of reliability/accuracy.

[b] Machen MS, Stevens PM: Should full-length weight-bearing anteroposterior radiographs replace the scanogram for measurement of limb-length discrepancy? *J Pediatr Orthop B* 2005;14:30-37.

[c] To calculate absorbed radiation dose measured in grays (SI unit), 1 gray = 0.1 mrad.

radiographic cassettes that may not be readily available and can be difficult to store. Some of these storage issues have been resolved with use of CR.

COMPUTED RADIOGRAPHY

CR is a relatively recent advance in the measurement of LLD[7,9] (**Figure 2**). The images are recorded with a long-length imaging system using a vertical cassette holder with three 35 × 43–cm CR storage phosphor cassettes. The composite image obtained is transferred digitally and can be manipulated with an automated system, such as a picture archiving and communication system, resulting in a film radiograph. The operator can enhance the final image by using the computer to adjust the image parameters; thus, quality radiographs can be obtained consistently with a significant reduction in the radiation dose, a feature that is extremely useful for patients who require repeated radiographic examination because of LLD.[7,10] Sabharwal et al[7] recently evaluated 111 patients with LLD who had undergone CR-based scanogram and CR teleoradiography performed on the same day. Despite a 4.6% magnification noted when measuring the absolute length of the lower extremity with the weight-bearing radiograph, the mean

difference in LLD measurements between the CR techniques was only 5 mm. The mean radiation dose was found to be 1.6 to 3.8 times greater for the CR-based scanogram study than for the teleoradiograph, and the costs for both studies were identical. In another study, excellent intraobserver and interobserver reliability were noted among five blinded observers with varying degrees of experience who assessed LLD using CR-based supine scanograms and weight-bearing teleoradiographs.[9]

MICRODOSE DIGITAL RADIOGRAPHY

Microdose digital radiography is a computer-aided imaging technique that substantially reduces the radiation exposure to patients compared with conventional radiographic techniques.[11] The patient stands still in front of the imaging assembly during the 20-second scanning process. A continuous series of photon beams collimated to act as a point source are projected through the patient to strike a computerized detector. The source assembly and detector move together, scanning the field in a line-by-line motion so that the beam is always horizontal to the patient, thus minimizing magnification

TABLE 1 (*continued*)

Approximate Charges ($ US)	Radiographic Deformity Analysis	Incorporation of Height of Foot and Pelvis?	Typical Availability in United States	Weight Bearing?
95[b]	Yes	Yes	Varies	Yes
110[b]	Minimal	No	Varies	No
110[b]	No	No	Varies	No
137[d]	Varies with technique (scanogram vs teleoradiograph)	Varies with technique	Varies	Varies with technique (scanogram vs teleoradiograph)
75[b]	Yes	Yes	No	Yes
Not reported	No	No	No	Yes
60[b]	Minimal	None	Varies	No
Not reported	Not reported	Not reported	No	No

[d] Sabharwal S, Zhao C, Mckeon JJ, McClemens E, Edgar M, Behrens F: Computed radiographic measurement of limb-length discrepancy: Full-length standing anteroposterior radiograph compared with scanogram. *J Bone Joint Surg Am* 2006;88:2243-2251.

(Adapted with permission from Sabharwal S, Kumar A: Methods for assessing limb-length discrepancy. *Clin Orthop Relat Res* 2008;466(12):2910-2922.)

error. In a study of 25 children with LLD, Altongy et al[11] found microdose digital radiography to be more accurate than orthoradiography; however, this technique has not gained popularity and is not readily available.

ULTRASONOGRAPHY

Several authors from European centers have reported on the use of ultrasonography for assessing LLD, with the bony landmarks at the hip, knee, and ankle joints identified using the ultrasound transducer.[12-14] Terjesen et al[14] compared the measurements of LLD in 45 patients obtained using real-time ultrasonography with the results obtained using weight-bearing radiographs. Although the ultrasonographic scan was slightly less reliable than the radiograph, given the lack of radiation, Terjesen recommended that ultrasonography be used as the initial screening tool for LLD. The benefits of ultrasonography are that it is inexpensive and does not involve any radiation exposure. The disadvantages are that, unlike a full-length weight-bearing radiograph, an ultrasonographic scan does not allow for a comprehensive analysis of the lower extremity, including angular deformities; it may be less accurate than radiographic methods and it is highly technician dependent. Use of ultrasonography to assess LLD may be a useful screening tool in the hands of experienced users.

CT SCANOGRAM

Digitized images obtained with CT scanning also have been used to measure LLD.[5,15-19] Typically, an AP scout view of both femora (**Figure 3**) and tibias is obtained, although use of lateral CT scanograms also has been reported.[5,16] Cursors are placed over the superior aspect of the imaged femoral head and the distal portion of the medial femoral condyle,[15,17,18] with the distance between these cursors representing the length of each femur. The tibial length is determined similarly by measuring the distance between cursors placed at the medial tibial plateau and the tibial plafond. To obtain femoral and tibial measurements, the patient lies supine on the CT scanner tabletop, which moves through a collimated x-ray beam from a stationary source. A CT scanogram has the advantages of displaying the entire length of the femurs and tibias and minimizing the measurement error related to patient movement and magnification.[18] A CT scanogram has similar costs and may be more accurate, with excellent reliability and less gonadal radiation, than some of the plain radiographic techniques;

FIGURE 1

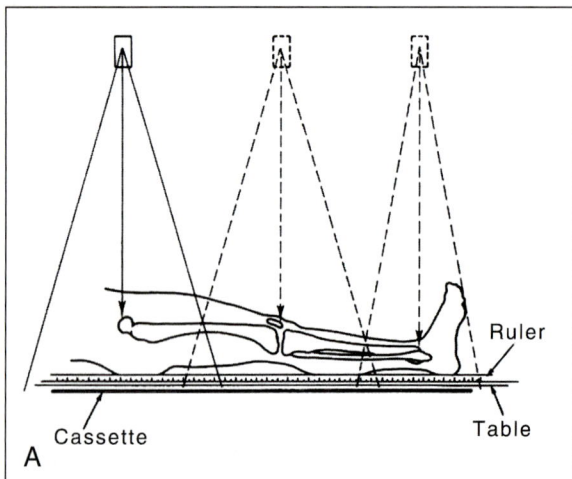

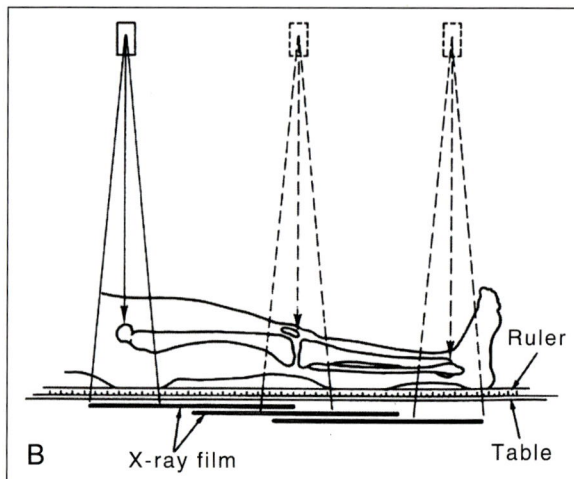

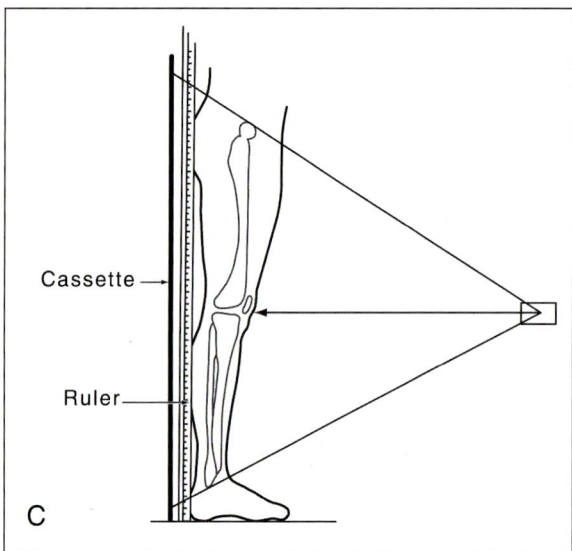

Plain radiographic techniques used for assessing LLD. **A,** An ortho-radiograph uses three radiographic exposures centered over the hip, knee, and ankle joints to minimize magnification error. A large cassette (35 × 110 cm) is placed under the patient, who remains still. **B,** The scanogram also uses three radiographic exposures centered over the hip, knee, and ankle joint to minimize magnification error. The patient remains supine next to a calibrated ruler and the standard-length radiographic cassette (35 × 43 cm) is moved. **C,** With teleoradiography, a long cassette (35 × 110 cm) is placed behind the patient while the x-ray beam is centered over the knee joint, preferably with the patient standing. (Reproduced with permission from Morrissy RT, Weinstein SL, eds: *Lovell and Winter's Pediatric Orthopaedics.* Philadelphia, PA, Lippincott Williams & Wilkins, 2006, pp 1213-1256.)

however, the CT scanogram may require a longer setup time.[5,6,15,17,18,20] For patients with flexion deformities of the hip or knee, especially those with overlying external fixators,[21] a lateral CT scanogram may be more accurate for assessing LLD.[5,18] For patients with limb shortening who also have associated torsional deformities, the CT scan can also be used to determine the version of the femur and tibia (**Figure 3**). Periarticular and diaphyseal angular deformities, as well as joint subluxation and mechanical axis deviations, are not as well ascertained on the supine images as on a weight-bearing full-length radiograph; moreover, the CT scanogram may not be readily available and usually requires prior scheduling in a radiology department or an imaging center.

MAGNETIC RESONANCE IMAGING

The use of MRI to determine LLD in cadaveric specimens has been reported. Leitzes et al[22] compared MRI scanogram with CT and plain radiography using 12

FIGURE 2

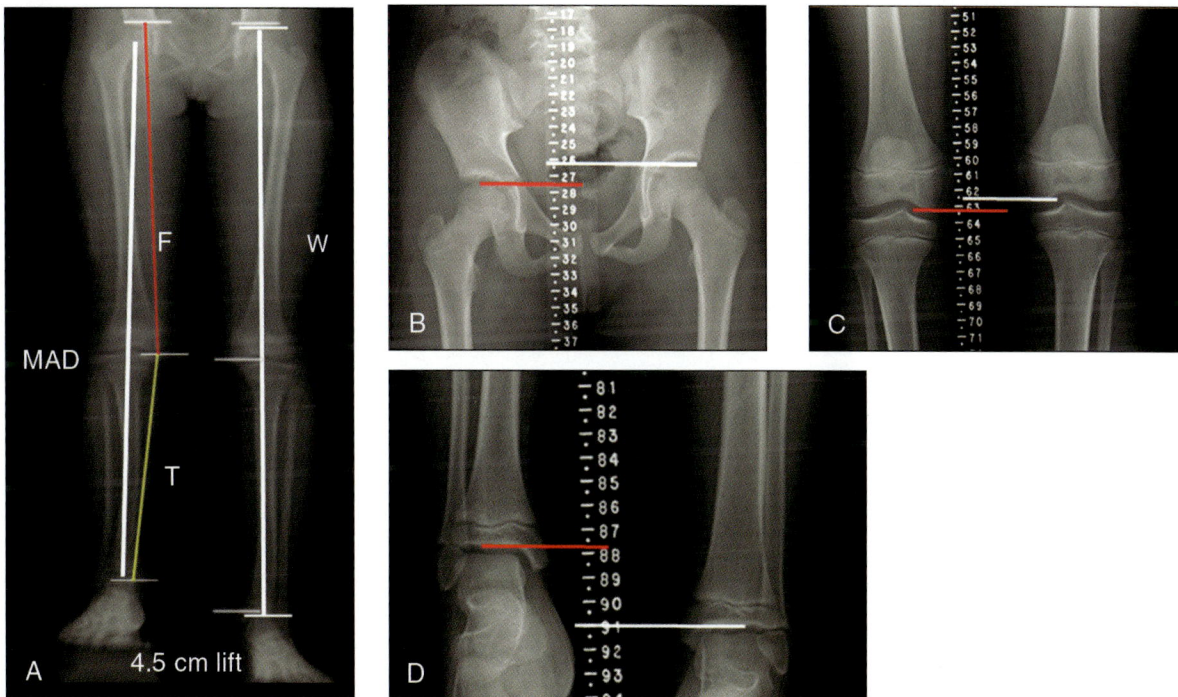

Images obtained using CR to assess LLD in a child with a congenital shortening of the tibia of approximately 4.5 cm. **A,** Weight-bearing AP radiograph (modified teleoradiograph) of the lower extremity. The child is standing on an appropriate-height lift under the short leg to level the pelvis. In addition to assessing LLD and length of the whole leg (W), femur (F, red line), and tibia (T, yellow line), CR can be used to measure mechanical axis deviation (MAD) and joint orientation angles around the knee. Modified scanogram obtained using CR requires three radiographic exposures, one each centered over the hip (**B**), knee (**C**), and ankle (**D**) joints. CR does not allow visualization of the entire length of the femur and tibia, and it fails to account for any shortening related to the foot. (Reproduced with permission from Sabharwal S, Zhao C, Mckeon JJ, McClemens E, Edgar M, Behrens F: Computed radiographic measurement of LLD: Full-length standing anteroposterior radiograph compared with scanogram. *J Bone Joint Surg Am* 2006;88:2243-2251.)

cadaveric femoral specimens to assess length. The intraobserver and interobserver reliability was excellent for all three techniques; however, MRI has not been well studied in the clinical setting, is likely to be more expensive, may require sedation, typically requires a longer time to schedule and to complete the study, and may be contraindicated in patients with certain implanted devices. Currently, supine MRI scanogram remains an investigational tool that requires clinical validation before it can be recommended for general use. Recently, MRI that allows the patient to remain upright has been introduced in the United States; upright MRI may be an attractive option in the future to comprehensively assess

LLD and alignment of the lower extremities, along with soft-tissue pathology, without radiation exposure; however, such emerging techniques will need to be critically evaluated and compared with already established imaging modalities.

SUMMARY
No ideal method exists for assessing LLD, but several imaging modalities are available. The ideal method for evaluating LLD would be readily available, accurate, reliable, and affordable, and it would allow visualization of the entire lower extremity, minimize radiation exposure, and have no magnification error. Although prone

FIGURE 3

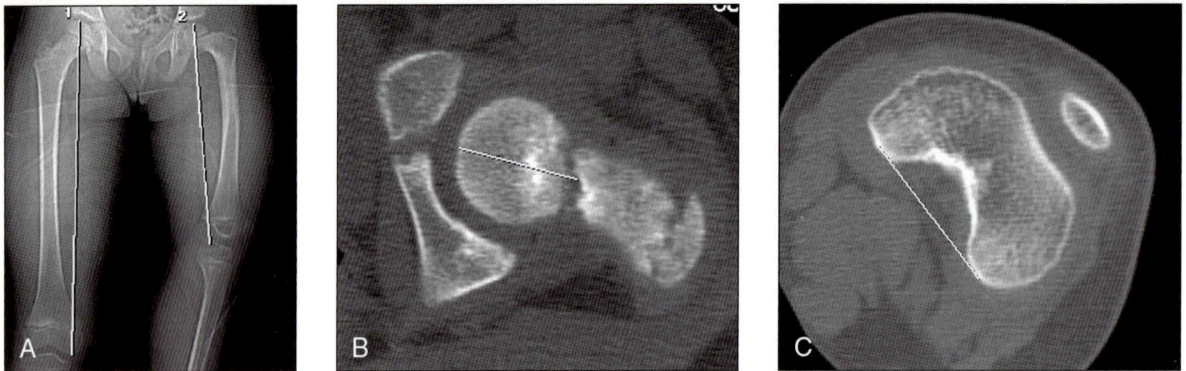

CT scans of a 3-year-old patient with congenital shortening of the left femur. **A,** AP scout view of the CT scan demonstrates a 9.3-cm LLD related to femoral shortening (1 = normal femur, 27.2 cm; 2 = short femur, 17.9 cm). Axial CT scans through the left femoral neck (**B**) and distal femoral condyle (**C**) demonstrate 37° of femoral retroversion (lines). The normal right femur had 17° of anteversion.

to slight magnification error, weight-bearing full-length AP CR of both lower extremities obtained with the pelvis level, along with use of a magnification marker, should be considered the primary imaging modality for the initial evaluation of LLD in most patients. Other techniques, such as a lateral scout CT scan, may be more useful in patients with flexion deformities around the knee. Ultrasonography may be a useful screening tool in the hands of experienced users. In the future, advanced imaging modalities such as a weight-bearing MRI of the lower extremities may prove a viable alternative without exposing patients to radiation hazards. A comprehensive imaging approach tailored to each patient, along with a careful physical examination, should be undertaken when evaluating for possible LLD.

REFERENCES

1. Cleveland RH, Kushner DC, Ogden MC, Herman TE, Kermond W, Correia JA: Determination of leg length discrepancy: A comparison of weight-bearing and supine imaging. *Invest Radiol* 1988;23(4):301-304.

2. Lampe HI, Swierstra BA, Diepstraten AF: Measurement of limb length inequality: Comparison of clinical methods with orthoradiography in 190 children. *Acta Orthop Scand* 1996;67(3):242-244.

3. Terry MA, Winell JJ, Green DW, et al: Measurement variance in limb length discrepancy: Clinical and radiographic assessment of interobserver and intraobserver variability. *J Pediatr Orthop* 2005;25(2):197-201.

4. Sabharwal S, Kumar A: Methods for assessing leg length discrepancy. *Clin Orthop Relat Res* 2008;466(12): 2910-2922.

5. Aaron A, Weinstein D, Thickman D, Eilert R: Comparison of orthoroentgenography and computed tomography in the measurement of limb-length discrepancy. *J Bone Joint Surg Am* 1992;74(6):897-902.

6. Machen MS, Stevens PM: Should full-length standing anteroposterior radiographs replace the scanogram for measurement of limb length discrepancy? *J Pediatr Orthop B* 2005;14(1):30-37.

7. Sabharwal S, Zhao C, McKeon JJ, McClemens E, Edgar M, Behrens F: Computed radiographic measurement of limb-length discrepancy: Full-length standing anteroposterior radiograph compared with scanogram. *J Bone Joint Surg Am* 2006;88(10):2243-2251.

8. Saleh M, Milne A: Weight-bearing parallel-beam scanography for the measurement of leg length and joint alignment. *J Bone Joint Surg Br* 1994;76(1): 156-157.

9. Sabharwal S, Zhao C, McKeon J, Melaghari T, Blacksin M, Wenekor C: Reliability analysis for radiographic measurement of limb length discrepancy: Full-length standing anteroposterior radiograph versus scanogram. *J Pediatr Orthop* 2007;27(1):46-50.

10. Kogutt MS: Computed radiographic imaging: Use in low-dose leg length radiography. *AJR Am J Roentgenol* 1987;148(6):1205-1206.

11. Altongy JF, Harcke HT, Bowen JR: Measurement of leg length inequalities by Micro-Dose digital radiographs. *J Pediatr Orthop* 1987;7(3):311-316.

12. Konermann W, Gruber G: Ultrasound determination of leg length. *Orthopade* 2002;31(3):300-305.

13. Krettek C, Koch T, Henzler D, Blauth M, Hoffmann R: A new procedure for determining leg length and leg length inequality using ultrasound: II. Comparison of ultrasound, teleradiography and 2 clinical procedures in 50 patients. *Unfallchirurg* 1996;99(1):43-51.

14. Terjesen T, Benum P, Rossvoll I, Svenningsen S, Fløystad Isern AE, Nordbø T: Leg-length discrepancy measured by ultrasonography. *Acta Orthop Scand* 1991;62(2):121-124.

15. Aitken AG, Flodmark O, Newman DE, Kilcoyne RF, Shuman WP, Mack LA: Leg length determination by CT digital radiography. *AJR Am J Roentgenol* 1985;144(3):613-615.

16. Glass RB, Poznanski AK: Leg-length determination with biplanar CT scanograms. *Radiology* 1985;156(3): 833-834.

17. Helms CA, McCarthy S: CT scanograms for measuring leg length discrepancy. *Radiology* 1984;151(3):802.

18. Huurman WW, Jacobsen FS, Anderson JC, Chu WK: Limb-length discrepancy measured with computerized axial tomographic equipment. *J Bone Joint Surg Am* 1987;69(5):699-705.

19. Tokarowski A, Piechota L, Wojciechowski P, Gajos L, Kusz D: Measurement of lower extremity length using computed tomography. *Chir Narzadow Ruchu Ortop Pol* 1995;60(2):123-127.

20. Temme JB, Chu WK, Anderson JC: CT scanograms compared with conventional orthoroentgenograms in long bone measurement. *Radiol Technol* 1987;59(1): 65-68.

21. Sabharwal S, Badarudeen S, McClemens E, Choung E: The effect of circular external fixation on limb alignment. *J Pediatr Orthop* 2008;28(3):314-319.

22. Leitzes AH, Potter HG, Amaral T, Marx RG, Lyman S, Widmann RF: Reliability and accuracy of MRI scanogram in the evaluation of limb length discrepancy. *J Pediatr Orthop* 2005;25(6):747-749.

PREDICTION OF LIMB-LENGTH DISCREPANCY AT SKELETAL MATURITY

MIHIR M. THACKER, MD

INTRODUCTION

Limb-length discrepancy (LLD) is common; an estimated 15% or more of the population has a discrepancy of at least 1 cm.[1,2] Considerable controversy exists regarding the symptoms and magnitude of LLD. Discrepancies of more than 2 cm at maturity or greater than 3% to 5% of the length of the contralateral side result in increased mechanical work during gait and use of compensatory strategies.[3,4] The association of smaller discrepancies with back pain is questionable, however, as is the association of LLD with hip and knee arthrosis. Equalization of large (>3 cm) discrepancies has been shown to result in improvement of back pain.[5]

Shapiro[6] described five patterns of progression of LLD in children (**Figure 1**). Most congenital cases of LLD in children follow the Shapiro type I (progressive) pattern. Developmental anomalies may not follow this pattern. Most of the available methods used to predict LLD are appropriate for cases that follow this progressive pattern. Prediction of rate and pattern of growth are critical in the prediction of LLD and also for appropriate timing of the growth modulation procedure used to correct LLD.

PREDICTION OF LLD

Various methods used to predict LLD are described in the literature.

Arithmetic (Rule-of-Thumb) Method

The arithmetic, or rule-of-thumb, method was initially described by White and Stubbins[7] in 1944 and subsequently popularized by Menelaus.[8] The arithmetic method is based on the following assumptions: (1) The distal femoral growth plate grows at a rate of 3/8 in (0.95 cm) per year, and the proximal tibial growth plate grows at a rate of 1/4 in (0.64 cm) per year; (2) boys stop growing at age 16 years and girls at age 14 years; (3) if one of the growth plates is completely arrested, the discrepancy will increase at a rate corresponding to the normal rate of growth for that plate (otherwise, it will increase at a rate of 1/8 in [0.32 cm] per year); and (4) chronologic age is adequate in assessing growth, and skeletal age is not used.

Advantages

No complex calculations, formulas, or growth charts are needed. This simple method has been used with reasonable accuracy to determine the timing of epiphyseodesis.[9]

Disadvantages

The arithmetic method should not be used for children younger than 8 years or for children with a difference of more than 1 year between their chronologic and skeletal ages.[8] This method also does not account for the individual's growth rate and maturation, the fact that growth

Neither Dr. Thacker nor any immediate family member has received anything of value from or owns stock in a commercial company or institution related directly or indirectly to the subject of this chapter.

FIGURE 1

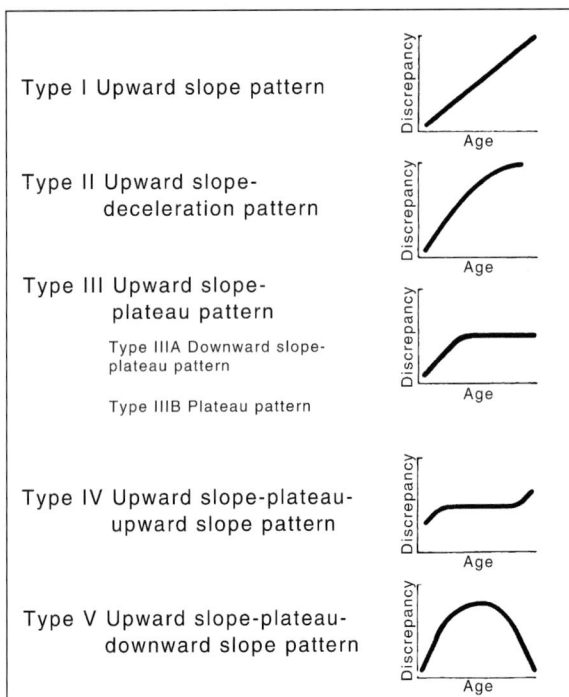

Type I Upward slope pattern

Type II Upward slope-
deceleration pattern

Type III Upward slope-
plateau pattern

Type IIIA Downward slope-
plateau pattern

Type IIIB Plateau pattern

Type IV Upward slope-plateau-
upward slope pattern

Type V Upward slope-plateau-
downward slope pattern

The Shapiro classification of development patterns. (Adapted with permission from Shapiro F: Developmental patterns in lower-extremity length discrepancies. *J Bone Joint Surg Am* 1982;64:639-651.)

velocity is not constant, or the fact that growth continues to different ages in different individuals. Moreover, the growth inhibition is assumed and not calculated. The arithmetic method also is not applicable in patients with incomplete closure of the growth plate.

Green-Anderson Growth Remaining Method

Anderson, Green, and Messner[10] developed graphs of average growth at the femur and tibia as well as another set of graphs showing the growth remaining at the epiphyses of the distal femur and the proximal tibia, which can then be used to determine the timing of epiphysiodesis (**Figure 2**).

Advantages

Unlike the arithmetic method, the Green-Anderson method is based on skeletal and not chronologic age,

and this reduces the degree of error in prediction. Also, the growth inhibition is calculated and not assumed, again leading to less error.

Disadvantages

The Green-Anderson growth remaining method is relatively cumbersome and depends on the availability of the graphs. The predictions are based on the most recent single measurement of skeletal age, which may be in error. Also, the method is based on limb growth measurements of Caucasian children in the 1940s and early 1950s, and growth patterns may vary somewhat by geography and race, and they may change over time.[11] In addition, this method assumes that the distal femur contributes 71% and the proximal tibia 57% to the growth of the individual bones. This is not true at all ages, however, and the contribution of the distal femoral and proximal tibial physes increases as the patient approaches skeletal maturity. For example, the proximal tibial contribution increases from 50% at 10 years to 80% at 14 years in girls and from 50% at 10 years to 80% at 16 years in boys. These differences can contribute to the error in growth prediction with epiphysiodesis.[12,13] Despite these disadvantages, the Green-Anderson data form the basis of most of the currently used prediction methods, including the straight-line graph and the multiplier methods.[14,15]

Straight-line Graph Method

Moseley[16] used the Green-Anderson[15] data and devised a straight-line graph by manipulating the abscissa (x axis) and creating a logarithmic plot. The length of the long (not the "normal") leg is plotted on the straight line and the length of the short leg is plotted along a vertical line at the same level. The skeletal age is plotted at the same time. This is done for a minimum of three data points (preferably as far apart as possible to increase the accuracy). A horizontal best-fit line is used to estimate the time of skeletal maturity, and a vertical line is drawn from this point to predict the lengths of the two extremities at skeletal maturity. This helps determine the growth rates of the two extremities and the age and LLD at skeletal maturity. The reference slopes for growth after a distal femoral, proximal tibial, or combined distal femoral and proximal tibial epiphysiodesis are available on the chart and can be used to determine the

FIGURE 2

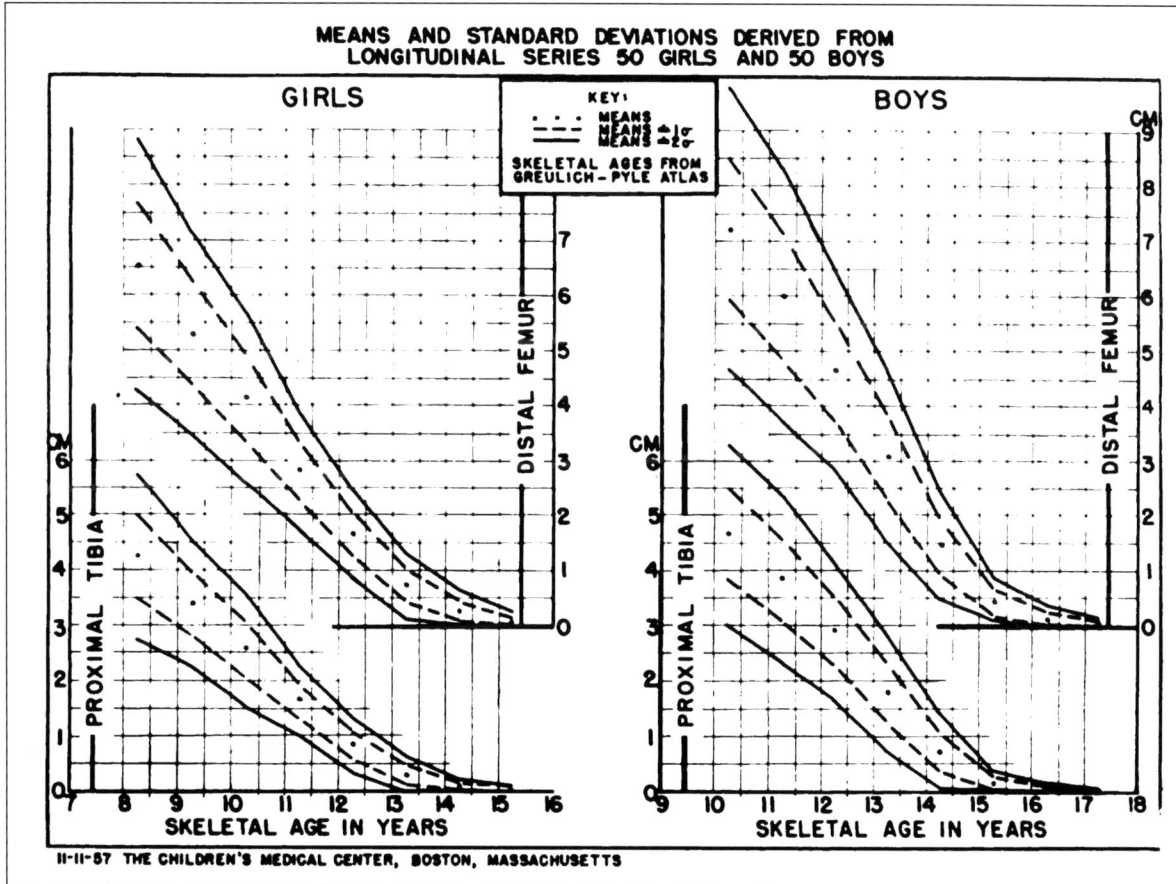

Green-Anderson growth remaining charts for the femur and tibia, for prediction of limb-length discrepancy (LLD). σ = standard deviation. (Reproduced from Anderson M, Green WT, Messner MB: Growth and predictions of growth in the lower extremities. *J Bone Joint Surg Am* 1963;45-A:1-14.)

appropriate timing of the procedure (**Figure 3**). The Moseley straight-line graph is widely used and seems to be the standard against which other methods are compared.

Advantages

The straight-line graph is easy to use and reduces the errors in calculations that are seen with the growth remaining method. Because serial measurements are taken, the growth percentile of the patient can be used to predict future growth rather than using the population mean.

Disadvantages

With the straight-line graph, multiple (preferably at least three) data points are required to determine the growth rates of the extremities and predict the difference at maturity. This method therefore cannot be used if a patient presents close to the time that the epiphysiodesis must be performed. Also, regional and present-day differences in skeletal maturation as well as the tendency of people in industrialized countries to grow taller may affect the results with this method.[11,13]

Although the straight-line graph uses skeletal age, it was prepared based on data that uses chronologic age.[10]

FIGURE 3

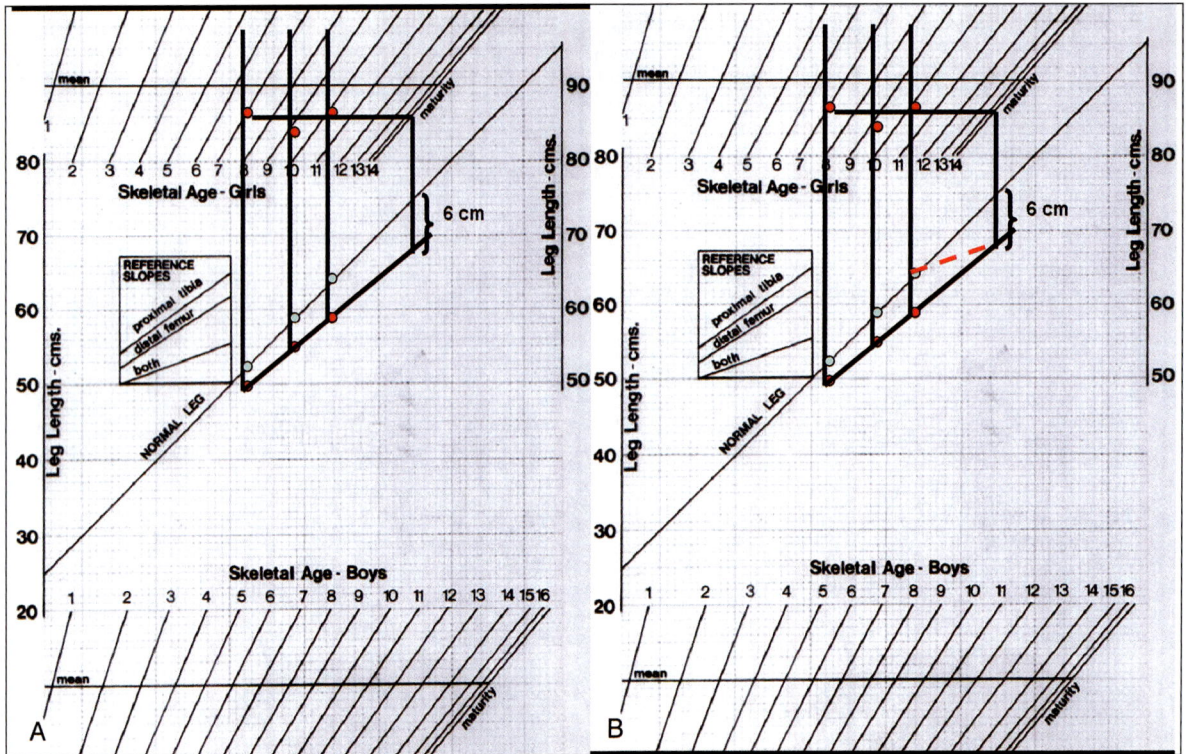

Use of the Moseley straight-line graph for predicting LLD at skeletal maturity and for predicting the timing and effects of epiphysiodesis. **A,** A minimum of three values of the length of the long leg (blue dots) and short leg (red dots) are plotted as shown along with the corresponding skeletal age values (red dots) for a female patient. The best fit skeletal age line is extended to the skeletal maturity line and the LLD at maturity is calculated. The predicted LLD at maturity in this case is 6 cm. **B,** A combined contralateral distal femoral and proximal tibial epiphysiodesis at skeletal age of 10 years (red dashed line) would result in equalization of limb lengths at maturity based on the straight-line graph prediction. (Adapted from Moseley CF: A straight-line graph for leg-length discrepancies. *J Bone Joint Surg Am* 1977;59[2]:174-179.)

Pritchett[12] studied sequential teleoradiograms of the lower and upper extremities in 244 healthy middle-class American children from age 7 years to skeletal maturity. These data suggest that more growth occurs in the femur and the tibia than is suggested by the Green-Anderson data. Pritchett found an average of approximately 1.3 cm of growth per year in the distal femur and 0.9 cm per year in the proximal tibia, except in the last 2 years of maturation, when the growth rate is one half of these rates. Using a combination of their straight-line graphs and the growth remaining charts, Pritchett and Bortel[13] reported results that were more accurate than those pro-

duced by the Moseley straight-line graphs or the Menelaus or Anderson-Green-Messner method. This method requires specialized graphs and growth remaining charts and hence may be a little cumbersome.

Multiplier Method

Paley et al[17] used the Green-Anderson data and divided the lengths of the tibia and the femur at skeletal maturity by the lengths of the tibia and femur at various ages and came up with the ratio that they termed the multiplier (**Table 1**). Paley et al used the data provided by Maresh et al[18] for children up to 1 year old (as this was not available in the Green-Anderson data). Age- and sex-related multipliers were then calculated using 18 other databases. They found that the multipliers were almost the same for similar percentiles at each age for both the femur and the tibia.

The predicted LLD at maturity (LLDm) in congenital discrepancies (congenital short femur, fibular hemimelia [longitudinal fibular deficiency], hemihypertrophy, etc) can be calculated as follows:

$$\text{LLDm} = \text{current LLD} \times \text{multiplier for the current chronologic age.}$$

For developmental discrepancies (Ollier disease, growth arrest, etc), the growth inhibition remains constant and the formula for prediction is as follows:

$$\text{LLDm} = \text{current LLD} + (I \times G),$$

where I is the growth inhibition calculated using the formula

$$I = 1 - (\text{growth of the short limb/growth of the long limb over the same period of time}),$$

and G is the growth remaining in the long leg and is calculated using the formula

$$G = L(M - 1),$$

where L is the current length of the long leg and M is the multiplier for the current age.

Advantages

The multiplier method is a quick, convenient, easy method for LLD prediction. This method is quite useful even if only a single data point is available, unlike the Moseley method, which requires at least three data points. The percentile group of the individual patient is not as important when using the multiplier method because the multipliers remain the same across the percentiles. This method also can be applied to very young children, unlike the Moseley and other methods. The multipliers for different races and growth periods as well as socioeconomic backgrounds are similar, although the heights may not be,[11] and this makes the multiplier method more universally applicable.

T A B L E 1 Multipliers for Boys and Girls

Age in Years, Months	Upper Limb Multiplier[a]		Lower Limb Multiplier[b]	
	Boys	Girls	Boys	Girls
Birth	3.14	3.00	5.080	4.630
0, 3			4.550	4.155
0, 6			4.050	3.725
0, 9			3.600	3.300
1, 0	2.37	2.38	3.240	2.970
1, 3			2.975	2.750
1, 6			2.825	2.600
1, 9			2.700	2.490
2, 0	2.08	1.97	2.590	2.390
2, 3			2.480	2.295
2, 6			2.385	2.200
2, 9			2.300	2.125
3, 0	1.89	1.79	2.230	2.050
3, 6			2.110	1.925
4, 0	1.74	1.65	2.000	1.830
4, 6			1.890	1.740
5, 0	1.63	1.54	1.820	1.660
5, 6			1.740	1.580
6, 0	1.54	1.45	1.670	1.510
6, 6			1.620	1.460
7, 0	1.46	1.37	1.570	1.430
7, 6			1.520	1.370
8, 0	1.39	1.31	1.470	1.330
8, 6			1.420	1.290
9, 0	1.33	1.25	1.380	1.260
9, 6			1.340	1.220
10, 0	1.28	1.20	1.310	1.190
10, 6			1.280	1.160
11, 0	1.23	1.15	1.240	1.130
11, 6			1.220	1.100
12, 0	1.19	1.09	1.180	1.070
12, 6			1.160	1.050
13, 0	1.15	1.05	1.130	1.030
13, 6			1.100	1.010
14, 0	1.10	1.03	1.080	1.000
14, 6			1.060	
15, 0	1.05	1.02	1.040	
15, 6			1.020	
16, 0	1.02	1.00	1.010	
16, 6			1.010	
17, 0	1.01	1.00	1.000	
18, 0	1.00	1.00		

The mature limb length = L (length of the limb) × M (multiplier, supplied by chart).
[a] From Paley D, unpublished data.
[b] Adapted from Reference 17.

Disadvantages

The multiplier method, like most of the other methods outlined above, is applicable only to Shapiro type I proportionate progression patterns. Also, it uses chronologic rather than skeletal age and this may lead to error if there is a large mismatch between the two. Also, the formulas do require calculation and are therefore subject to error.

Upper Extremity Length Predictions

Whereas a small LLD in the upper extremity is well tolerated and is not usually a functional impediment, larger discrepancies may need to be addressed surgically. Straight-line graphs are available for individual segments of the upper extremity.[19] The multiplier method[20] also can be used to predict LLD in the upper extremity and to plan appropriate timing of surgical intervention.

CONTROVERSIES IN LLD PREDICTION
Chronologic or Skeletal Age

Considerable differences may exist between the skeletal and chronologic ages. Cundy et al[21] found that 10% of their patients had a discrepancy of greater than 2 years between the chronologic and skeletal ages. Diméglio et al[22] found that only about one third of their patients had a difference of less than 6 months between their chronologic and skeletal ages. Prediction methods also may be less accurate in patients with significantly delayed skeletal age, as the skeletal age seems to accelerate and approaches the chronologic age closer to maturity.

Little et al[9] found no advantage in accurate timing of epiphysiodesis using skeletal age as opposed to chronologic age when they compared the methods of Green-Anderson, Moseley, and Menelaus.

LLD is difficult to predict with accuracy in children younger than 10 years. Kasser and Jenkins[23] followed 35 children aged 5 to 10 years. They found that the use of skeletal age (as opposed to choronologic age) in this cohort did not improve the accuracy of LLD prediction, except in five girls with advanced skeletal age.

Skeletal Age Assessment

Various methods are available for prediction of skeletal age. The Greulich and Pyle method utilizes ossification centers in the wrist and hand and is most commonly used, but it has the disadvantages of wide standard deviations and considerable interobserver variation.[21,24]

The Tanner method[25] of skeletal age assessment also uses wrist radiography, but it relies mainly on the distal ossification centers rather than the carpal ones. It is more complicated, but one study found it resulted in a more accurate prediction of LLD.[23]

The Sauvegrain method[26] and its modification by Diméglio et al[22] are based on AP and lateral radiographs of the elbow. The advantage of this method is that it breaks down the crucial time around puberty into 6-month intervals. It also divides the pubertal growth spurt into an accelerating phase and a decelerating phase (the latter of which begins once the ossification of the elbow growth centers is complete). Epiphysiodesis performed in the decelerating phase provides very little correction, as most of the growth is complete by this time.

Limb Growth After Lengthening

The growth of long bones after lengthening may be unpredictable. Lengthening of long bones may be associated with growth stimulation (femoral diaphyseal lengthening) or growth retardation (tibial metaphyseal and diaphyseal lengthening).[27,28] This phenomenon is not well understood and may be a result of increased forces generated during lengthening across an unhealthy growth plate. This makes prediction of LLD at maturity unreliable.

REFERENCES

1. Gross RH: Leg length discrepancy: How much is too much? *Orthopedics* 1978;1(4):307-310.
2. Rush WA, Steiner HA: A study of lower extremity inequality. *Am J Roentgenol Radium Ther* 1946;56(5):616-623.
3. Gurney B, Mermier C, Robergs R, Gibson A, Rivero D: Effects of limb-length discrepancy on gait economy and lower-extremity muscle activity in older adults. *J Bone Joint Surg Am* 2001;83-A(6):907-915.
4. Song KM, Halliday SE, Little DG: The effect of limb-length discrepancy on gait. *J Bone Joint Surg Am* 1997;79(11):1690-1698.
5. Tjernström B, Rehnberg L: Back pain and arthralgia before and after lengthening: 75 patients questioned after 6 (1-11) years. *Acta Orthop Scand* 1994;65(3):328-332.

6. Shapiro F: Developmental patterns in lower-extremity length discrepancies. *J Bone Joint Surg Am* 1982;64(5): 639-651.

7. White JW, Stubbins SG Jr: Growth arrest for equalizing leg lengths. *J Am Med Assoc* 1944;126:1146-1149.

8. Menelaus MB: Correction of leg length discrepancy by epiphysial arrest. *J Bone Joint Surg Br* 1966;48(2): 336-339.

9. Little DG, Nigo L, Aiona MD: Deficiencies of current methods for the timing of epiphysiodesis. *J Pediatr Orthop* 1996;16(2):173-179.

10. Anderson M, Green WT, Messner MB: Growth and predictions of growth in the lower extremities. *J Bone Joint Surg Am* 1963;45-A:1-14.

11. Beumer A, Lampe HI, Swierstra BA, Diepstraten AF, Mulder PG: The straight line graph in limb length inequality: A new design based on 182 Dutch children. *Acta Orthop Scand* 1997;68(4):355-360.

12. Pritchett JW: Longitudinal growth and growth-plate activity in the lower extremity. *Clin Orthop Relat Res* 1992(275):274-279.

13. Pritchett JW, Bortel DT: Single bone straight line graphs for the lower extremity. *Clin Orthop Relat Res* 1997(342):132-140.

14. Anderson M, Messner MB, Green WT: Distribution of lengths of the normal femur and tibia in children from one to eighteen years of age. *J Bone Joint Surg Am* 1964;46:1197-1202.

15. Green WT, Anderson M: Epiphyseal arrest for the correction of discrepancies in length of the lower extremities. *J Bone Joint Surg Am* 1957;39-A(4):853-872.

16. Moseley CF: A straight-line graph for leg-length discrepancies. *J Bone Joint Surg Am* 1977;59(2):174-179.

17. Paley D, Bhave A, Herzenberg JE, Bowen JR: Multiplier method for predicting limb-length discrepancy. *J Bone Joint Surg Am* 2000;82-A(10):1432-1446.

18. Maresh MM: Linear growth of long bones of extremities from infancy through adolescence; continuing studies. *AMA Am J Dis Child* 1955;89(6):725-742.

19. Bortel DT, Pritchett JW: Straight-line graphs for the prediction of growth of the upper extremities. *J Bone Joint Surg Am* 1993;75(6):885-892.

20. Paley D, Gelman A, Shualy MB, Herzenberg JE: Multiplier method for limb-length prediction in the upper extremity. *J Hand Surg Am* 2008;33(3):385-391.

21. Cundy P, Paterson D, Morris L, Foster B: Skeletal age estimation in leg length discrepancy. *J Pediatr Orthop* 1988;8(5):513-515.

22. Diméglio A, Charles YP, Daures JP, de Rosa V, Kaboré B: Accuracy of the Sauvegrain method in determining skeletal age during puberty. *J Bone Joint Surg Am* 2005;87(8):1689-1696.

23. Kasser JR, Jenkins R: Accuracy of leg length prediction in children younger than 10 years of age. *Clin Orthop Relat Res* 1997(338):9-13.

24. Greulich WW, Pyle SI: *Radiographic Atlas of Skeletal Development of the Hand and Wrist*, ed 2. Stanford, CA, Stanford University Press, 1959.

25. Tanner JM, Whitehouse RH, Marshall WA, Healy MJ, Goldstein H: *Assessment of Skeletal Maturity and Prediction of Adult Height (TW2 Method)*. London, United Kingdom, Academic Press, 1975.

26. Sauvegrain J, Nahum H, Bronstein H: Study of bone maturation of the elbow. *Ann Radiol (Paris)* 1962;5: 542-550.

27. Shapiro F: Longitudinal growth of the femur and tibia after diaphyseal lengthening. *J Bone Joint Surg Am* 1987;69(5):684-690.

28. Sharma M, MacKenzie WG, Bowen JR: Severe tibial growth retardation in total fibular hemimelia after limb lengthening. *J Pediatr Orthop* 1996;16(4):438-444.

CHAPTER 5

TREATMENT OF LIMB-LENGTH DISCREPANCY WITH EPIPHYSIODESIS

NEIL SARAN, MD, FRCSC
KARL E. RATHJEN, MD

HISTORY

In 1933, Phemister[1] described his epiphysiodesis technique in his seminal paper on a series of patients in whom he performed "epiphyseodiaphyseal fusions" for limb-length and angular deformities. At that time, only crude estimates of growth potentials of the different anatomic physes were available; therefore, Phemister was unable to time the epiphysiodesis so that the limbs would equalize at skeletal maturity. In 1945, Haas[2] described the effects of tethering the growth plate. Shortly afterward, Blount and Clarke[3] described the use of staples to treat both angular and limb-length deformities. In his 1949 paper, Blount described the extraperiosteal technique that was used to temporarily arrest the physis with staples. Although these techniques for temporary epiphysiodesis decreased problems with the timing of epiphysiodesis, problems with hardware migration, implant failure, unpredictable rebound growth, and the risk of permanent physeal damage became evident and continue to be of concern.[3,4] With time, the Anderson-Green-Messner growth charts enabled surgeons to better predict the timing of epiphysiodesis to equalize the limb-length discrepancy (LLD) by the time skeletal maturity was reached, making permanent epiphysiodesis more attractive for many surgeons treating children close to skeletal maturation.[5]

INDICATIONS

The primary indication for epiphysiodesis is an LLD measuring 2 to 5 cm in a skeletally immature child with adequate growth remaining. The "2-cm rule" is based primarily on the results of a four-question survey performed by Gross[6] in 74 skeletally mature patients with an LLD of 1.5 cm or greater. Gross concluded that there was little evidence to support equalizing discrepancies less than 2 cm. More quantitative studies have elaborated that the 2-cm cutoff may be too small. Song et al[7] used gait analysis to evaluate 37 patients with LLDs from 0.6 to 11 cm. They found no correlation between the actual discrepancy or the percentage of discrepancy and any of the dependent kinematic or kinetic variables. Discrepancies less than 3% of the length of the longer extremity were not associated with compensatory strategies, whereas discrepancies 5.5% or more resulted in increased mechanical work performed by the longer extremity and greater vertical displacement of the center of body mass. Vitale et al[8] performed a study of 76 patients that showed that differences in quality of life (measured with the Child Health Questionnaire) became more apparent with increasing LLD; however, no statistically significant data supported the 2-cm cutoff proposed by Gross.[6] Despite the evidence presented by these quantitative reports, concerns over future problems related to the back, hip, or knee lead most par-

Dr. Saran or an immediate family member has received research or institutional support from Stryker. Dr. Rathjen or an immediate family member serves as an unpaid consultant to Orthopediatrics.

ents—and physicians—to opt for epiphysiodesis to treat skeletally immature patients with LLDs greater than 2 to 2.5 cm. Although there is no maximum-size LLD that can be treated with epiphysiodesis, concerns over lowering final adult height make it uncommon to treat an LLD greater than 5 or 6 cm with epiphysiodesis.

Timing of Surgery

The timing of surgery is the most challenging component of epiphysiodesis. The surgery must be timed so that the LLD equalizes at skeletal maturity. Different methods for determining the amount of growth remaining include the Anderson-Green-Messner distal femur and proximal tibia growth remaining charts, the Anderson-Messner-Green lengths of normal femur and tibia charts, the Menelaus method, the Moseley straight-line graph, and the Paley multiplier method.[5,9-14] Each method has advantages and disadvantages, and the main constraint is that they rely on the assumption of linear growth patterns. For a more detailed description, see chapter 4. Regardless of which method is used, parents must be educated that estimating growth is at best an imprecise science and that close clinical follow-up in the postoperative period is critical to allow early identification and treatment of undercorrection, overcorrection, or asymmetric correction.

Surgical Options

The two main types of surgical procedures used to perform epiphysiodesis are permanent and temporary. The open and most percutaneous epiphysiodeses are permanent; staples, tension-bond plates, and percutaneous epiphysiodesis using transphyseal screws can be used in a temporary fashion.

Permanent Epiphysiodesis

Open epiphysiodesis as originally described by Phemister[1] entails three steps: (1) removal of a 3-cm-long and 1- to 1.5-cm-wide cortical window of bone eccentrically positioned around the physis to include 1 cm of epiphysis; (2) using a chisel or curet to remove the physis anterior and posterior to the window to a depth of 1 cm; and (3) replacement of the cortical window rotated 180° so that the physis is no longer in continuity. Variations, including square- or diamond-shaped windows rotated 90°, have been suggested.[15] We prefer to use a 90° bone block rotation with the physeal curettage (**Figure 1**).

The depth of cartilage removal also has been debated, with recommendations ranging from a 1-cm depth to all the way across the central physis, leaving the anterior and posterior peripheral rings intact to keep the distal femur or proximal tibia stable. The most important aspect of the procedure is to ensure that the physis is removed both anteriorly and posteriorly at both the medial and lateral sites to provide an adequate surface area for physeal closure.

In 1984, Bowen and Johnson[16] published results of a percutaneous method of epiphysiodesis. Their method involves curetting the physis under fluoroscopic imaging to a depth of one third the width of the physis on each side through a 3-mm incision after entering the physis to a depth of 5 mm with a 3-mm osteotome. In their original procedure, Bowen and Johnson did not perform percutaneous epiphysiodesis of the proximal fibula because of proximity to the peroneal nerve. Physeal arrest occurred within 4 months in all 12 patients, and the only complication was one keloid scar. Since Bowen and Johnson's initial report, multiple modifications have been made to the percutaneous technique.[17-19] Some reports of percutaneous epiphysiodeses of the fibula include instances of peroneal nerve injury.[17] More recently, Inan et al[20] reported on a series of 97 patients treated with percutaneous epiphysiodesis timed using the Moseley chart predictions and described only three incomplete arrests. Surdam et al[21] retrospectively analyzed 40 open and 56 percutaneous epiphysiodeses and found no angular deformities or epiphysiodesis failures in the open group; however, two failed arrests and one postoperative angular deformity occurred in the percutaneous group, but these differences were not statistically significant. Scott et al[22] reviewed 24 cases of percutaneous epiphysiodesis and 24 cases of open epiphysiodesis and found failure-of-arrest rates of 12% and 15%, respectively. Although studies support the use of percutaneous epiphysiodesis for improved cosmesis, shorter hospital stays, less physical therapy, and equal physeal arrest, we prefer to perform open epiphysiodesis because we believe that, even under the best circumstances, incomplete or partial arrest may occur, and we are more confident in our ability to perform an adequate physeal curettage, thus decreasing the likelihood of angular deformity and/or further surgery, when using an open technique with direct visualization of the physis.[18]

FIGURE 1

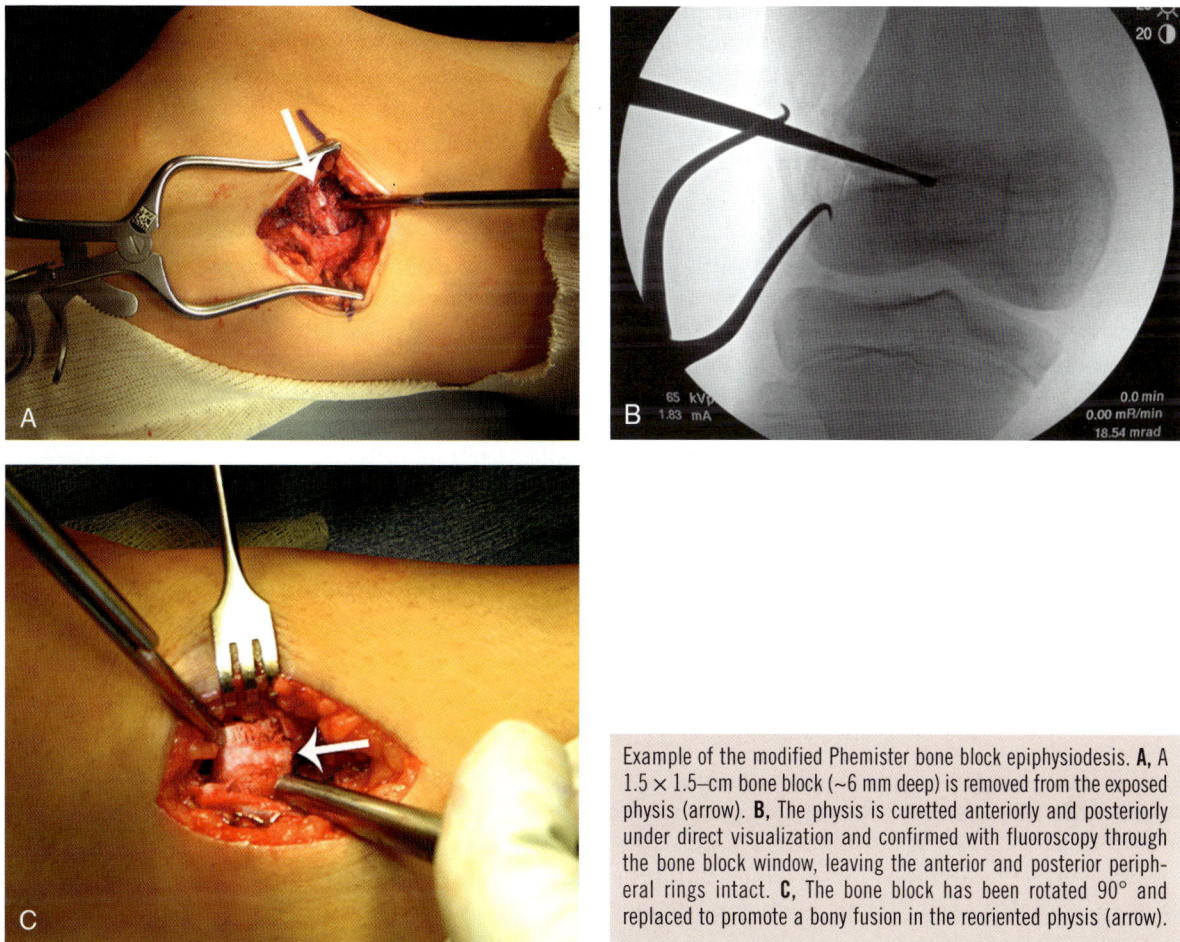

Example of the modified Phemister bone block epiphysiodesis. **A,** A 1.5 × 1.5–cm bone block (~6 mm deep) is removed from the exposed physis (arrow). **B,** The physis is curetted anteriorly and posteriorly under direct visualization and confirmed with fluoroscopy through the bone block window, leaving the anterior and posterior peripheral rings intact. **C,** The bone block has been rotated 90° and replaced to promote a bony fusion in the reoriented physis (arrow).

Temporary Epiphysiodesis

The first method of temporary epiphysiodesis was a wire loop experiment performed by Haas,[2] which was followed by use of staples by Blount and Clarke.[3] Although staples have been previously used to equalize limb lengths, the advent of better predictive tools to determine the timing of permanent epiphysiodesis as well as problems with implant breakage and hardware migration have made this technique less common for LLD although it remains a popular and viable option to treat angular deformities. More recently, Stevens[23] developed a plate-and-screw construct known as an 8-plate that is a similar alternative but with fewer appar-

ent hardware-related complications.[24] Because screws accidentally placed across the physis can cause angular deformity, Métaizeau et al[25] described a new technique of percutaneous epiphysiodesis using transphyseal screws (PETS), which entails placing screws across the growth plate to inhibit growth. The technique worked well in the 18 limbs with postfracture limb overgrowth, with LLD corrections from 20.14 to 4.3 mm in 14 femurs and from 14.11 to 2.33 mm in 9 tibias. The two main advantages of the PETS method are the cosmetically appealing percutaneous insertion of the screws and its potential reversibility. Khoury et al[26] reported on 30 patients undergoing PETS for LLD in which the multiplier method was used to determine the timing of epiphysiodesis. The difference between the average final length and the predicted length of the femur and tibia were 0.15 and 0.05 cm, respectively. Recurvatum developed in one patient who underwent tibial PETS as a result of the screws being placed too far anteriorly, and seven patients required implant removal for mild hardware irritation. Although PETS is an aesthetically attractive and theoretically reversible epiphysiodesis, the results are not as predictable as with a permanent epiphysiodesis; therefore, we do not routinely use this technique for treatment of LLD. Although we do not routinely use physeal tethering techniques (staples, tension-bond plates, or PETS) to treat LLD, we feel that they may be indicated to treat LLD in very young patients who cannot wait for correction until they are close to skeletal maturity or in a child with growth abnormalities that are unpredictable (eg, a child on growth hormones).

COMPLICATIONS

Epiphysiodesis is a relatively straightforward procedure; however, potential complications include hemarthrosis and knee stiffness; incomplete, asymmetric, or partial physeal closure producing angular deformity; and undercorrection and overcorrection. Hemarthrosis and knee stiffness occur more commonly with open epiphysiodesis of the distal femur and may be limited by immobilizing the knee in extension or avoiding prolonged periods of knee flexion until the hemarthrosis resolves. Partial physeal closure producing angular deformity can occur even with close attention to detail. Incomplete, asymmetric, or partial arrest, which usually can be diagnosed at the 4- or 8-month follow-up examination, may require further imaging and repeat epiphysiodesis. Undercorrection and overcorrection are largely the result of incorrect timing of the epiphysiodesis secondary to difficulty in predicting future growth. Although the appropriate use of predictive methods as discussed previously can minimize undercorrection or overcorrection, parents must understand that growth cannot be predicted with complete certainty and that occasionally, a contralateral epiphysiodesis may be required to prevent excessive overcorrection or shortening osteotomies or distraction osteogenesis may be required to treat undercorrection.

SUMMARY

Epiphysiodesis is a viable option for treating LLDs of approximately 2 to 5 cm in skeletally immature patients. Many methods exist to calculate the optimum time for an epiphysiodesis, and many surgical techniques may be used to achieve permanent or temporary growth cessation. Although we most commonly use a modified open Phemister epiphysiodesis timed using the Menelaus method, good results can be achieved with any of the described techniques. A skilled surgeon is aware of and practiced in all options and uses them when clinically indicated. Undoubtedly, the most important aspect of using epiphysiodesis to treat LLD is to spend adequate time with the family to ensure a well-educated and compliant patient who returns for regularly scheduled visits, which limits the likelihood of overcorrection or undercorrection or significant angular deformity from unintended or iatrogenic partial physeal arrest.

REFERENCES

1. Phemister DB: Operative arrestment of longitudinal growth of bones in the treatment of deformities. *J Bone Joint Surg Am* 1933;15:1-15.

2. Haas SL: Retardation of bone growth by a wire loop. *J Bone Joint Surg Am* 1945;27:25-36.

3. Blount WP, Clarke GR: Control of bone growth by epiphyseal stapling: A preliminary report. *J Bone Joint Surg Am* 1949;31A(3):464-478.

4. Zuege RC, Kempken TG, Blount WP: Epiphyseal stapling for angular deformity at the knee. *J Bone Joint Surg Am* 1979;61(3):320-329.

5. Anderson M, Green WT, Messner MB: Growth and predictions of growth in the lower extremities. *J Bone Joint Surg Am* 1963;45-A:1-14.

6. Gross RH: Leg length discrepancy: How much is too much? *Orthopedics* 1978;1(4):307-310.

7. Song KM, Halliday SE, Little DG: The effect of limb-length discrepancy on gait. *J Bone Joint Surg Am* 1997;79(11):1690-1698.

8. Vitale MA, Choe JC, Sesko AM, et al: The effect of limb length discrepancy on health-related quality of life: Is the '2 cm rule' appropriate? *J Pediatr Orthop B* 2006;15(1):1-5.

9. Anderson M, Messner MB, Green WT: Distribution of lengths of the normal femur and tibia in children from one to eighteen years of age. *J Bone Joint Surg Am* 1964;46(6):1197-1202.

10. Menelaus MB: Correction of leg length discrepancy by epiphysial arrest. *J Bone Joint Surg Br* 1966;48(2): 336-339.

11. Westh RN, Menelaus MB: A simple calculation for the timing of epiphysial arrest: A further report. *J Bone Joint Surg Br* 1981;63-B(1):117-119.

12. Moseley CF: A straight line graph for leg length discrepancies. *Clin Orthop Relat Res* 1978(136):33-40.

13. Moseley CF: A straight-line graph for leg-length discrepancies. *J Bone Joint Surg Am* 1977;59(2):174-179.

14. Paley D, Bhave A, Herzenberg JE, Bowen JR: Multiplier method for predicting limb-length discrepancy. *J Bone Joint Surg Am* 2000;82-A(10):1432-1446.

15. White J, Stubbins S: Growth arrest for equalizing leg lengths. *J Am Med Assoc* 1944;126:1144.

16. Bowen JR, Johnson WJ: Percutaneous epiphysiodesis. *Clin Orthop Relat Res* 1984(190):170-173.

17. Canale ST, Christian CA: Techniques for epiphysiodesis about the knee. *Clin Orthop Relat Res* 1990(255):81-85.

18. Liotta FJ, Ambrose TA II, Eilert RE: Fluoroscopic technique versus Phemister technique for epiphysiodesis. *J Pediatr Orthop* 1992;12(2):248-251.

19. Gabriel KR, Crawford AH, Roy DR, True MS, Sauntry S: Percutaneous epiphyseodesis. *J Pediatr Orthop* 1994;14(3):358-362.

20. Inan M, Chan G, Littleton AG, Kubiak P, Bowen JR: Efficacy and safety of percutaneous epiphysiodesis. *J Pediatr Orthop* 2008;28(6):648-651.

21. Surdam JW, Morris CD, DeWeese JD, Drvaric DM: Leg length inequality and epiphysiodesis: Review of 96 cases. *J Pediatr Orthop* 2003;23(3):381-384.

22. Scott AC, Urquhart BA, Cain TE: Percutaneous vs modified phemister epiphysiodesis of the lower extremity. *Orthopedics* 1996;19(10):857-861.

23. Stevens PM: Guided growth for angular correction: A preliminary series using a tension band plate. *J Pediatr Orthop* 2007;27(3):253-259.

24. Stevens PM, Pease F: Hemiepiphysiodesis for posttraumatic tibial valgus. *J Pediatr Orthop* 2006;26(3): 385-392.

25. Métaizeau JP, Wong-Chung J, Bertrand H, Pasquier P: Percutaneous epiphysiodesis using transphyseal screws (PETS). *J Pediatr Orthop* 1998;18(3):363-369.

26. Khoury JG, Tavares JO, McConnell S, Zeiders G, Sanders JO: Results of screw epiphysiodesis for the treatment of limb length discrepancy and angular deformity. *J Pediatr Orthop* 2007;27(6):623-628.

CHAPTER 6

TREATMENT OF LIMB-LENGTH DISCREPANCY WITH SHORTENING

JAMES J. MCCARTHY, MD

INTRODUCTION

Limb shortening for the treatment of limb-length discrepancy (LLD) has been shown to be a reliable method of obtaining limb equalization with few complications.[1-5] Although closed intramedullary femoral shortening is the most common technique, other options, including subtrochanteric shortening with plate fixation, step-cut osteotomy, and shortening of the tibia, have been used.[6-9] This chapter delineates preoperative considerations such as patient selection, education, and preoperative planning; outlines surgical techniques, with an emphasis on closed femoral shortening; and describes postoperative results, care, and complications.

The ultimate goal of any method of treating LLD is to obtain limb-length equality in the safest and least invasive manner. Lifts and other orthotic devices may provide satisfactory correction and patient satisfaction, but they are required indefinitely and may have functional and cosmetic disadvantages. If the patient is skeletally immature, an appropriately timed epiphysiodesis may result in limb-length equality by means of a simpler outpatient procedure, but timing of the procedure is critical and the results are not completely predictable even with careful preoperative assessment.[10,11] Limb lengthening is an attractive option. It is performed on the shorter limb, which is often the affected limb, and it adds height. It is commonly associated with significant complications, however, even when performed by experienced surgeons.[12-14]

PATIENT SELECTION

A shortening procedure should not be considered for a small LLD that will produce no long-term functional deficits, or for one for which a simpler procedure such as an epiphysiodesis can be performed. Larger LLDs (>6 to 7 cm) cannot be fully equalized with a shortening procedure alone; therefore, other techniques should be considered.

Limb shortening is an accurate method of providing limb equalization in skeletally mature patients with LLDs of 2 to 6 cm.[1-5] Although the procedure is as technically demanding as lengthening, shortening is an accurate technique and involves a much shorter convalescence when compared with lengthening techniques; in addition, rotational and angular corrections also can be incorporated in the procedure.[6,15,16] Shortening can be performed in the proximal femur using a blade plate or hip screw, in

Dr. McCarthy or an immediate family member is a member of a speakers' bureau or has made paid presentations on behalf of EBI and Biomet and has received research or institutional support from EBI and Biomet.

FIGURE 1

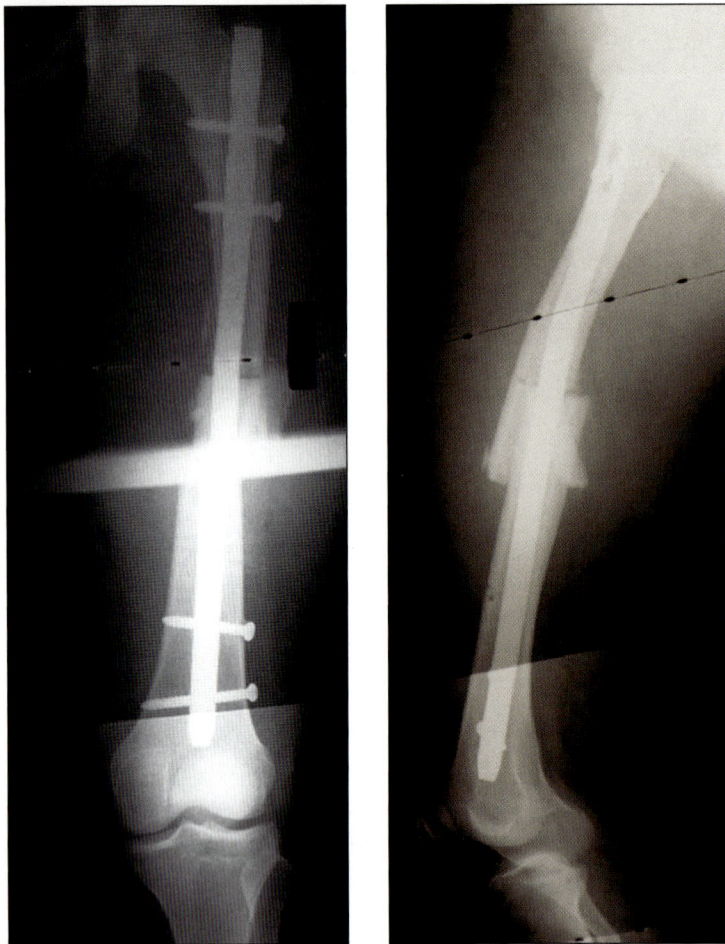

AP **(A)** and lateral **(B)** radiographs of the femur after a closed femoral shortening over an intramedullary nail.

FIGURE 2

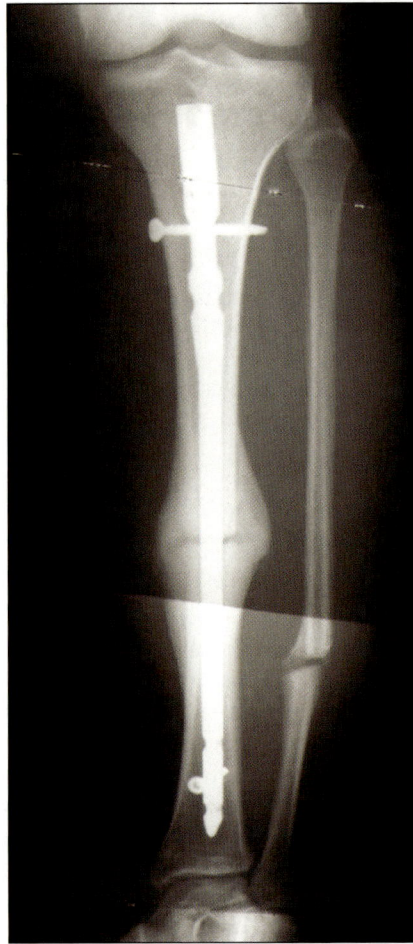

AP radiograph of a tibia after a shortening over an intramedullary nail. An intramedullary saw was not used.

the mid diaphysis of the femur using a closed intramedullary technique (**Figure 1**), or in the tibia also using a closed intramedullary (**Figure 2**) or an open technique. Quadriceps weakness may occur with femoral shortening procedures, especially if a mid diaphyseal shortening greater than 10% is performed. If the femoral shortening is performed proximally, less significant weakness may result. Tibial shortenings can be performed, but there may be a residual bulkiness to the leg, and the risks of nonunion and compartment syndrome are higher.[6,16]

If a tibial shortening is performed, shortening over an intramedullary nail and prophylactic compartment release is suggested.

PREOPERATIVE PATIENT EDUCATION

Patient education is critical for the treatment of LLD, and the consequences and risks of surgery should be balanced against the long-term issues associated with an LLD. It is important that the patient and his or her family understand the available options; discussion with former patients can be helpful. Patient information is available online (http://orthoinfo.AAOS.org/), and recent research information and a directory of Limb Lengthening and Reconstruction Society members are also available (http://www.llrs.org/).

PREOPERATIVE PLANNING

Preoperative planning is critical for any limb reconstruction procedure, including what may initially seem to be a simple limb shortening. First, accurate assessment of limb length is critical. Several pitfalls should be avoided when assessing the LLD clinically and radiographically. Hip and knee flexion contractures, hip adduction or abduction contractures, and technical errors in clinical or radiographic evaluation all can result in significant errors in limb-length measurements. Limb-length (from the pelvis to the bottom of the foot) and leg-length (from the proximal femur to the distal tibia) inequalities may be different as a result of pelvic or foot size asymmetry. Functionally, some patients may prefer a small residual LLD, such as patients with motor weakness who may actually benefit from a small LLD to aid in clearance. Multiple measurements obtained over time, an accurate physical examination, and a trial orthotic lift should all be used to ensure that radiographic and clinical measurements correspond and that the clinical picture is clear.

Rotational and angular assessment also is important. Angular deformities can be corrected during limb shortening but may have significant implications for the technique used and may alter limb length. It is extremely important to assess rotation in both limbs to ensure that symmetric rotation is obtained at the time of limb shortening.

SURGICAL TECHNIQUE

Closed intramedullary shortening is the most common technique used to perform limb shortening, and it has the advantage of providing an extremely stable postoperative construct so the patient can bear weight as tolerated immediately after surgery. Surgical incisions are small and discreet, and most orthopaedic surgeons are familiar with intramedullary fixation. Complications can occur, and care must be taken to avoid these issues. The closed intramedullary shortening technique is already well described by several authors[1-5] and so is outlined only briefly here.

FIGURE 3

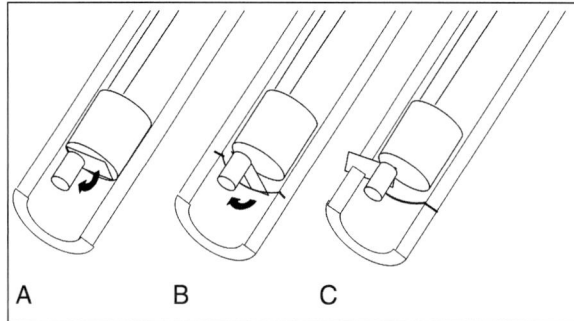

Schematic of the intramedullary saw technique. **A,** After appropriate reaming, the saw is inserted in the femoral canal with the blade fully retracted. **B,** The blade is gradually deployed, and the entire saw is rotated with each deployment. **C,** The blade is fully deployed, dividing the cortex of the femur.

Patient positioning and the incision and entry point are similar to those used for a standard intramedullary rod placement. I do not use a fracture table for this procedure. Rotation should be evaluated and marked preoperatively. Accurate assessment of the contralateral hip rotation is made with preoperative fluoroscopy, and rotational markers are placed.

Prior to reaming, a distal vent hole must be created to prevent fat emboli. Unlike fracture fixation, with shortening, there is no egress to dissipate intramedullary pressure during reaming. I drill multiple holes at the location of the planned distal osteotomy, so that the extruded bone marrow may aid in healing. Additional vent holes also can be made in the distal metaphysis. The intramedullary canal is reamed to 1.5 to 2 mm larger than the planned rod. The diaphyseal portion should be reamed fully, especially in patients with a thick cortex; otherwise, the osteotomy will be difficult to perform with the intramedullary saw. I prefer a mid diaphyseal shortening so that the span of removed bone is the narrowest possible; slight overreaming will not interfere with bone healing because this section of bone will be split and will rest outside the femoral canal.

The intramedullary saw is an eccentrically based saw that rotates around a cam. The surgeon should conduct a careful preoperative review of saw function to ensure that all pieces are available and working. The blade is gradually deployed until the cortical osteotomy is completed (**Figure 3**).

FIGURE 4

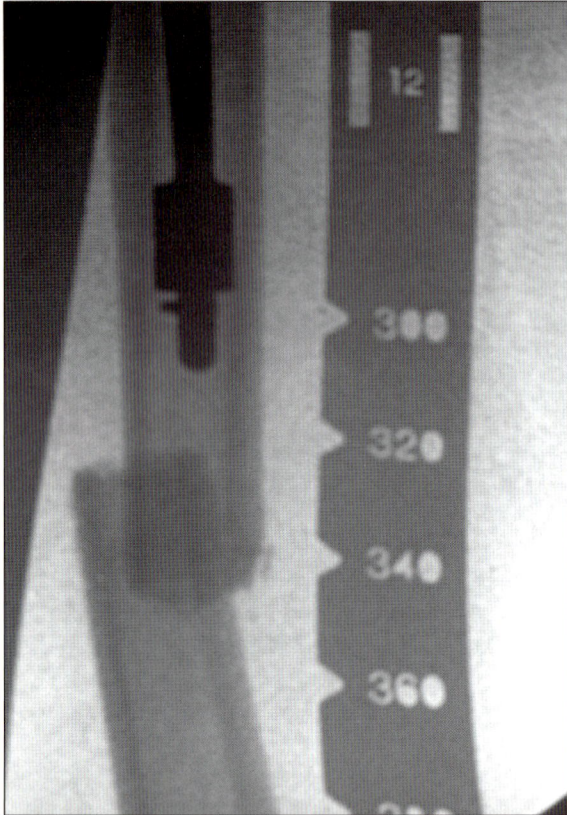

Intraoperative AP fluoroscopic view of a femur shows the completed initial distal cut. The saw has been retracted 4 cm, as measured by the radiolucent ruler.

FIGURE 5

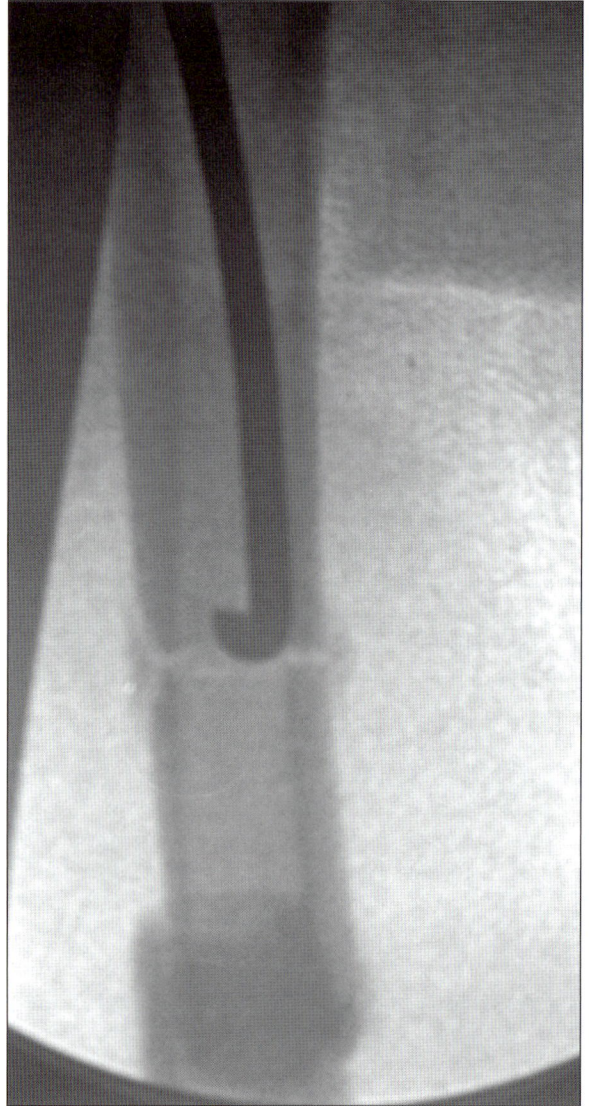

Intraoperative AP fluoroscopic view shows the reverse cutting osteotome hooked on the distal edge of the napkin ring of bone. The osteotome is then backslapped in an attempt to divide the bone.

The distal osteotomy is completed first and is typically distal to the mid diaphysis. The osteotomy can be completed by producing a gentle torsion moment (much like completing a corticotomy when lengthening) and is usually a straightforward procedure. The saw is then retracted a specified amount, typically 0.5 cm less than the LLD, and the position is confirmed with a radiolucent ruler (**Figure 4**). A shortening of more than 6 cm can result in poor compression across the osteotomy site and may lead to quadriceps weakness.[9] The second osteotomy is then made. This may be more difficult to complete, as the rotational maneuver cannot be used because of the previous osteotomy. If needed, an osteotome can be inserted percutaneously to help complete the proximal osteotomy. What remains is a "napkin ring" of bone that must be divided using the hooked osteotomes (**Figure 5**), which are used to hook the distal end of the bone fragment and backslapped so that the ring is divided and the two ends of the femur can be approximated. A guidewire and rod are then inserted in standard fashion, the distal interlocking screws are placed, and the rod is backslapped to provide compression across the osteotomy. Careful attention to rotation is necessary before placing the proximal interlocking screws.

Other techniques used to perform limb shortening include a step-cut open femoral subtrochanteric shortening with blade plate fixation. Most of these techniques enable early return to weight bearing. Subtrochanteric femoral shortening may result in reduced quadriceps weakness postoperatively.[9]

POSTOPERATIVE CARE

One advantage of closed femoral shortening is that the patient can begin weight bearing as tolerated immediately postoperatively. Patient activities can be advanced as strength and motor control improve. Radiographic healing usually occurs by 3 months, and full activity can be initiated at that time.

RESULTS/COMPLICATIONS

In general, patients respond well to closed femoral shortening and experience few significant complications. In a review of five papers that evaluated 118 patients, only three significant complications were reported: two were related to rotational asymmetry and one was a delayed union that required additional surgery.[1-5] It should be noted that these were all retrospective studies, so the complications are most likely underrepresented. Fat emboli resulting in significant pulmonary injury or death are a possibility and all steps must be taken to reduce this risk, including creating a vent hole distal to the diaphysis and maintaining its patency throughout the reaming process.

Rotation must be carefully assessed preoperatively by means of fluoroscopy. The nonoperated knee is placed in a neutral position and an image of the nonoperated hip is saved. At the end of the procedure, before securing the proximal interlocking screws, the saved fluoroscopic image of the nonoperated hip can be compared with the operated hip. Adjustments in rotation are made, if needed, before placement of the proximal locking screws. Another technique is to place threaded guide pins laterally in the femur, one distal to the planned tip of the intramedullary rod and one proximally, posterior to the entry site of the intramedullary rod, to act as a guide; alignment should remain unchanged postoperatively.

SUMMARY

Limb shortening is an accurate method of providing limb equalization in skeletally mature patients with LLDs of 2 to 6 cm. The procedure is technically demanding, and careful assessment and familiarity with the instrumentation is important. Significant complications are uncommon, and weight bearing can begin immediately postoperatively.

REFERENCES

1. Blair VP III, Schoenecker PL, Sheridan JJ, Capelli AM: Closed shortening of the femur. *J Bone Joint Surg Am* 1989;71(10):1440-1447.

2. Chapman ME, Duwelius PJ, Bray TJ, Gordon JE: Closed intramedullary femoral osteotomy: Shortening and derotation procedures. *Clin Orthop Relat Res* 1993;(287):245-251.

3. Eyres KS, Douglas DL, Bell MJ: Closed intramedullary osteotomy for the correction of deformities of the femur. *J R Coll Surg Edinb* 1993;38(5):302-306.

4. Peters JD, Friermood TG: Closed intramedullary femoral shortening. *Orthop Rev* 1990;19(8):709-713.

5. Winquist RA, Hansen ST Jr, Pearson RE: Closed intramedullary shortening of the femur. *Clin Orthop Relat Res* 1978(136):54-61.

6. Coppola C, Maffulli N: Limb shortening for the management of leg length discrepancy. *J R Coll Surg Edinb* 1999;44(1):46-54.

7. Gulsen M, Ozkan C: Angular shortening and delayed gradual distraction for the treatment of asymmetrical bone and soft tissue defects of tibia: A case series. *J Trauma* 2009;66(5):E61-E66.

8. Johansson JE, Barrington TW: Femoral shortening by a step-cut osteotomy for leg-length discrepancy in adults. *Clin Orthop Relat Res* 1983(181):132-136.

9. Nordsletten L, Holm I, Steen H, Bjerkreim I: Muscle function after femoral shortening osteotomies at the subtrochanteric and mid-diaphyseal level: A follow-up study. *Arch Orthop Trauma Surg* 1994;114(1):37-39.

10. Horton GA, Olney BW: Epiphysiodesis of the lower extremity: Results of the percutaneous technique. *J Pediatr Orthop* 1996;16(2):180-182.

11. Little DG, Nigo L, Aiona MD: Deficiencies of current methods for the timing of epiphysiodesis. *J Pediatr Orthop* 1996;16(2):173-179.

12. Dahl MT, Gulli B, Berg T: Complications of limb lengthening: A learning curve. *Clin Orthop Relat Res* 1994(301):10-18.

13. Herzenberg JE, Scheufele LL, Paley D, Bechtel R, Tepper S: Knee range of motion in isolated femoral lengthening. *Clin Orthop Relat Res* 1994(301):49-54.

14. Naudie D, Hamdy RC, Fassier F, Duhaime M: Complications of limb-lengthening in children who have an underlying bone disorder. *J Bone Joint Surg Am* 1998;80(1):18-24.

15. Hasler CC: Leg length inequality: Indications for treatment and importance of shortening procedures. *Orthopade* 2000;29(9):766-774.

16. Kempf I, Grosse A, Abalo C: Locked intramedullary nailing: Its application to femoral and tibial axial, rotational, lengthening, and shortening osteotomies. *Clin Orthop Relat Res* 1986(212):165-173.

THE ILIZAROV METHOD OF DISTRACTION OSTEOGENESIS

STUART A. GREEN, MD

INTRODUCTION

Distraction osteogenesis is a method used to lengthen bone in which the bone is cut and the ends are moved apart gradually, causing new bone to form in the gap. The observation that bone could form in a region devoid of osseous tissue was made by Codivilla[1] and others at the beginning of the 20th century, but not until the 1950s did Ilizarov discover the requirements for the formation of bone tissue during limb lengthening without the production of an intermediate cartilaginous precursor (as happens in fracture healing).[2]

Ilizarov[3,4] and his colleagues, working in Kurgan, Russia (the former U.S.S.R.), employed a canine model to ascertain the ideal environment for rapid bone formation and maturation in distracted tissue. Given the appropriate conditions, virtually any bone can be stimulated to form new osseous tissue in a widening distraction gap. Distraction osteogenesis is most commonly used to lengthen long tubular bones, but it also works well in tarsal and carpal bones, as well as in flat bones of the cranium, mandible, and maxilla. Currently, maxillofacial surgeons use Ilizarov's method of bone formation as often as orthopaedic surgeons do.

Distraction osteogenesis was initially associated with circular tension-wire external skeletal fixators, but bone will form in an appropriate environment regardless of the means used to establish stability; for example, circular fixators mounted with half pins rather than thin wires are as effective as Ilizarov's original construct[5] (**Figures 1** and **2**). Likewise, monolateral tubular fixators can be readily used in place of circular frames for distraction osteogenesis;[6] in certain anatomic locations, monolateral fixators are better tolerated by patients than are complicated circular devices.

Ilizarov warned that damaging the intramedullary blood supply of a bone during implant insertion inhibits distraction osteogenesis. Recent studies have shown, however, that distraction osteogenesis reliably produces bone around an intramedullary nail when the bone is distracted by an external device mounted on the same bone containing the nail.[7] Other authors have described self-lengthening nails that eliminate the need for transcutaneous implants. These nails lengthen by means of a variety of devices, including mechanical ratchets,[8] friction clutches,[9] and internal motors.[10] Bone forms in the osseous tissue surrounding the implant.

REQUIREMENTS FOR DISTRACTION OSTEOGENESIS

Ilizarov identified several factors that are required for successful formation of bone with distraction osteogenesis. The factors are stable fixation, appropriate osteotomy, a properly timed latency interval, rate and rhythm of distraction, and use of the limb after distraction.

Dr. Green or an immediate family member has received royalties from Smith & Nephew and owns stock or stock options in Amgen and Johnson & Johnson.

FIGURE 1

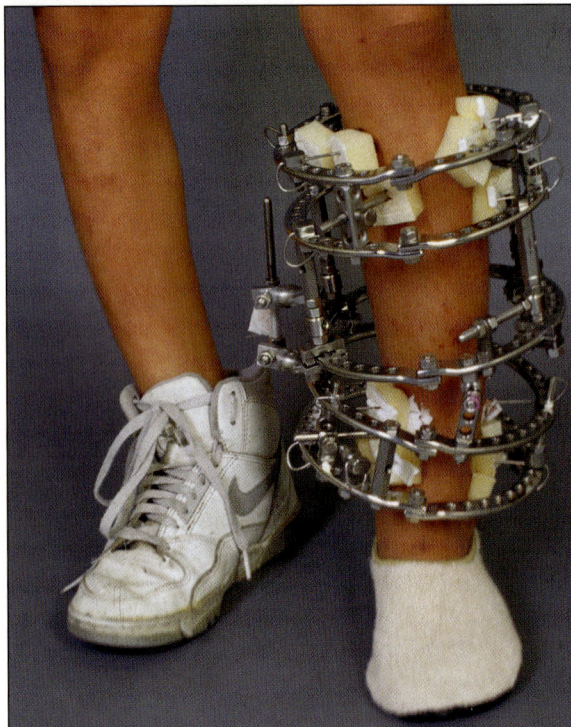

Classic Ilizarov external skeletal fixator for correction of a deformity. (Courtesy of Stuart A. Green, MD, Los Alamitos, CA.)

FIGURE 2

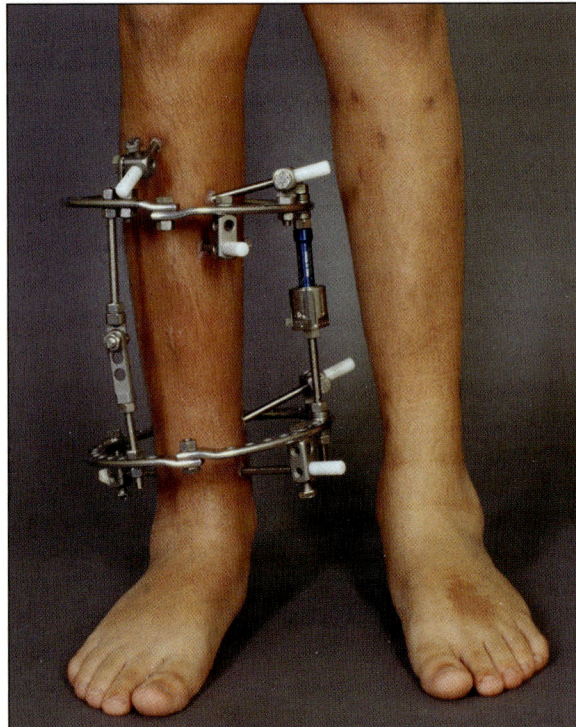

American modification of an Ilizarov fixator on the same patient as in Figure 1. (Courtesy of Stuart A. Green, MD, Los Alamitos, CA.)

Fixation

Ilizarov[3] conducted several experiments to confirm the importance of stable fixation to the quality of bone that forms during distraction. He performed identical osteotomies in three groups of dogs. Similar fixator configurations were applied to all three groups; the only difference was the degree of stability provided. In the first group, a two-ring fixator was applied with loosely tensioned wires. In the second group, the same two-ring fixator was applied but the wires were tensioned to increase stability. The third group of animals had four-ring fixators, with each ring secured to bone with tensioned wires.

All animals underwent identical postoperative management. In the group with the least stable fixation, the distraction gap filled with poorly differentiated connective tissue containing large islands of cartilage. In the second group, with more stable fixation, more osteogenic activity occurred in the distracted zone; however, the upper and lower ends of the zone were filled with cone-shaped segments of regenerated osseous tissue separated by a fibrocartilaginous layer. In the group with the most stable fixation, a high level of osteogenic activity occurred, with the trabecular bone formation parallel to the direction of distraction; little or no fibrous tissue or cartilage formed in these stable configurations.

Osteotomy

Ilizarov also investigated the influence of osteotomy technique on the formation of bone in the distraction zone. Ilizarov performed three kinds of osteotomies in dogs.[3] In the first group, Ilizarov performed a typical open osteotomy of the bone; in the second group, he used a percutaneous technique that preserved marrow circulation by cutting the bone cortex without crossing the medullary canal (a so-called corticotomy); and in the third group, he used a percutaneously placed tension wire to bend the bone until it broke. The most stable type of fraction, the four-ring configuration with crossed tension wires, was used in all three groups. As with the stability study, Ilizarov determined that the more sparing the osteotomy was of both the periosteal and intramedullary blood supplies, the more vigorous was the new bone formation.

Latency Interval

No studies have been performed specifically to confirm the importance of the latency interval, but Ilizarov's success with distraction osteogenesis clearly depended to a considerable extent on the delay before distraction. Following osteotomy, the bone is left at its original length for several days before elongation; this latency interval permits primary healing of the osteotomy. With other limb-lengthening methods such as the Wagener technique, the bone is lengthened immediately after osteotomy, usually to the limit of soft-tissue tolerance; therefore, the patient would leave the operating room with an osseous defect about 1 cm long. Distraction follows immediately after, at a rate of about 1 mm/d in one step. Bone rarely formed under such circumstances.

The latency interval is usually 5 days after osteotomy, during which time the limb is not elongated nor is any deformity corrected; instead, the first stages of osseous healing commence in a stable environment. When distraction begins, the healing tissue on one side of the osteotomy gap continually tries to connect with healing tissue on the opposite side.

In some cases, Ilizarov recommended prolonging the latency interval. For example, if the osteotomy was performed through an open rather than a percutaneous technique, or if the soft tissues surrounding the osteotomy site are damaged by trauma, infection, or radiation, it may be advisable to lengthen the latency interval to 7, 10, or even up to 21 days.[1] The latency interval may have to be shortened for young children, especially for bones completely surrounded by healthy soft tissues.

Rate and Rhythm of Distraction

Ilizarov's observation that the rate and rhythm of distraction influence the quality of bone formation during distraction osteogenesis may have been his most signif-

icant contribution to limb lengthening. Ilizarov[4] conducted a series of experiments on 120 dogs to confirm the importance of the rate and rhythm of distraction. Ilizarov divided the animals into two groups; in the first, the bone was distracted at a rate of 0.5 mm/d; in the second, the bone was distracted at a rate of 1.0 mm/d. The animals in each group were further subdivided into three groups, each with a different rhythm of distraction. In the first subgroup, the bone was distracted at a rate of one step per day; in the second subgroup, the bone was distracted at a rate of four steps per day (one distraction every 6 hours); and in the final subgroup, the bone was distracted with a motorized lengthener that elongated the limb in 60 steps per day.

Ilizarov found that the more fractioned the distraction rhythm, the better the quality of the bone that formed in the distraction gap. Ilizarov also determined that a rate of distraction of 1 mm/d ensured good regenerate bone formation, whereas lengthening the limb at a rate of 0.5 mm/d often led to premature consolidation. Considering the normal rate of biologic growth, it is not surprising that a rate of 1 mm/d is optimal; hair grows at that rate, as does regenerating nerve tissue.

Ilizarov also investigated limb lengthening at a rate faster than 1 mm/d and found that the bone can tolerate a higher elongation rate, but the soft tissues are negatively affected by overly rapid distraction. Ilizarov examined the effect distraction has on skin, nerves, muscles, and other periosseous tissues; as with the bone, the more fractionated the distraction, the better was the tissue tolerance.[3,4]

Limb Use

Ilizarov asserted that functional use of a limb is important for the maturation and ossification of the regenerate bone once the distraction phase ends and the consolidation phase of the process of osteogenesis begins.[1] Regenerate bone takes at least twice as long to mature as it does to form; thus, if limb elongation of 60 mm is planned, it will take 60 days to distract the limb at a rate of 1.0 mm/d and an additional 120 days for the bone to mature. This rapid rate of maturation is seen in children but is unlikely in adults, so the minimum number of days of treatment in adults is usually far longer than three times the planned lengthening (measured in millimeters). To encourage maturation of the regenerate bone, the surgeon should encourage the patient to use the limb in as normal a manner as possible, given the constraints of the fixation apparatus, which means weight bearing on lower extremities and functional use of the upper limbs.

Osteogenesis During Distraction

Ilizarov believed he had discovered a previously hidden capacity within bone to form new bone under appropriate conditions of stability, rate and rhythm of distraction, and functional use during elongation and maturation. He asserted that the new bone that formed under such circumstances was a unique tissue not present in nature. Aronson and Harrison,[11] however, proved Ilizarov wrong regarding the unique nature of this new bone. They showed that bone with the same histologic appearance as the distraction regenerate exists in a growing child just beneath the ring of Ranvier, adjacent to the physeal plate. A growing bone is surrounded by a periosteum that widens the cortex and a physeal plate that elongates the bone. The physeal plate also widens to keep up with the growing size of the osseous structure by means of a perichondreum that surrounds the physis, increasing the diameter of the growth plate as the cortex enlarges transversely.

In the enlarging cortex, bone forms by means of an intramembranous mechanism, whereas the longitudinal growth from the physis undergoes an enchondral ossification process. In regions at the top and bottom of the cortex, however, intramembranous bone formed from the underside of the periosteum is acted upon by the longitudinal growth forces of the adjacent physeal plate. The newly forming bone has the histologic appearance of typical intramembranous bone, but because the bone is lengthening as this tissue forms, its trabeculae assume the orientation of the axis of elongation of the underlying bone. The bone at the ring of Ranvier therefore has an appearance identical to Ilizarov's regenerate bone. Rather than creating an entirely new type of tissue, therefore, the Ilizarov technique establishes conditions that permit any bone to display properties it had during natural rapid growth.

Bone Widening

Ilizarov observed that during distraction osteogenesis, new bone forms parallel to the vector of elongation even if that vector is perpendicular to the longitudinal axis of the bone. This discovery allowed Ilizarov to design surgical procedures to widen bones for cosmetic or functional reasons; for instance, a limb shortened as a result of poliomyelitis also has an underdeveloped appearance as a consequence of lack of muscle bulk. Ilizarov developed a strategy to widen the bone in places where added bulk would improve the cosmetic contour of the limb. To achieve this, Ilizarov designed several surgical procedures that involve splitting off a cortical fragment of bone and distracting that piece sideways to widen the limb.[1]

Neovascularization

Ilizarov[1] performed vascular injection studies using bone widening techniques in laboratory animals and learned that neovascularization takes place in the widening bone tissue as readily as it does in elongated new bone. Ilizarov reasoned that one could create a type of bypass graft in the newly formed bone to help provide circulation to distal parts of the limb with arterial insufficiency. In cases of arterial insufficiency, limb elongation would be undesirable because most dysvascular limbs are at normal length; Ilizarov therefore developed an operation to split off the posterior cortex of the tibia in a region of the limb where vascular blockage had occurred. Ilizarov claimed that this technique of creating a bypass graft of newly formed vascular tissue successfully cured thromboangiitis obliterans in a large series of patients, thereby avoiding amputation.

Vascular surgeons in Western nations have not adopted Ilizarov's method of limb revascularization through laterally directed distraction osteogenesis. This may be because of concerns about the bulkiness and inconvenience associated with wearing a circular external skeletal fixator modified for lateral distraction of a fragment split off the tibia. Adventurous surgeons in countries with limited access to modern techniques of vascular reconstruction have attempted this method.

Tissue Histiogenesis

Fractionated distraction in a stable mechanical environment creates new bone and permits the safe elongation of many other tissues in a limb. Ilizarov and other researchers developed methods of tissue expansion for a variety of purposes; one such method involves placing a balloon under the skin and gradually inflating it with saline,[12] causing the skin to expand, creating redundant tissue that can be used for plastic reconstruction of cutaneous defects.

Ilizarov initially devised strategies to overcome large soft-tissue defects by slowly pulling distracting skin and underlying structures transversely across open wounds. He inserted multiple wires in the free edge of skin lining an open defect and connected these wires to an external plate that was then secured to components of a circular external fixator attached to the limb with transosseous wires. Gradual movement of the external plate, accomplished by turning threaded rods connected to the assembly, pulls the plate away from the skin edge, gradually drawing the skin and underlying soft tissues across the defect.

MEDULLARY BLOOD SUPPLY
Ilizarov contended that both the medullary and periosteal blood supplies must be preserved for regenerate bone to form properly. Delloye et al,[13] however, confirmed in a series of experiments that the periosteal blood supply is more important than marrow vascularity for distraction osteogenesis. They demonstrated this by filling the intramedullary canal with absorbable bone wax in some experimental animals. Bone formed during distraction, provided that the researchers maintained appropriate conditions of stability, latency interval, and a rate and rhythm of the distraction. This work led to the acceptance of using intramedullary nails as part of the limb elongation hardware.

Some surgeons perform lengthening over an intramedullary nail placed at the time of fixator application and osteotomy.[7] More recently, one group of researchers has proposed lengthening with an external skeletal fixator followed by insertion of an intramedullary nail as soon as elongation or conformity correction is complete but before full maturation of the regenerate bone.[14] This strategy allows removal of the external fixator when the limb reaches its corrected length and alignment. The fixator, therefore, is left on for a much shorter time than would be required if the device were left on until the regenerate bone consolidated fully.

STIMULATION AND INHIBITION OF REGENERATE FORMATION
As one might expect, external factors that stimulate maturation of bone have a favorable effect on the regenerate bone in a widening distraction gap, either while the bone is forming or during the maturation phase. Electromagnetic stimulation,[15] ultrasound,[16] and the addition of bone growth–stimulating factors[17] all may accelerate maturation of the regenerate bone. On the other hand, exogenous factors such as alcohol consumption[18] and cigarette smoking,[19] as well as intrinsic factors such as diabetes mellitus,[20] have been shown to inhibit regenerate maturation.

APPLICATIONS OF DISTRACTION OSTEOGENESIS
Although bone elongation to overcome a limb-length discrepancy is the most common application of Ilizarov's discoveries, distraction osteogenesis also can be used to achieve elective stature increase for vanity or other purposes. Because of the great plasticity of regenerate bone as it forms, deformity correction is easily accomplished with Ilizarov's methods without the need for wedge resection and concomitant shortening typically used for such problems in the past.

The Ilizarov intercalary bone transport method is being used with increasing frequency to eliminate skeletal defects as the result of a birth malformation, traumatic bone loss, or surgical débridement for osteomyelitis or tumor.[21] Bone on one or both sides of the defect is osteotomized and lengthened, creating intercalary fragments that traverse and eliminate the defect. For a bone defect accompanied by a soft-tissue deficiency, the method of intercalary bone transport can fill in the soft-tissue loss as well. Other applications of Ilizarov's discoveries include maxillofacial defects, plastic surgery applications, and any condition in which new tissue needs to be created to overcome a deficiency.

REFERENCES
1. Codivilla A: On the means of lengthening, in the lower limbs, the muscles and tissues which are shortened through deformity. *J Bone Joint Surg Am* 1905;2(2):353-369.
2. Ilizarov GA: *Transosseous Osteosynthesis*. Berlin, Germany, Springer-Verlag, 1991.

3. Ilizarov GA: The tension-stress effect on the genesis and growth of tissues: I. The influence of stability of fixation and soft-tissue preservation. *Clin Orthop Relat Res* 1989(238):249-281.

4. Ilizarov GA: The tension-stress effect on the genesis and growth of tissues: II. The influence of the rate and frequency of distraction. *Clin Orthop Relat Res* 1989(239):263-285.

5. Green SA: The Ilizarov method: Rancho technique. *Orthop Clin North Am* 1991;22(4):677-688.

6. McCarthy JJ, Ranade A, Davidson RS: Pediatric deformity correction using a multiaxial correction fixator. *Clin Orthop Relat Res* 2008;466(12):3011-3017.

7. Paley D, Herzenberg JE, Paremain G, Bhave A: Femoral lengthening over an intramedullary nail: A matched-case comparison with Ilizarov femoral lengthening. *J Bone Joint Surg Am* 1997;79(10):1464-1480.

8. Guichet JM: Leg lengthening and correction of deformity using the femoral Albizzia nail. *Orthopade* 1999;28(12):1066-1077.

9. Cole JD, Justin D, Kasparis T, DeVlught D, Knobloch C: The intramedullary skeletal kinetic distractor (ISKD): First clinical results of a new intramedullary nail for lengthening of the femur and tibia. *Injury* 2001; 32(Suppl 4):SD129-SD139.

10. Baumgart R, Zeiler C, Kettler M, Weiss S, Schweiberer L: Fully implantable intramedullary distraction nail in shortening deformity and bone defects: Spectrum of indications. *Orthopade* 1999;28(12):1058-1065.

11. Aronson J, Harrison B: Mechanical induction of osteogenesis: Preliminary studies. *Ann Clin Lab Sci* 1893;169(203):1988.

12. Houpt P, Dijkstra R: Tissue expansion in reconstructive surgery. *Neth J Surg* 1988;40(1):13-16.

13. Delloye C, Delefortrie G, Coutelier L, Vincent A: Bone regenerate formation in cortical bone during distraction lengthening: An experimental study. *Clin Orthop Relat Res* 1990(250):34-42.

14. Rozbruch SR, Kleinman D, Fragomen AT, Ilizarov S: Limb lengthening and then insertion of an intramedullary nail: A case-matched comparison. *Clin Orthop Relat Res* 2008;466(12):2923-2932.

15. Taylor KF, Inoue N, Rafiee B, Tis JE, McHale KA, Chao EY: Effect of pulsed electromagnetic fields on maturation of regenerate bone in a rabbit limb lengthening model. *J Orthop Res* 2006;24(1):2-10.

16. Chan CW, Qin L, Lee KM, Zhang M, Cheng JC, Leung KS: Low intensity pulsed ultrasound accelerated bone remodeling during consolidation stage of distraction osteogenesis. *J Orthop Res* 2006;24(2):263-270.

17. Hu J, Qi MC, Zou SJ, Li JH, Luo E: Callus formation enhanced by BMP-7 ex vivo gene therapy during distraction osteogenesis in rats. *J Orthop Res* 2007;25(2):241-251.

18. Wahl EC, Aronson J, Liu L, et al: Chronic ethanol exposure inhibits distraction osteogenesis in a mouse model: Role of the TNF signaling axis. *Toxicol Appl Pharmacol* 2007;220(3):302-310.

19. Ueng SW, Lin SS, Wang CR, Liu SJ, Tai CL, Shih CH: Bone healing of tibial lengthening is delayed by cigarette smoking: Study of bone mineral density and torsional strength on rabbits. *J Trauma* 1999;46(1):110-115.

20. Liu Z, Aronson J, Wahl EC, et al: A novel rat model for the study of deficits in bone formation in type-2 diabetes. *Acta Orthop* 2007;78(1):46-55.

21. Green SA, Jackson JM, Wall DM, Marinow H, Ishkanian J: Management of segmental defects by the Ilizarov intercalary bone transport method. *Clin Orthop Relat Res* 1992(280):136-142.

CHAPTER 8

DISTRACTION OSTEOGENESIS: LENGTHENING WITH EXTERNAL FIXATORS

DAVID S. FELDMAN, MD

SONIA CHAUDHRY, MD

INTRODUCTION

External fixation is a versatile and powerful tool used for both limb deformity correction and limb lengthening. External fixation allows gradual distraction osteogenesis with minimal soft-tissue disruption and juxta-articular osteotomies. External fixation has drawbacks, however, such as difficulty with patient acceptance, binding of soft tissues, joint stiffness, and pin-tract infection. Many of these concerns have been addressed as external fixation has evolved over the past three decades, and surgeons now have numerous weapons in their arsenal to solve both simple and complex problems. Limb lengthening has been practiced for more than a century,[1] but external fixation has been used longer, since before the invention of plaster,[2] beginning with transcutaneous metal prongs and clamps.[3] The later development of wires and half pins along with more sophisticated constructs has allowed for more treatment options. Today, many combinations of techniques and devices are available. Once the decision to undertake lengthening or deformity correction has been made, the external fixator can be tailored to the patient and his/her deformity factors and the surgeon's experience.

PINS AND WIRES

Most external fixations use half pins to connect the frame to the bone. Half pins achieve bicortical fixation in bone just as transfixation pins do; however, they protrude through the skin and soft tissues on only one side of the limb. Pins have certain advantages over alternative fixation devices such as wires in that they have intrinsic rigidity from an increased core diameter, are more familiar to surgeons, and are relatively well tolerated by patients. Additionally, their strategic use in certain areas where they can achieve large crossing angles and a greater anterior-posterior orientation without invading muscle compartments, such as in the tibial shaft, provides superior fixation. In each segment, an attempt should be made to gain control in multiple planes by achieving 90° crossing angles or as close to that as possible, allowing safe corridors.[4,5] Each construct is unique and should be thoughtfully planned. Each frame generally should have at least three pins per segment

Dr. Feldman or an immediate family member serves as a board member, owner, officer, or committee member of the Limb Lengthening and Reconstruction Society; is a member of a speakers' bureau or has made paid presentations on behalf of Stryker; serves as a paid consultant to or is an employee of Biomet; serves as an unpaid consultant to Orthopediatrics; and has received research or institutional support from EBI, Smith & Nephew, and Stryker. Neither Dr. Chaudhry nor any immediate family member has received anything of value from or owns stock in a commercial company or institution related directly or indirectly to the subject of this chapter.

FIGURE 1

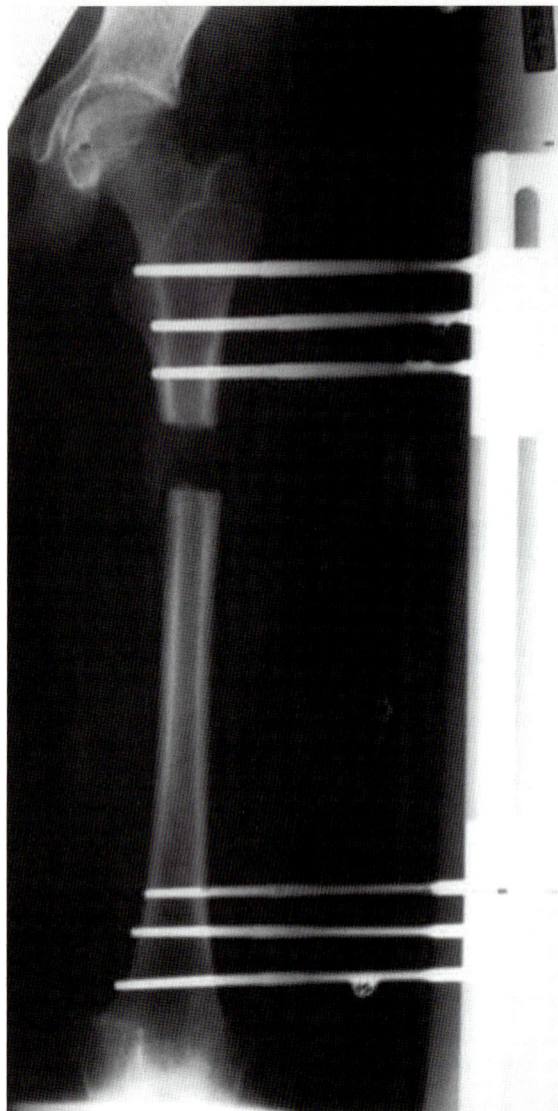

AP radiograph shows femoral lengthening with a rail system using pin fixation with three proximal and three distal pins. This system is easy to place and is used for lengthening along the mechanical axis.

provides adequate fixation such that if a pin needs to be removed because of infection, the construct is stable enough that additional surgery is not necessary.

Selection of pin size requires a balance between achieving increased rigidity with increased pin diameter and minimizing bone violation with decreased pin diameter. Pin diameter should be less than one third of bone diameter to minimize pin-site fracture, which typically translates to 4-mm pins for the upper extremity and 5-mm pins for the tibia and femur. Proportionately smaller pins are used for smaller pediatric patients. Pins are available in interval sizes such as 3.5 and 4.5 mm in some systems. Most pins are stainless steel that is ion plasma–coated with hydroxyapatite. This material has the desirable stiffness of traditional steel without its relatively high infection rates. Pins made from titanium are less likely to become infected but have less stiffness.[2] The hydroxyapatite coating allows pins to osteointegrate, although the resultant strength of fixation achieved often requires the removal of pins under general anesthesia. Another decision is pin shape. Tapered pins achieve slightly stronger cortical fixation, but bicylindrical pins are easier to back out without significant loosening if found to be too proud.

Pin insertion technique is as important as the construct itself because it can minimize pin-site infection, the most common adverse occurrence with external fixators. All pins sites should be predrilled to reduce bone temperature by approximately 50%. Osteocyte damage occurs after exposure to 55°C for 1 minute.[2] When a high-speed drill bit builds heat by passing through hard cortical bone, it necrotizes the bone and causes thermal damage to the skin and soft tissue as it emerges from the opposite side. Tourniquets should not be inflated before drilling because the passing circulation cools the drill and the implant. A sharp drill bit should be used with a start/stop drilling rhythm, along with frequent irrigation, to prevent thermal necrosis. Stopping the drill to allow the cutting tip to cool also prevents the osseous tissue from "work hardening" and resisting further advancement. After removing the drill, the flutes should be wiped clean before being used again, and if the bone removed is black or brown or the drill tip is too hot to be held comfortably for 15 to 20 seconds, another hole should be considered. During drilling, the surrounding soft tissues should be protected with a sleeve.

(Figure 1), with the exception of stagnant segments, which at times can be managed with two. This pin configuration reduces the soft-tissue tension on each pin, allows control of the segment in multiple planes, and

The sleeve should be left in place for pin insertion because deep soft-tissue necrosis ensues when tissues are compressed by implant insertion. Along with thermal injury, relative motion contributes to the risk of pin-tract infection. Reducing motion between the pin and the tissue decreases pin-tract infections, as evidenced by the decreased incidence when pins are in plaster casts that immobilize the skin. Selecting areas for pin insertion that avoid muscle transfixion and wrapping the portion of the pin between the skin and the fixator pins with bulky wads of gauze dressing can decrease motion at this interface.

Wires often are used in circular fixators in addition to pins. These transosseous implants, usually less than 2 mm in diameter, are not stiff enough to provide stability until tensioned and bolted to the fixator, requiring them to be transfixed on both ends. The advantage of this additional soft-tissue violation is the significantly smaller bony defect created by wires compared with pins.[6] In soft bone with little potential for remodeling, such as bone with congenital pseudarthrosis, this is clinically important. Additionally, using wires for periarticular fixation is advantageous because it avoids muscle compartments and allows placement of reference wires to guide application of rings on bony segments. Last, wires are easily removed in a clinical setting, making them ideal for temporary fixation of joints during lengthening. For example, during tibial lengthening, wires can be used to span the midfoot and forefoot initially and can be removed in the clinic once the patient is mobile and pain free, before undergoing surgery for frame removal.

As with pins, wire insertion technique is important to prevent loosening and subsequent infection. Motion at the wire-skin interface should be minimized by avoiding transcompartmental wires, which also tend to be more uncomfortable. Incisions and drill sheaths are not necessary for 1.5- and 1.8-mm wires, but they should be used for the larger 2-mm wires. Necrosis due to tissue windup should be avoided by pushing the wire through tissue, down to the cortex, before drilling. Sponges soaked in normal saline can be used to cool and direct the wire during drilling. Once the far bony cortex is penetrated, drilling should be stopped. The wire is then stabilized with pliers as it is tapped through the skin of the opposite side of the limb with a mallet. Once the wire is placed, the skin should be checked for tension at the wire interface and the skin hole incised if necessary to prevent undue pressure. The frame is then attached to the wire, not vice versa,[4] and tensioned to 110 to 130 kg or until the ring deflects. Open rings withstand less force, in the range of 70 to 100 kg.

Pin sites should be cleaned daily with a washcloth and soap and water, usually in a shower, to remove the crust from the skin, and then covered by a light pressure dressing to minimize pin-skin motion. If an infection does ensue, empiric antibiotics and aggressive local pin care are used. If this does not resolve the infection, culture-specific antibiotics and eventual removal of the implant may be necessary. Surgery for pin replacement or bone débridement for osteomyelitis is rarely necessary.

Another consideration is for skin tension that interferes with the local circulation of the subdermal capillary plexus and leads to skin necrosis. Skin tension is minimized by aligning the osteotomy site before pin insertion to avoid pinching the skin on the convex side and tensioning skin on the concave side. With larger lengthening, soft-tissue pressure at fixation sites can be minimized with bifocal corticotomy, allowing the tensioning and regenerate bone to be spread over multiple sites, minimizing the amount at each site.[7] Additionally, skin should be assessed after frame assembly is complete, and if pressure on the skin at any fixation point is evident, the wire or pin hole should be enlarged on the compression side and sutured on the tension side with nylon if necessary. Finally, when using transfixation wires, the adjacent joint should be near its end range of motion to prevent excessive soft-tissue pressure. For example, in a distal tibiofibular wire, the foot should be in dorsiflexion when breaching the posterolateral skin and in plantar flexion before exiting the anteromedial side. Similarly, every joint adjacent to a transfixed segment should be taken through passive range of motion before leaving the operating room to assess for soft-tissue binding. If fixation through muscle compartments limits joint mobility in the operating room before distraction has begun, the increased tension on muscles and the effect this has on joints can be expected to worsen once lengthening is initiated.

JOINT PROTECTION

In lengthening procedures, adjacent joints are exposed to excessive forces and may be at risk for cartilage dam-

FIGURE 2

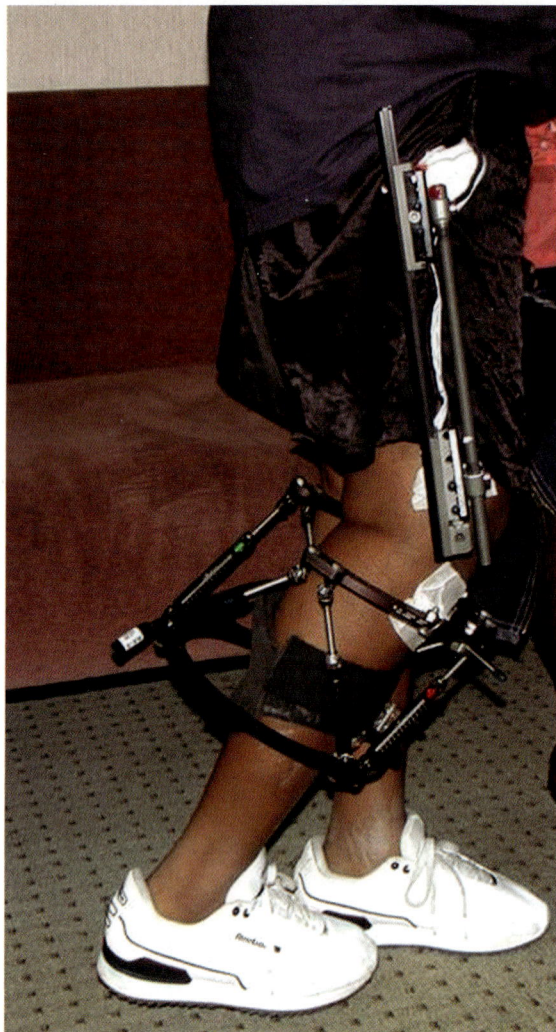

Clinical photograph shows circular external fixator for femoral lengthening with knee-spanning extension to protect the joint during distraction.

age or joint dislocation.[8] No absolute indications for external fixation spanning the hip, knee, or ankle exist, but consideration should be given to external fixation for a hip that is dysplastic or unstable, a knee that is anterior cruciate ligament–deficient, or an ankle with a tight Achilles tendon. Specific conditions in which the common lack of a competent anterior cruciate ligament

requires additional stabilization to prevent dislocation, such as a congenitally short femur, may require spanning of the knee during femoral lengthening[9] (**Figure 2**). Adjacent joints also can be bridged to prevent contractures (eg, equinus) with tibial lengthening. Circular frames, with their modular designs, more easily enable attaching foot plates to the rings, or fixing the foot through metatarsal/cuneiform pins or wires. As mentioned above, the wires can be used for temporary fixation and are removed in the office once the patient is ambulating.

Soft-tissue releases also can protect joints during the lengthening. In addition to incorporating the ankle into a tibial frame, the expected tensioning of the Achilles tendon with tibial lengthening justifies a preemptive or subsequent Achilles tendon lengthening. Similarly, when lengthening the femur, a hamstring and iliotibial band release is often prudent to prevent both knee flexion contracture and destabilizing forces across the knee. Adjacent joints are subject to tremendous joint reaction forces—up to 64 N with just 25 mm of tibial lengthening.[10] The osteotomy site influences these forces, with the closer joint bearing most of the increased force. These forces remain high even into the consolidation phase,[11] often requiring protective joint spanning for the entire treatment period.

NERVE PROTECTION

Tension on neurovascular structures can be anticipated with lengthening or deformity correction. The common peroneal nerve is the most sensitive to stretch injury, and it should be routinely released when correcting valgus deformity in excess of 20° or while lengthening if early symptoms such as pain on the dorsum of the foot develop. The medial plantar nerve also can be trapped in the tarsal tunnel and may require release during foot corrections. Nerve release should be performed before frank nerve injury, such as a foot drop.

BONE CONSIDERATIONS

Certain anatomic segments are prone to predictable deformity during limb lengthening with external fixation, depending on the type of fixator used. For example, using a monolateral fixator on the lateral side of the femur may cause the lengthening to drift into varus with preferential lengthening on the lateral side. Using at least three pins in each segment and placing the fixator as close to the thigh as possible may counteract this drift. In the leg, fibular distraction progresses at a slower rate and to a lesser degree than tibial lengthening with a monolateral fixator, which may lead to ankle valgus.[12,13] A distal syndesmotic screw often is used to prevent relative proximal migration of the lateral malleolus when the lengthening is more than 2.5 cm. A proximal tibiofibular screw also may be used to counteract the tendency of the fibular head to migrate distally,[14,15] but this may be less important because distal migration of the proximal fibula has limited clinical significance.

The osteotomy site also should be strategically chosen with consideration given to both bone and soft tissue. For example, proximal osteotomy in the femur allows for better regenerate bone and less quadriceps binding. In the case of a congenitally short femur, however, a distal osteotomy should be performed because proximal regenerate bone is not as strong, although decreased knee range of motion is then inevitable. If impending malunion of the osteotomy site is observed, revision surgery occasionally can be avoided by adjusting the alignment of the external fixation in the office.

Dynamization is an important part of distraction osteogenesis, as all fixators should provide initial rigid fixation[16] that gradually can transfer axial load to the regenerate bone.[17] Dynamization prevents stress shielding and allows for greater callus formation. Unilateral frames can be destabilized by sliding bars farther from bone, removing bars, moving half pins, and releasing tension or compression. This is not biomechanically ideal because the regenerate bone will experience shear and torsional forces in addition to the desired axial load. Circular fixators allow for a "trampoline effect" from wires, allowing some degree of axial compression, which can be increased further by releasing tension on wires, removing connecting rods between rings, or even removing rings. The enhancement of osteogenesis by weight bearing is common to all methods, but if weight bearing is allowed in an uncontrolled manner, it risks delayed union, refracture through the osteotomy, and secondary deformity.

FIXATOR TYPES
Thoughtful preoperative planning is required for any lengthening or deformity correction. Two main types of external fixators are used: uniplanar and circular. The uniplanar external fixator usually sits on the lateral side of the thigh and the medial or anteromedial aspect of the leg. In some unusual circumstances, a medial or anterior thigh fixator and a lateral leg fixator can be used. The uniplanar system may consist of balls, joints, and translational devices or simply may be connected by a rail or pin to the bars.[18] Although these fixators are uniplanar, meaning they are on one side of the limb in a single plane, several systems are available that allow for multiplanar correction using a uniplanar frame (**Figure 3**). These systems use distractors for lengthening and angulators or translators for deformity correction. These constructs are lighter and occupy less space than circular fixators, so they are better tolerated by patients; however, they may not resist the tendency toward deformity. Strut position controls the most significant clinical forces at the osteotomy site; however, when loaded with out-of-plane varus/valgus and torsional forces, motion occurs at the osteotomy site and cantilever bending occurs, with resultant asymmetric loading at the osteotomy site. A multiplanar system provides more stability.

Circular fixators work on a different principle than uniplanar fixators, creating an exoskeleton surrounding the limb consisting of connecting rods, struts, and rings; the rings can be fully closed, partially open, or arches.[19] Partial rings are used around the knee to allow greater flexion. They are also used around the shoulder and proximal femur, where full rings would be uncomfortable. The classic Ilizarov construct involves tensioned wires; however, the modern Ilizarov fixator refers to a circular ring with any combination of tensioned wires, half pins, and full pins. Hybrid fixation refers to a unilateral fixator with an attached ring.[2,20] A true hybrid frame is rarely used for lengthening or deformity correction. Frame stability directly affects osteogenesis. Ideally, external fixators are rigid in torsion, bending, and shear but allow for axial movement. The advantage of circular frames is that unlike monolateral fixators, they demonstrate load-dependent axial stiffness, allowing more axial motion to stimulate fracture callus at lower loads and preventing excessive motion at increased loads to protect the healing fracture. Circular frames allow uniform compression/distraction, which enhances healing and prevents malunion (**Figure 4**). The modular

FIGURE 3

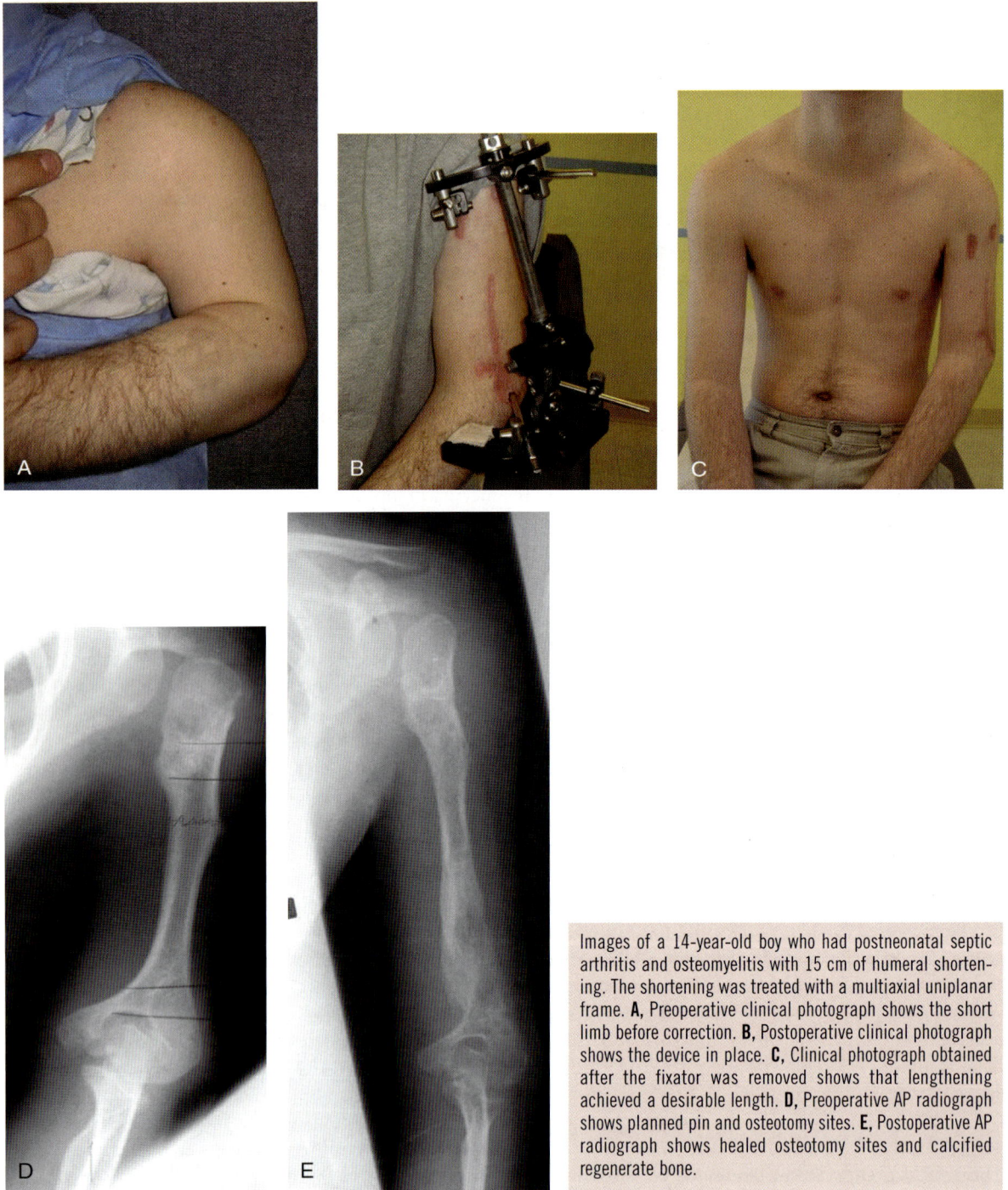

Images of a 14-year-old boy who had postneonatal septic arthritis and osteomyelitis with 15 cm of humeral shortening. The shortening was treated with a multiaxial uniplanar frame. **A,** Preoperative clinical photograph shows the short limb before correction. **B,** Postoperative clinical photograph shows the device in place. **C,** Clinical photograph obtained after the fixator was removed shows that lengthening achieved a desirable length. **D,** Preoperative AP radiograph shows planned pin and osteotomy sites. **E,** Postoperative AP radiograph shows healed osteotomy sites and calcified regenerate bone.

FIGURE 4

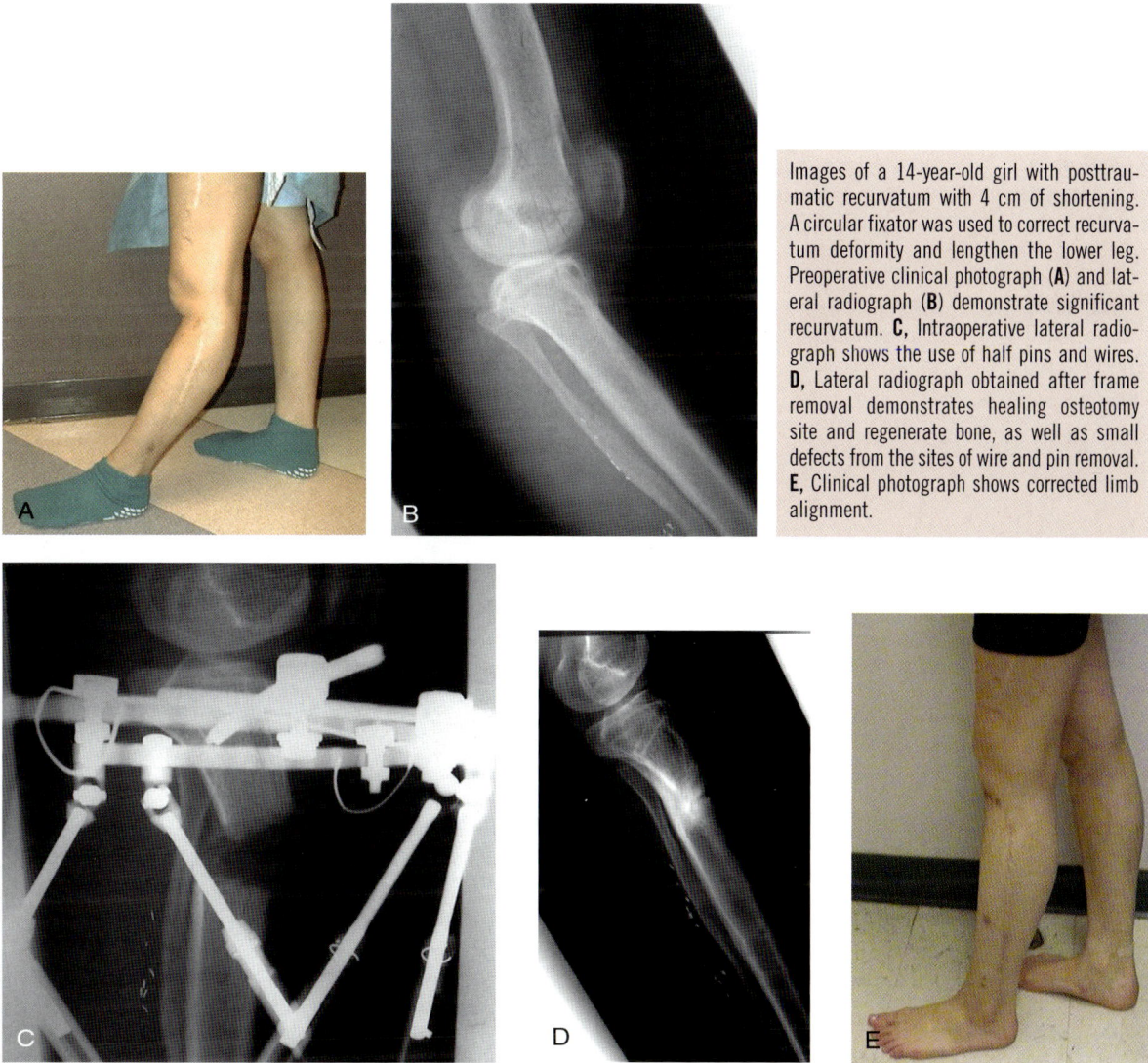

Images of a 14-year-old girl with posttraumatic recurvatum with 4 cm of shortening. A circular fixator was used to correct recurvatum deformity and lengthen the lower leg. Preoperative clinical photograph (**A**) and lateral radiograph (**B**) demonstrate significant recurvatum. **C,** Intraoperative lateral radiograph shows the use of half pins and wires. **D,** Lateral radiograph obtained after frame removal demonstrates healing osteotomy site and regenerate bone, as well as small defects from the sites of wire and pin removal. **E,** Clinical photograph shows corrected limb alignment.

nature of circular fixators allows for re-creation of both simple hinge joints, such as the elbow, and oblique joints, such as the ankle. Three-dimensional configurations allow for deformity correction in virtually any plane, with the advantage of periarticular fixation with wires. This increased versatility, however, mandates a thorough knowledge of safe corridors for implant placement.[21] Additionally, circular frames are bulkier, more difficult to ambulate with, and harder to care for; however, these disadvantages are offset by advantages, including the decrease in cortical violation with wire placement compared with pins and the ease with which frames can be built upon or debulked as necessary. Table 1 compares the types of fixators.

Fixator Examples
Monolateral Rail Fixation
Monolateral rail fixation is one of the simplest methods of lengthening a long bone. A monolateral rail fixator can be used as a stand-alone device for limb lengthen-

TABLE 1: Characteristics of Uniplanar Versus Circular External Fixators for Limb Lengthening

Parameter	Uniplanar	Circular	Considerations for Both
Ease of application	Conceptually simpler, with easier assembly and application of components	More components, requires familiarity and extensive knowledge of safe corridors for pin/wire placement	Thoughtful preoperative planning is required for lengthening or deformity correction
Indications	Simple lengthening with or without minor deformity correction	Lengthening and major deformity correction are possible through three-dimensional construct. Wires can traverse closer to joints than pins. Modular design allows hinges in multiple axes.	External fixators are fixed-angle devices, giving superior fixation in compromised bone. This optimizes stability while minimizing tissue damage. Both types offer gradual correction in any limb segment.
Soft-tissue effects	Uses pins, which create larger bone defects than wires	Tensioned wires offer strength without drilling large holes in the bone.	Safe corridors should be respected. Soft-tissue damage can be minimized by insertion technique. All external fixation causes less disruption of soft tissues, osseous blood supply, and periosteum compared with internal fixators or intramedullary devices.
Patient tolerance	Well tolerated because constructs are light and occupy less space, reduced bulk facilitates hygiene	Heavier and bulkier, more difficult to ambulate with and to care for	All external fixators have significant physical and psychologic effects, which should be addressed both before and during lengthening.
Disadvantages/ complications	Weight bearing produces cantilever bending, delivering asymmetric compression to the osteotomy site.	Multiple pin and wire sites in addition to bulky construct make pin care more difficult.	All external fixators are subject to pin/wire-site infections; any lengthening can create instability in the adjacent joints.

ing or for lengthening over a rail or lengthening with a plate. For example, in the femur, three half pins are placed proximally in the lateral thigh and three are placed distally in parallel alignment. Ideally, the pins are placed perpendicular to the mechanical axis of the femur so that when the lengthening device is placed and the rail is applied, the lengthening occurs along that axis. Most rail systems have a pin clamp that allows pins to be placed in parallel alignment. Because of the anterior bow of the femur, this alignment is sometimes not possible, in which case outriggers can be placed to attach the pins to each other. In the tibia, lengthening with a monolateral fixator is performed medially, and, as in the femur, the rail needs to be applied perpendicular to the mechanical axis of the tibia. If inadequate fixation is used or the pins are placed off axis, an anteromedial bow often develops.

When lengthening with a rail system, the knee must be protected during femoral lengthening and the ankle must be protected during tibial lengthening. This protection can be accomplished with pin or rail attachments that allow for crossing a joint. Other measures also can be used, such as extra-articular screw fixation of the ankle in neutral position during tibial lengthening.

Complex Monolateral Systems

Modern monolateral systems allow for correction and lengthening of a long bone in multiple planes. These monolateral fixators consist of pin clamps, arches, angulators, rotators, and translators and can be used to treat complex deformities that require lengthening. These fixators are applied on the lateral side of the femur and humerus and are applied anteromedially on the tibia. They also can be used on the foot. The advantage of these systems is that they avoid the cumbersome circular fixator but allow correction in the axial, coronal, and sagittal planes.

Circular Fixators

In the 1980s, circular fixators became the standard for limb lengthening. The Ilizarov and Monticelli-Spinelli systems are circumferential devices that were used to perform distraction osteogenesis. Circular fixation is a powerful tool that allows for correction in all planes. Secondary deformities may develop during lengthening even when using circular fixation. Procurvatum of the proximal tibia often occurs.[22,23] Most circular systems allow for corrections of these iatrogenic deformities. Altering translation or rotation with circular fixation is cumbersome and requires a thorough knowledge of the system, and intensive changes that require additional surgery are often needed. For this reason, over the past two decades most surgeons opted for the more user-friendly monolateral fixator systems.

Computer-assisted circular fixation has developed over the last decade. With the rings attached using six adjustable struts, the system can readily adapt to primary or secondary deformities without the need for major construct adjustments, thereby avoiding additional surgery.[24] The surgeon has to learn how to describe the deformity in six axes and understand the method of describing the frame in relation to the deformity. The advantage of this system has led to its widespread use for complex lengthening and deformity correction (**Figure 5**).

CONCLUSION

External fixation remains an important tool in the correction of limb deformity and limb-length discrepancies. Used in combination with plating and intramedullary rods, external fixation is steadily decreasing the time required for frame wear. The use of external fixation requires adherence to some basic principles that allow for optimal patient outcome and minimal complications.

FIGURE 5

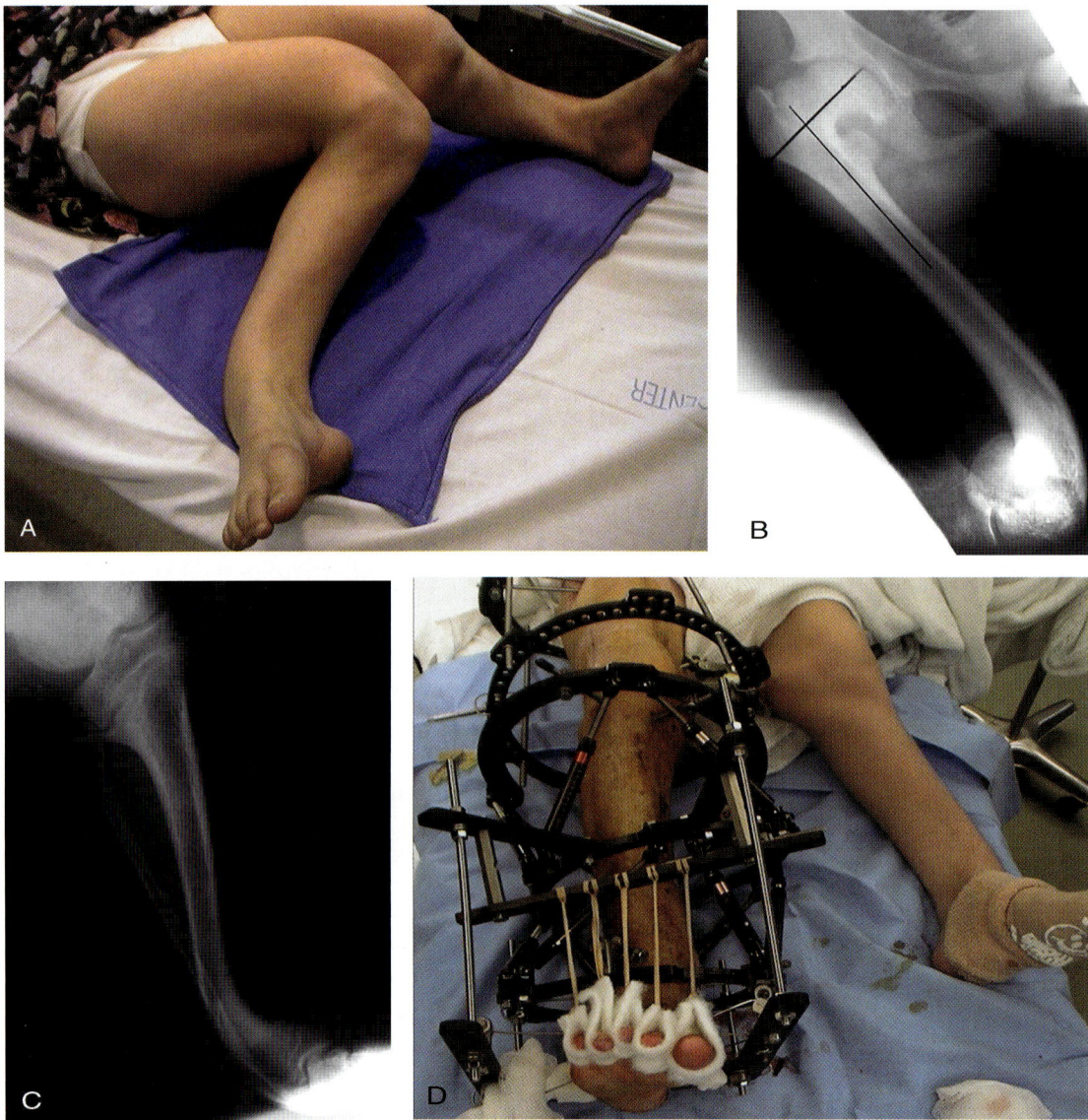

Images of a 12-year-old girl with severe limb deformity from pseudopseudohypoparathyroidism. The deformity was corrected and the limb was lengthened using a computerized ring fixator. Preoperative clinical photograph (**A**) and AP radiographs demonstrate femoral valgus (**B**) and tibia vara (**C**). **D,** Frontal photograph shows the ring fixator extending from the femur to the foot.

(continued)

FIGURE 5 (*continued*)

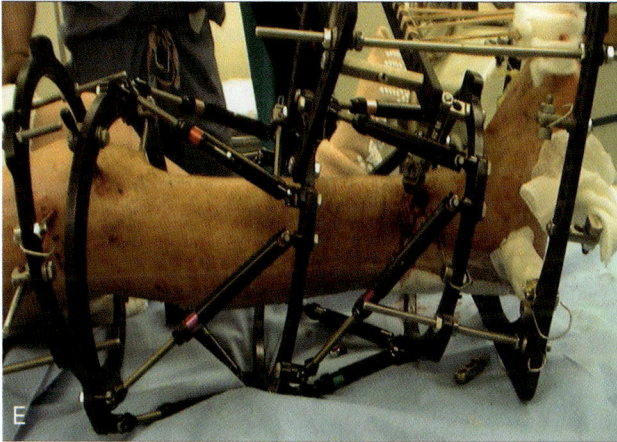

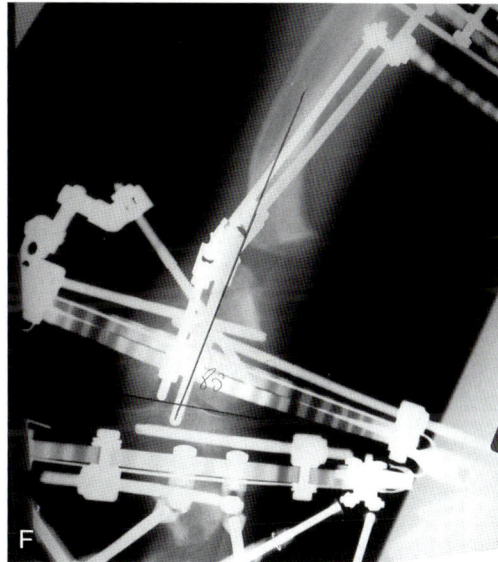

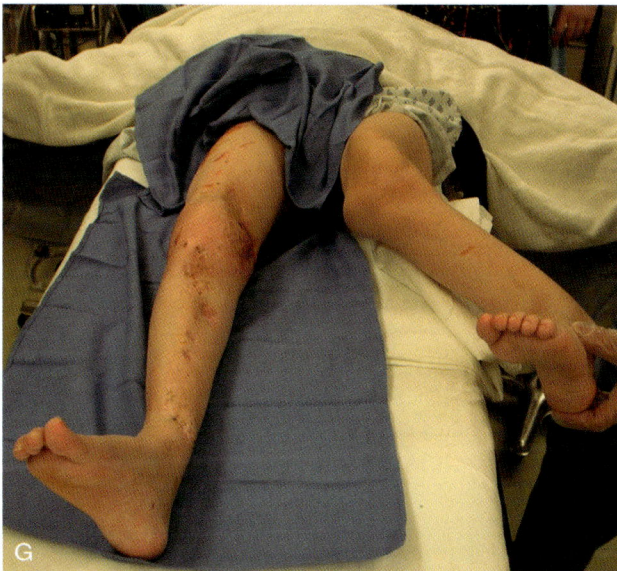

E, Side photograph shows the ring fixator extending from the femur to the foot. **F,** AP radiograph shows multiple osteotomies and adjustments. **G,** Postoperative clinical photograph shows a good functional outcome was realized.

REFERENCES

1. Codivilla A: On the means of lengthening in lower limb, the muscles and tissues which are shortened through deformity. *Am J Orthop Surg* 1905;2:353-369.

2. Green SA: Principles and complications of external fix-ation, in Browner BD, Jupiter JB, Levine AM, Trafton PG, Krettek C, eds: *Skeletal Trauma: Basic Science, Management, and Reconstruction,* ed 4. Philadelphia, PA, Saunders, 2008, p 2768.

3. Malgaigne J: *Treatise on Fractures.* Philadelphia, PA, Lippincott, 1859.

4. Paley D: Biomechanics of the Ilizarov external fixator, in Maiocchi AB, Aronson J, eds: *Operative Principles of Ilizarov: Fracture, Treatment, Nonunion, Osteomyelitis, Lengthening Deformity Correction.* Baltimore, MD, Williams & Wilkins, 1991, pp 33-41.

5. Orbay GL, Frankel VH, Kummer FJ: The effect of wire configuration on the stability of the Ilizarov external fixator. *Clin Orthop Relat Res* 1992(279):299-302.

6. Bronson DG, Samchukov ML, Birch JG, Browne RH, Ashman RB: Stability of external circular fixation: A multi-variable biomechanical analysis. *Clin Biomech* 1998;13(6):441-448.

7. Paley D: Current techniques of limb lengthening. *J Pediatr Orthop* 1988;8(1):73-92.

8. Paley D: Problems, obstacles, and complications of limb lengthening by the Ilizarov technique. *Clin Orthop Relat Res* 1990(250):81-104.

9. Aston WJ, Calder PR, Baker D, Hartley J, Hill RA: Lengthening of the congenital short femur using the Ilizarov technique: A single-surgeon series. *J Bone Joint Surg Br* 2009;91(7):962-967.

10. Olney BW, Jayaraman G: Joint reaction forces during femoral lengthening. *Clin Orthop Relat Res* 1994(301): 64-67.

11. Yang L, Cai G, Coulton L, Saleh M: Knee joint reaction force during tibial diaphyseal lengthening: A study on a rabbit model. *J Biomech* 2004;37(7):1053-1059.

12. Coleman SS, Noonan TD: Anderson's method of tibial-lengthening by percutaneous osteotomy and gradual distraction: Experience with thirty-one cases. *J Bone Joint Surg Am* 1967;49(2):263-279.

13. Kashiwagi N, Seto Y: Tibio-fibular fixation in lower limb lengthening. *Journal of the Japanese Association of External Fixation and Limb Lengthening* 2003;(14): 79-84.

14. Hatzokos I, Drakou A, Christodoulou A, Terzidis I, Pournaras J: Inferior subluxation of the fibular head following tibial lengthening with a unilateral external fixator. *J Bone Joint Surg Am* 2004;86-A(7):1491-1496.

15. Shyam AK, Song HR, An H, Isaac D, Shetty GM, Lee SH: The effect of distraction-resisting forces on the tibia during distraction osteogenesis. *J Bone Joint Surg Am* 2009;91(7):1671-1682.

16. Yasui N, Kojimoto H, Sasaki K, Kitada A, Shimizu H, Shimomura Y: Factors affecting callus distraction in limb lengthening. *Clin Orthop Relat Res* 1993(293): 55-60.

17. Gardner TN, Evans M, Simpson H: Temporal variation of applied inter fragmentary displacement at a bone fracture in harmony with maturation of the fracture callus. *Med Eng Phys* 1998;20(6):480-484.

18. Ziran BH, Smith WR, Anglen JO, Tornetta P III: External fixation: How to make it work. *J Bone Joint Surg Am* 2007;89(7):1620-1632.

19. Behrens F: General theory and principles of external fixation. *Clin Orthop Relat Res* 1989(241):15-23.

20. Khalily C, Voor MJ, Seligson D: Fracture site motion with Ilizarov and "hybrid" external fixation. *J Orthop Trauma* 1998;12(1):21-26.

21. Watson MA, Mathias KJ, Maffulli N: External ring fixators: An overview. *Proc Inst Mech Eng H* 2000;214(5): 459-470.

22. Ilizarov GA: Clinical application of the tension-stress effect for limb lengthening. *Clin Orthop Relat Res* 1990(250):8-26.

23. Catagni M: Lengthening of the tibia, in Maiocchi AB, Aronson J, eds: *Operative Principles of Ilizarov: Fracture, Treatment, Nonunion, Osteomyelitis, Lengthening Deformity Correction.* Baltimore, MD, Williams & Wilkins, 1991, pp 288-309.

24. Naqui SZ, Thiryayi W, Foster A, Tselentakis G, Evans M, Day JB: Correction of simple and complex pediatric deformities using the Taylor-Spatial Frame. *J Pediatr Orthop* 2008;28(6):640-647.

CHAPTER 9

DISTRACTION OSTEOGENESIS: LENGTHENING WITH INTERNAL DEVICES

ALEC C. STALL, MD, MPH

SHAWN C. STANDARD, MD

JOHN E. HERZENBERG, MD, FRCSC

INTRODUCTION

Distraction osteogenesis performed using Ilizarov's principles and an external fixator is a widely accepted practice; however, complications from prolonged use of an external fixator are associated with this technique. Minor setbacks are expected with prolonged treatment; in fact, the most common morbidity associated with external fixation, pin-site infection, occurs in as many as 80% of patients.[1,2] Lengthening with external fixators can lead to secondary axial deformity and to the risk of osteoporotic or regenerate fracture after external fixator removal. Additional drawbacks include the sequelae of prolonged soft-tissue transfixion by means of wires and pins, including muscle contracture, joint stiffness, and pain.[3-6] The technical difficulties and complications associated with prolonged use of an external fixator are compounded by patient dissatisfaction with the devices, which are bulky, uncomfortable, and can interfere with normal daily activities.

FULLY IMPLANTABLE DEVICES

In an attempt to decrease the morbidity associated with limb lengthening and to improve patient satisfaction, recent technical refinements have focused on minimizing or eliminating the role of external fixation in limb lengthening. The ideal situation would be a completely implantable internal lengthening nail that would eliminate the need for any external fixation device. Initial attempts to develop such an implant included some devices that were activated either mechanically or hydraulically via cables or tubes that penetrated the skin. Recently, completely implantable telescopic intramedullary nails have become available. These internal lengthening devices have inherent risks, including mechanical failure and difficulty controlling and/or monitoring the rate of lengthening.

Bliskunov[7-9] devised the first totally implantable telescopic nail in the early 1980s; it coupled hip rotation to femoral lengthening. Bliskunov's device included a complex direct mechanical linkage between the proxi-

Dr. Herzenberg or an immediate family member is a member of a speakers' bureau or has made paid presentations on behalf of Biomet; serves as an unpaid consultant to Intramed; has received research or institutional support from Orthofix, Smith & Nephew, and Synthes; and owns stock or stock options in Orthogon and Orthocrat. Neither of the following authors nor any immediate family member has received anything of value from or owns stock in a commercial company or institution related directly or indirectly to the subject of this chapter: Dr. Stall and Dr. Standard.

mal femur and the iliac wing whereby hip rotation activated a gear box to lengthen the femoral component. Reports on Bliskunov's device cite frequent complications, including pain and device failure; however, it is still in use in limited areas of Russia and India.

More recent designs for mechanically telescoping intramedullary devices have obviated the need to link to the pelvis. Both the Albizzia nail (designed by Guichet and Grammont [DePuy, Saint-Priest, France]) and the Intramedullary Skeletal Kinetic Distractor (ISKD; Orthofix, McKinney, TX) use torsional movements at the osteotomy site to activate a ratchet mechanism in the nail, which results in lengthening through the callus.[10-13] The Albizzia nail consists of telescoping tubes connected by a double-ratchet mechanism. A rotation arc of 20° is required to unscrew the ratchet mechanism and lengthen the nail. Because of the large degree of rotation required to distract the nail, many patients experience severe pain during lengthening; this has been the major drawback to this design. In a series by Guichet et al,[12] 39% of patients required readmission to the hospital and a general anesthetic for ratcheting during the lengthening. The Albizzia nail is available in Europe and the Far East but is not currently approved for use in the United States. The ISKD also uses torsional motion at the osteotomy site to induce lengthening; however, it has a double reverse-clutch mechanism that requires only a 3° to 9° arc of rotation to induce nail distraction. The reduced rotational requirements for lengthening have made the ISKD more tolerable for patients.[14]

In contrast to mechanically driven devices like the Albizzia nail and ISKD, complex motorized lengthening nails offer precise control over the rate of lengthening. To date, the only fully motorized lengthening nail commercially available for human use is the Fitbone nail (Wittenstein, Igersheim, Germany). This device, developed by Baumgart et al,[15] uses a totally implantable, motorized, programmable sliding mechanism for limb lengthening. Early clinical results are promising, but the Fitbone is not currently available for use in the United States and has limited availability elsewhere.[15,16] Currently, the size of the Fitbone device limits its application to adults of normal or large osseous morphology. The ISKD is the only completely implantable intramedullary device currently approved for use by the US Food and Drug Administration; therefore, much of

this chapter focuses on this device, including indications for use, surgical technique, postoperative care, and complications (**Table 1**).

INTRAMEDULLARY SKELETAL KINETIC DISTRACTOR

Design

The ISKD, which is available in both femoral and tibial nail models, is designed to lengthen during physiologic movement by mechanically converting rotational oscillations to linear distraction. The ISKD includes two telescoping sections, a drive mechanism, and a length indication feedback mechanism. There are four interlocking peg holes, similar to standard intramedullary nail designs. The drive mechanism consists of two roller clutches and a threaded rod. The distraction is unidirectional and irreversible. The length indication feedback mechanism consists of a magnet in the threaded rod of the drive mechanism. The rotation and relative position of the magnet are monitored with an external sensor that calculates the magnitude of lengthening on the basis of changes in the magnetic pole.

Both femoral and tibial nails are offered in models capable of lengthening either 50 or 80 mm (80-mm nails are rarely used). Each nail can be preset to shorter lengths before insertion. The nails are noncannulated and the locking screws are solid pegs with threads in the near cortex only. The femoral nails are manufactured in lengths from 255 to 345 mm, with a diameter of either 12.5 or 14.5 mm; tibial nails are produced in lengths from 215 to 300 mm, with a diameter of 10.7, 12.5, or 13.5 mm. The locking screws are partially threaded with a 4.8-mm shaft diameter (4.0 mm for the distal holes in the 10.7-mm tibial nail) and are available in lengths from 20 to 75 mm. The 10.7-mm tibial nail is commonly used as an antegrade trochanteric femoral nail, which provides a smaller-diameter nail with a safe entry point.

Preoperative Planning

Careful patient selection and preoperative planning are essential for successful limb lengthening with the ISKD. The preoperative physical examination should note muscle strength, joint range of motion, and preexisting instability or contracture. Accurate radiographic measurements of limb-length discrepancy (LLD) are essential because the nail length is preset before insertion and

T A B L E 1 Complications of the Intramedullary Skeletal Kinetic Distractor

Complication	Resolution
Implant-related	
Runaway length	Bracing (hip-knee-ankle-foot orthosis)
	Reduced activity, reduced physical therapy
	Two-pin external fixator
Failure to distract	Walking epidural
	Manual manipulation
Fatigue	Observation
	Exchange nail
Soft-tissue–related	
Iliotibial band contracture	Proximal and distal iliotibial band release
Knee flexion contracture	Physical therapy
	Dynamic splinting
	Surgical lengthening/release of soft tissues
Ankle equinus contracture	Extra-articular calcaneotibial screw
Knee subluxation	Knee extension splint
	Dynamic splinting
	Soft-tissue releases
Muscle spasm	Botox injections
Peroneal nerve entrapment	Peroneal nerve decompression
Sciatic nerve entrapment	Proximal iliotibial band release
Bone-related	
Failure of formation	Allograft (modified Wasserstein)
	Autograft
	Exchange nailing
Premature consolidation	Re-osteotomy

cannot be altered. Mechanical alignment and joint orientation angles also should be obtained. Essential radiographs include long weight-bearing AP views with appropriate blocks under the short limb, and lateral views. The ISKD nails are straight in the sagittal plane and do not mirror the normal femoral anterior bow; therefore, careful assessment of the lateral views is especially important for preoperative planning before femoral lengthening.

The ISKD size must be determined and ordered for each patient, which requires careful measurement of canal length and diameter before surgery. Both the amount of lengthening needed and the starting length of nail that the bone will accommodate dictate the ISKD length. The nail length will determine the level of osteo-

tomy, and the canal width must be able to accommodate the nail size plus 2 mm of planned overreaming.

SURGICAL TECHNIQUE

The femoral surgical technique is described here in detail (**Figure 1**). Owing to the limited scope of this chapter, the discussion of the tibial surgical technique is limited to surgical caveats and tips.

Femoral Insertion

The patient is placed supine with a bump under the sacrum. The level of the greater trochanter (trochanteric entry) or the piriformis fossa (adult femoral nail) is marked on the skin. The length of the nail is then marked from this starting point distally. The nail must

FIGURE 1

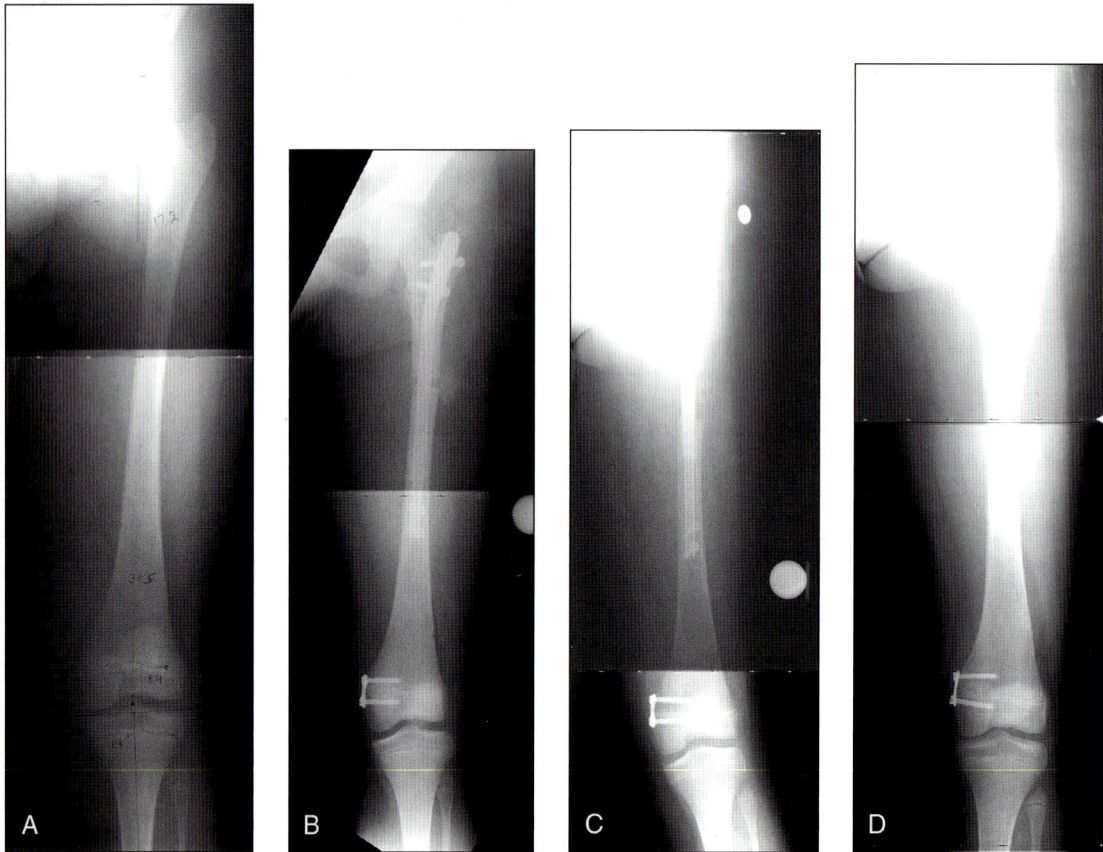

AP radiographs demonstrate the use of the tibial ISKD for femoral lengthening in a child with congenital femoral deficiency and fibular hemimelia. **A,** Preoperative radiograph. **B,** Immediate postoperative radiograph shows reamings at osteotomy site. **C,** Radiograph obtained at completion of the lengthening procedure. **D,** Radiograph obtained 1 year postoperatively, after consolidation of regenerate bone. (© 2009, Rubin Institute for Advanced Orthopedics, Sinai Hospital of Baltimore, Baltimore, MD.)

be set to the actual lengthening amount before this line is drawn. For example, if a 305- to 355-mm femoral nail is used for a 3-cm lengthening, then the nail must be dialed to a starting length of 325 mm, which is marked distally from the entry point. The osteotomy site is marked 11 cm proximal to this point to prevent excessive force at the nail junction. For a 5-cm lengthening, the smaller distal rod protrudes 3 cm from the distal aspect of the rod, the rod will lengthen 5 cm, and at least 3 cm of the proximal thicker rod needs to remain in the distal lengthening fragment for stability; therefore, 3 + 5 + 3 cm = 11 cm. For the previous example of a

3-cm lengthening using a 305-mm femoral nail, the osteotomy site is still 11 cm proximal to the end of the nail. Because the nail was set for a 3-cm lengthening, the small-diameter nail now protrudes 5 cm from the distal end of the nail, the nail will lengthen 3 cm, and 3 cm of the larger proximal rod needs to remain in the distal lengthening fragment; therefore, 5 + 3 + 3 cm = 11 cm. At a point 11 cm proximal to the distal end of the nail, multiple drill holes are created at the planned osteotomy site through a small stab incision. These drill holes allow for venting during the intramedullary reaming and also allow fragments to accumulate as bone graft. A percu-

taneous Steinmann pin is inserted at the starting position in the proximal femur and confirmed using fluoroscopy. The starting hole is then created with a
cannulated 8-mm anterior cruciate ligament reamer. A
beaded guide rod is inserted in the starting hole and
driven to the distal aspect of the planned femoral nail
length. The femur is sequentially reamed in 0.5-mm
increments, starting with an 8-mm end-cutting reamer
to 2 mm more than the implant diameter. Some surgeons insert proximal and distal reference pins behind
the nail channel to control for rotation. After the reaming is completed, the guide rod is removed. The preset
ISKD nail is inserted in the starting hole and driven to
the preplanned osteotomy site. At this point, the proximal and distal aspects of the femur are supported and
the surgeon completes the osteotomy with an
osteotome. Without losing reduction or rotational alignment, the nail is driven across the osteotomy site and to
its final position. The proximal nail is locked with a
proximal locking guide and the distal aspect of the nail
is locked using the "perfect circle" technique.

The magnet in the distal aspect of the nail is visualized using fluoroscopy and the site is marked on the
skin. The monitoring device is placed in a sterile plastic
bag and activated. The osteotomy site is visualized with
fluoroscopy and the leg is manipulated to activate the
nail. Usually, 15 to 20 rotations are required to create a
pole change. A single pole change equals 0.337 mm. The
leg is checked after each manipulation to determine if a
pole change has occurred. Pole changes are recorded
by the hand-held monitor. Six to 10 pole changes are
performed intraoperatively to ensure the nail is functioning properly and that the osteotomy is complete. A 2- to
4-mm distraction gap should be readily visualized on the
final fluoroscopic view of the osteotomy.

Tibial Insertion
The proximal and distal tibiofibular joints require stabilization, which is achieved by inserting percutaneous
4.5-mm solid screws both proximally and distally across
the tibiofibular joints. The fibula is cut at the mid level
to avoid neurologic complications from osteotomies in
the proximal third of the fibula. The longest possible
ISKD rod should be planned for the tibial lengthening
to allow the osteotomy site to be more diaphyseal, which
prevents a secondary valgus/procurvatum deformity

from occurring during the lengthening process. The foot
and ankle must be controlled to prevent significant equinus contracture. A gastrocnemius-soleus recession may
be required for patients with significant soft-tissue tightness before lengthening. An extra-articular calcaneotibial screw is placed from the posterior plantar aspect of
the calcaneus, bypassing the posterior aspect of the talus
and entering the posterolateral portion of the tibia. This
screw holds the foot in a rigid and neutral position without harming the ankle joint.[17] Casting or bracing is
another option but has potential complications and failures. Routine prophylactic percutaneous anterior and
lateral compartment fasciotomies are performed to prevent compartment syndrome.

POSTOPERATIVE CARE
Postoperatively, patients are braced in a hip-knee-ankle-
foot orthosis for the femoral ISKD and a removable cast
boot for the tibial ISKD; the bracing avoids inadvertent
rotations and pole changes. Patients who have no pole
changes without bracing can avoid these restrictions.
Rapid distraction, however, is a common postoperative
problem. If this occurs, bracing may be initiated to keep
pole changes at less than two to three per day during the
first 5 days. Physical therapy begins immediately to
maintain range of motion of the hips, knees, and ankles,
with monitoring of pole changes. The patient is allowed
50% weight bearing with assistive devices. Physical therapy continues 5 days per week during the distraction
phase. One week postoperatively, the patient and family review use of the hand-held monitor and manipula-
tions. If rapid distraction occurs, then bracing is
increased and physical therapy is decreased. If pole
changes are difficult to achieve, however, then more
aggressive physical therapy and increased weight bearing can be instituted to drive the nail. Radiographs are
obtained to ensure that preconsolidation of the regenerate site has not occurred. Repeat manipulation under
either general anesthesia or epidural anesthesia is used
to "jump-start" the nail distraction. A slowly distracting
nail can convert to a "runaway" nail after a manipulation. A brace should be ready for the patient undergoing a reactivation of the ISKD.

During the consolidation phase, physical therapy sessions are reduced to two to three times per week and
weight bearing is increased as the regenerate thickens

radiographically. Once the distraction gap is filled on one cortex of the bone, the patient may resume full weight bearing with no assistive devices. Physical therapy continues until the patient has regained preoperative range of motion and strength.

CLINICAL RESULTS

Few published clinical series exist that document the results of ISKD limb lengthening.[10,14,18-20] These clinical series universally report encouraging clinical results, but most also advise caution in ISKD use, emphasizing the importance of careful preoperative planning, patient selection, and close postoperative follow-up. Our clinical experience with the ISKD includes more than 200 procedures performed in more than 170 patients treated from 2001 to 2008. The average lengthening achieved in our series is 5.0 cm (range, 1.0 to 8.0 cm). In our practice, indications for lengthening with the ISKD included both posttraumatic/infectious and congenital LLDs. Our experience suggests that the ISKD is an excellent device to correct posttraumatic and developmental LLDs less than 5.0 cm, but great care and extensive limb-lengthening experience is needed to correct congenital LLDs.

SUMMARY

Implantable devices (such as the ISKD) reduce external fixator–related complications, are generally less painful, and protect the regenerate bone during the lengthening and consolidation phases. Disadvantages of the ISKD include the inability to accurately control the rate and rhythm of distraction; the size limitations of the device, which preclude its use in smaller individuals; and the limited ability to allow for concurrent deformity correction at the time of lengthening.

REFERENCES

1. Eldridge JC, Bell DF: Problems with substantial limb lengthening. *Orthop Clin North Am* 1991;22(4): 625-631.

2. Green SA: Complications of external skeletal fixation. *Clin Orthop Relat Res* 1983(180):109-116.

3. García-Cimbrelo E, Olsen B, Ruiz-Yagüe M, Fernandez-Baíllo N, Munuera-Martínez L: Ilizarov technique: Results and difficulties. *Clin Orthop Relat Res* 1992(283):116-123.

4. Herzenberg JE, Scheufele LL, Paley D, Bechtel R, Tepper S: Knee range of motion in isolated femoral lengthening. *Clin Orthop Relat Res* 1994(301):49-54.

5. Kristiansen LP, Steen H: Lengthening of the tibia over an intramedullary nail, using the Ilizarov external fixator: Major complications and slow consolidation in 9 lengthenings. *Acta Orthop Scand* 1999;70(3):271-274.

6. Paley D: Problems, obstacles, and complications of limb lengthening by the Ilizarov technique. *Clin Orthop Relat Res* 1990(250):81-104.

7. Bliskunov AI: Intramedullary distraction of the femur (preliminary report). *Ortop Travmatol Protez* 1983 (10):59-62.

8. Bliskunov AI: Lengthening of the femur using implantable appliances. *Acta Chir Orthop Traumatol Cech* 1984;51(6):454-466.

9. Bliskunov AI: Implantable devices for lengthening the femur without external drive mechanisms. *Med Tekh* 1984;(2):44-49.

10. Cole JD, Justin D, Kasparis T, DeVlught D, Knobloch C: The intramedullary skeletal kinetic distractor (ISKD): First clinical results of a new intramedullary nail for lengthening of the femur and tibia. *Injury* 2001;32 (Suppl 4):SD129-SD139.

11. Guichet JM, Casar RS: Mechanical characterization of a totally intramedullary gradual elongation nail. *Clin Orthop Relat Res* 1997(337):281-290.

12. Guichet JM, Deromedis B, Donnan LT, Peretti G, Lascombes P, Bado F: Gradual femoral lengthening with the Albizzia intramedullary nail. *J Bone Joint Surg Am* 2003;85-A(5):838-848.

13. Guichet JM, Grammont PM, Trouilloud P: A nail for progressive lengthening: An animal experiment with a 2-year follow-up. *Chirurgie* 1992;118(6-7):405-410.

14. Hankemeier S, Pape HC, Gosling T, Hufner T, Richter M, Krettek C: Improved comfort in lower limb lengthening with the intramedullary skeletal kinetic distractor: Principles and preliminary clinical experiences. *Arch Orthop Trauma Surg* 2004;124(2):129-133.

15. Baumgart R, Betz A, Schweiberer L: A fully implantable motorized intramedullary nail for limb lengthening and bone transport. *Clin Orthop Relat Res* 1997(343):135-143.

16. Singh S, Lahiri A, Iqbal M: The results of limb lengthening by callus distraction using an extending intramedullary nail (Fitbone) in non-traumatic disorders. *J Bone Joint Surg Br* 2006;88(7):938-942.

17. Belthur MV, Paley D, Jindal G, Burghardt RD, Specht SC, Herzenberg JE: Tibial lengthening: Extraarticular calcaneotibial screw to prevent ankle equinus. *Clin Orthop Relat Res* 2008;466(12):3003-3010.

18. Hankemeier S, Gösling T, Pape HC, Wiebking U, Krettek C: Limb lengthening with the Intramedullary Skeletal Kinetic Distractor (ISKD). *Oper Orthop Traumatol* 2005;17(1):79-101.

19. Potaczek T, Kacki W, Jasiewicz B, Tesiorowski M, Lipik E: Femur lengthening with a telescopic intramedullary nail ISKD: Method presentation and early clinical results. *Chir Narzadow Ruchu Ortop Pol* 2008;73(1):10-14.

20. Leidinger B, Winkelmann W, Roedl R: Limb lengthening with a fully implantable mechanical distraction intramedullary nail. *Z Orthop Ihre Grenzgeb* 2006; 144(4):419-426.

COMPLICATIONS OF DISTRACTION OSTEOGENESIS

JANET D. CONWAY, MD

INTRODUCTION

Complication rates for distraction osteogenesis are among the highest in orthopaedic surgery and have discouraged many surgeons from performing these techniques. Krishnan et al[1] documented 71 complications in 20 patients with infected femoral nonunions; and Paley[2] reported 73 "problems, obstacles, and other complications" in 46 patients (60 limbs). Surgeons who use the technique frequently, however, benefit from their experience and are able to decrease the number of complications.[3-6] Distraction osteogenesis techniques include the use of external fixation only, lengthening over a nail with external fixation, and completely internal intramedullary lengthening. The complications associated with distraction osteogenesis are similar for each of the techniques.

The main categories of orthopaedic complications are regenerate bone and healing difficulties, joint subluxation and stiffness, axial deviation and residual limb-length discrepancy (LLD), nerve and vascular injuries, pin- and wire-tract infections, systemic and life-threatening complications, and soft-tissue envelope compromise.

Defining the complications associated with distraction osteogenesis is difficult because of the dynamic nature of the techniques and the long periods of treatment. The external fixator is a dynamic device that causes soft-tissue trauma with lengthening, muscle tightness with the potential for contractures, pressure and motion around the pins with resultant infection and loosening, and potential nerve palsies. Difficulties are encountered to varying degrees based on the severity of the deformity, the compliance of the soft-tissue envelope, and the quality of the host and bone. Anticipating adverse events and taking steps to aggressively manage them can maximize the overall result. If the desired outcome is achieved, it is difficult to label an adverse event as a true complication. The Paley classification, which distinguishes among problems, obstacles, and true complications, is the best tool for defining the adverse events associated with distraction osteogenesis.[2] Paley defines problems as issues that occur during the period of external fixation and are resolved nonsurgically by the end of treatment. Obstacles are issues that occur during the period of external fixation and require surgical intervention but are fully resolved by the end of treatment. True complications are issues that occur during the period of external fixation and are unresolved at the end of treatment. Major complications interfere with the original goals of the surgery, and minor complications do not.[2,4,7]

Dr. Conway or an immediate family member has received royalties from Quantum Medical Concepts; is a member of a speakers' bureau or has made paid presentations on behalf of Smith & Nephew; serves as a paid consultant to or is an employee of Smith & Nephew; and has received research or institutional support from Synthes and Medtronic.

FIGURE 1

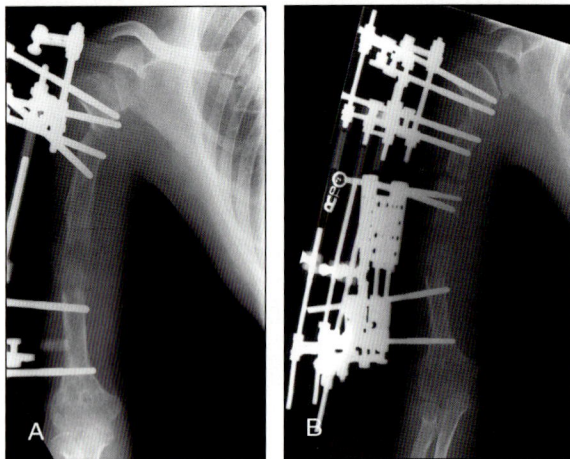

Images of the humerus in a 28-year-old man with sequelae of neonatal sepsis. A proximal humeral valgus osteotomy was performed, and the patient underwent midshaft lengthening. The regenerate bone consolidated prematurely after achieving 5 cm of length. The patient felt a pop during the daily distraction of the external fixator; this was caused by acute distraction of the regenerate bone, resulting in radial nerve palsy. Radial nerve decompression was performed, and the nerve recovered. **A,** AP radiograph obtained during lengthening. **B,** AP radiograph obtained approximately 4 weeks after repeat corticotomy for additional length at a different level. Additional pins were inserted. (© 2009, Rubin Institute for Advanced Orthopaedics, Sinai Hospital of Baltimore, Baltimore, MD.)

PREOPERATIVE CONSIDERATIONS

Several conditions increase the risk of complications during distraction osteogenesis: vascular disease, smoking, congenital diseases such as Ollier disease and proximal femoral focal deficiency (PFFD, also called longitudinal deficiency of the proximal femur), and metabolic bone diseases such as renal osteodystrophy and hypophosphatemic rickets. Metabolically abnormal bone heals at a slower rate than healthy bone, and patients with any of these conditions should be prepared to spend several additional months with the external fixator in place. Age is an important factor: it affects both the psychologic impact of the procedure and the ability to form regenerate bone.[8] At our center, any lengthening procedure is delayed for children between 4 and 7 years of age because children in that age range have an emerging sense of

self-awareness and body awareness, but they cannot appreciate the long-term goal of making their limbs more functional for the future.[9] Limb lengthening in that age group is difficult because the children do not cooperate with physical therapy and do not understand the inconvenience of wearing an external fixator. The social situation and mental status of the adult patient also must be considered preoperatively. Patients who are unable to tolerate wearing a frame are better served by another method of limb reconstruction. Assessment of the social support structure is crucial because many patients are unable to transport themselves to the surgeon's office for frequent postoperative follow-up visits. In such cases, the preoperative assistance of a social worker is critical to ensure that the patient is treated at a facility that can care for the external fixator (eg, pin care, daily distraction with the external fixator), provide physical therapy, and arrange transportation to follow-up visits. Close follow-up examination at least every 2 weeks allows the orthopaedic surgeon to conduct clinical and radiographic evaluations and prevent the complications of contracture, poorly grown regenerate bone, and axial deviation.

Patients with comorbid conditions such as diabetes and those who smoke are not ideal candidates for distraction osteogenesis because they are at increased risk for complications. Counseling and resources should be provided for these patients, as optimized blood glucose levels and smoking cessation can improve regenerate bone formation and decrease the risk of pin-tract infections.

Another preoperative consideration is the amount of lengthening planned. Lengthening greater than 30% of the initial bone length is associated with more complications than lengthening of 10%.[4,10] For lengthening greater than 20%, the Ilizarov circular fixator is associated with fewer complications than are other fixators, according to Maffulli et al.[10] Optimizing the patient's condition preoperatively and anticipating problems before surgery can prevent true complications.

TYPES OF COMPLICATIONS
Regenerate Bone Problems
Premature Consolidation

Premature consolidation occurs when the regenerate bone heals too quickly and lengthening cannot progress because a solid bridge of bone exists (**Figure 1**). Premature consolidation that occurs early, during the distraction phase, usually is caused by an incomplete osteotomy or a prolonged latency phase.[2] Premature consolidation that occurs later, during lengthening, is a result of rapid bone formation. Obtaining AP and lateral radiographs at frequent follow-up visits allows the surgeon to assess the quality of the regenerate bone. Premature consolidation is associated with young age, Ollier disease, and lengthening over an intramedullary nail[11,12] and is treated with repeat osteotomy. Maffulli et al[10] reported on 19 of 240 patients with premature consolidation who were treated with repeat osteotomy. In cases with abundant bone formation, the rate of distraction can be increased for a short time to 1.25 mm/d to prevent premature healing. Debate is ongoing as to whether repeat osteotomy should be performed through the healed regenerate bone or through healthy normal bone. At our center, we prefer performing repeat osteotomy through adjacent normal bone because of the difficulty in passing an osteotome through soft regenerate bone and because of the considerable blood loss associated with this procedure.[2] Occasionally, premature consolidation occurs and is not noticed until the regenerate bone fractures through the prematurely consolidated bone. The "popping" that occurs is painful and is accompanied by a noticeable gap in the regenerate bone. The gap occurs because the tension in the frame has been relieved. Correction consists of closing the gap by compressing the external fixator and then beginning distraction 3 to 4 days later. Tjernström et al[13] reported six premature consolidations (three femoral and three tibial): three of the patients were treated with open repeat corticotomy, one was treated with closed repeat corticotomy while under anesthesia, one was treated with forced distraction, and the treatment of one patient was not reported.

Failure of Regenerate Bone to Heal

Failure of regenerate bone to heal can occur for a variety of reasons, including an unstable frame, rapid lengthening, smoking, and infection. The location of the osteotomy affects healing potential. Metaphyseal osteotomies have the best healing potential; therefore, when possible, the corticotomy should be performed in metaphyseal bone. Maffulli et al[10] and Paley and Tetsworth[14] documented that statistically, a metaphyseal osteotomy heals significantly faster than does a diaphy-

seal osteotomy. If a diaphyseal osteotomy is necessary, a Gigli saw should not be used, both because the periosteum must be stripped and because the saw generates heat. When using diaphyseal osteotomy for lengthening, the initial rate of distraction should be less than 1 mm/d to ensure that the osteotomy site is generating bone. The corticotomy site must be free of any surrounding soft-tissue trauma because this often is a sign that the underlying bone and periosteum have been damaged, rendering the site less than ideal for new bone formation. It also is important to adjust the rate of lengthening based on the quality of the regenerate bone. If the regenerate bone is "wispy," the rate should be decreased to 0.5 mm/d until it appears more robust. Jochymek and Gal[15] found that if no periosteal callus is present by 5 weeks after femoral lengthening surgery, a bone graft will be necessary.

A stable frame is the key to preventing nonunion. Micromotion at the healing site promotes nonunion. García-Cimbrelo et al[6] reported a 4% (4 of 100 cases) nonunion rate and attributed the complications to technical errors, such as traumatic corticotomy or early removal of the frame. Healing index and age are directly related to longer healing time of regenerate bone[8] (**Figure 2**). This is true even in younger patient populations, with a statistically significant decrease in bone healing reported for girls older than 12 years and boys older than 14 years.[15]

Refracture

Tjernström et al[13] treated four cases of refracture after external fixator removal from three femora and one tibia among 53 lengthening cases. Among the 281 lengthenings for congenital, posttraumatic, or postinfection in 240 patients in the series reported by Maffulli et al,[10] 22 fractures occurred through the new regenerate bone after fixator removal. The author now treats congenital LLD by using splints for 4 to 8 weeks after removal of the fixator. Based on our clinical experience with refracture after lengthening in congenitally deficient femora, it is our practice to insert a Rush rod (Zimmer, Warsaw, IN) into the femur at the time of fixator removal. This method has been very successful in preventing refracture and has not been associated with intramedullary infections (**Figure 3**).

FIGURE 2

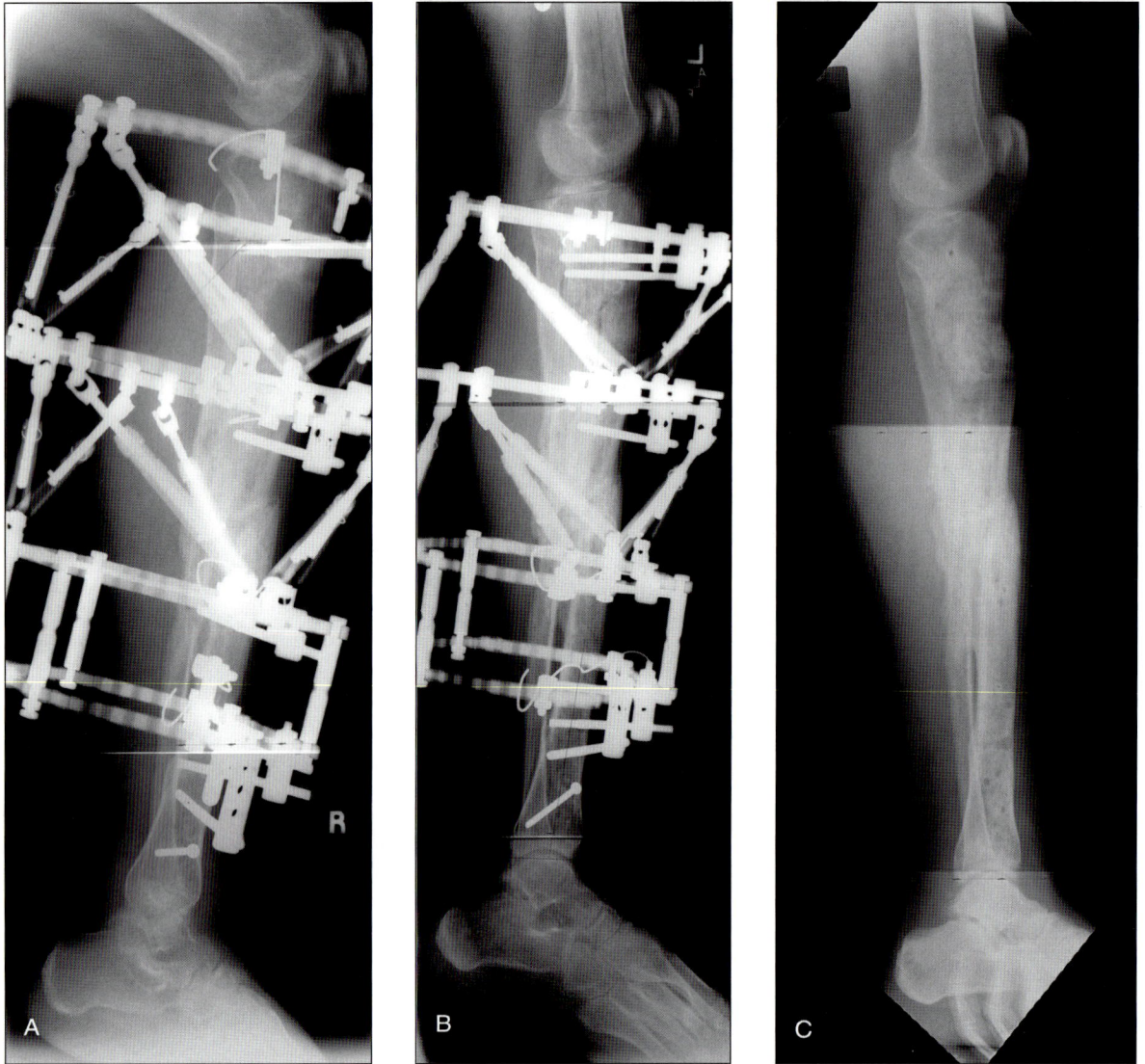

Images of the tibia of a 41-year-old man who smoked. He underwent nonunion correction and proximal lengthening. **A,** Lateral radiograph shows the large anterior gap at the proximal regenerate site. **B,** Lateral radiograph obtained after bone grafting and insertion of bone morphogenetic protein (BMP)-2. **C,** Lateral radiograph obtained after complete healing of the regenerate site and removal of the frame. (© 2009, Rubin Institute for Advanced Orthopaedics, Sinai Hospital of Baltimore, Baltimore, MD.)

FIGURE 3

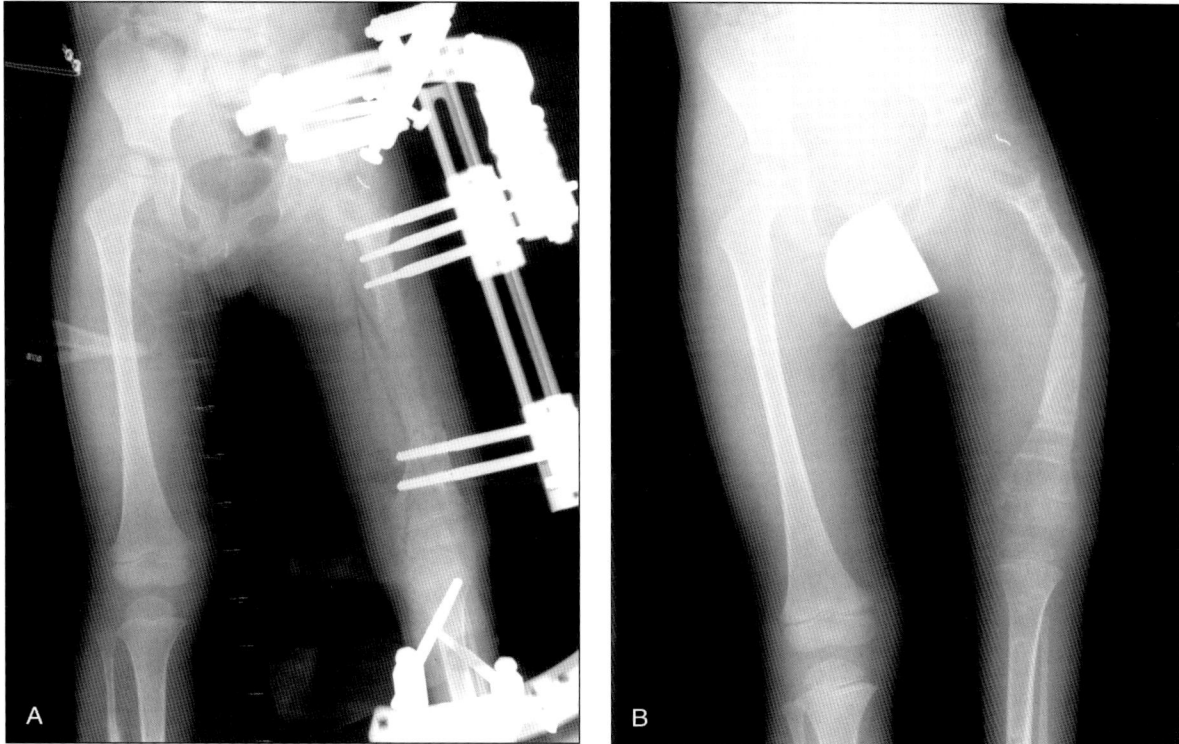

Images of a 4-year-old boy who underwent lengthening for a congenitally short femur. **A,** AP radiograph obtained after lengthening shows the hinged external fixation spanning the knee and the hip. **B,** AP radiograph obtained after the fixator was removed shows a fracture through the proximal regenerate bone with deformity. The fracture was treated with the insertion of a Rush rod (Zimmer, Warsaw, IN) and application of a spica cast. (© 2009, Rubin Institute for Advanced Orthopaedics, Sinai Hospital of Baltimore, Baltimore, MD.)

Joint Stiffness and Subluxation

Joint stiffness commonly occurs during lengthening procedures. Tjernström et al[13] reported decreased range of motion in 49 of 53 patients who underwent lengthening. Many of these symptoms resolved, but minor restrictions persisted in 14 patients.

Knee range of motion decreases by approximately 37% during femoral lengthening, as documented by Herzenberg et al.[16] Aggressive physical therapy can be prescribed to manage range of motion. A minimum of 45° of knee flexion must be maintained during femoral lengthening. If knee flexion decreases to less than 45°, lengthening should be discontinued. The remaining lengthening can be accomplished with a second procedure at a much later date.

Zhang et al[17] reported on 27 cases of distraction osteogenesis for treatment of nonunion and femoral shortening. Twelve of 27 patients (44%) had 20° of additional stiffness postoperatively; 11 of those responded to physical therapy, and one required manipulation. Maffulli et al[10] reported on 13 patients who underwent simultaneous femoral and tibial lengthening procedures and in whom more that 15° of flexion contracture developed. The contractures were treated with cessation of lengthening for 5 to 8 days, knee splinting, and aggressive physical therapy. Final length was achieved in all patients without persistent knee problems.

Knee subluxation is a problem, particularly in patients with congenital femoral deficiency secondary to lack of cruciate ligaments. In a study by Maffulli et al,[10] seven

FIGURE 4

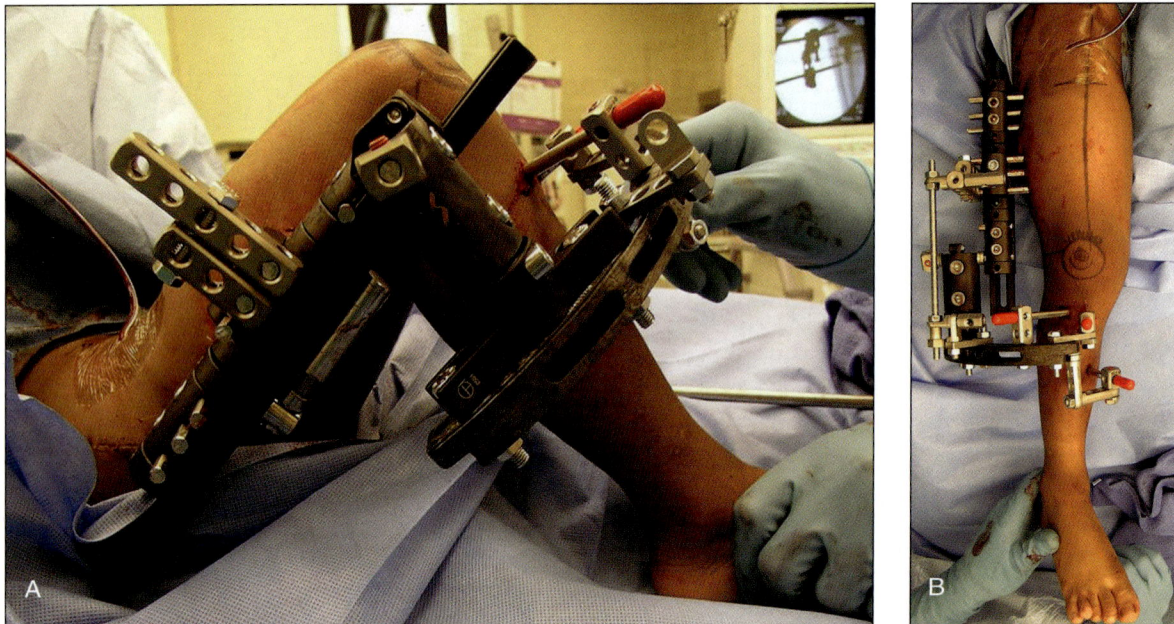

Lateral (**A**) and frontal (**B**) clinical photographs of a patient with a monolateral external fixator for femoral lengthening. Note the hinged fixation spanning the knee joint to prevent contractures and subluxation. (© 2009, Rubin Institute for Advanced Orthopaedics, Sinai Hospital of Baltimore, Baltimore, MD.)

patients experienced knee subluxation during tibial lengthening and two experienced knee subluxation during femoral lengthening. At our center, knee subluxation during lengthening has been virtually eliminated with prophylactic spanning of the knee with an external fixator (**Figure 4**). The construct allows the knee range of motion during physical therapy, and the frame can be locked in extension at night to prevent knee flexion contractures.

Zhang et al[17] reported on three patients with previous acetabular dysplasia who experienced subluxation of the hip joint. Tjernström et al[13] reported on hip subluxation occurring after 14 cm of lengthening in the femur; the subluxation was treated with cessation of the femoral lengthening and surgical release of the hip contracture. Maffulli et al[10] reported on nine patients who experienced hip subluxation after femoral lengthening. Most cases were congenital. The hip subluxation was treated with fixator adjustment with the patients under anesthe-

sia and with reduction of the rate of lengthening. In two of the nine cases, the hip subluxation was persistent and progressed to a painful stiff hip. To prevent this catastrophic consequence, especially in patients with congenital femoral deficiency, the acetabulum and hip joint need to be evaluated carefully before lengthening. If any evidence of dysplasia is present, a Dega acetabular osteotomy should be performed and allowed to fully heal before any femoral lengthening procedure is started (**Figure 5**).

Ankle equinus is a problem that can occur after tibial lengthening. Maffulli et al[10] reported on 27 of 240 patients with ankle equinus after tibial lengthening. None of the patients underwent spanning of the joint, all underwent lengthening greater than 20% of the initial bone length, and all were treated with Achilles tendon lengthening. At our center, the foot is held in a neutral position by including it in the frame during lengthening. This technique is used for any lengthening

FIGURE 5

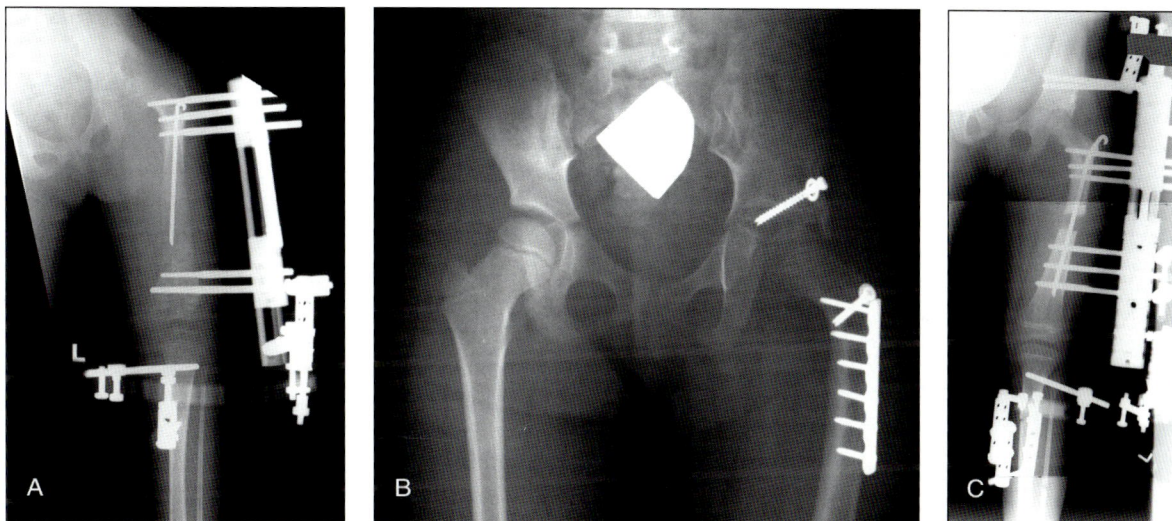

Images of a 4-year-old boy with congenital femoral deficiency. **A,** AP radiograph shows the hip subluxation the patient sustained while undergoing lengthening. **B,** AP radiograph obtained after the patient underwent a Dega osteotomy of the acetabulum and a femoral shortening to allow relocation of the hip joint. **C,** AP radiograph obtained during a subsequent lengthening. Note the fixation across the acetabulum to prevent subluxation. (© 2009, Rubin Institute for Advanced Orthopaedics, Sinai Hospital of Baltimore, Baltimore, MD.)

of the tibia greater than 4 cm. Used in combination with recession of the gastrocnemius-soleus complex, this method has eliminated equinus contractures and decreased the occurrence of stiff ankles.

Another technique uses botulinum toxin to weaken the muscles. For tibial lengthening, the botulinum toxin usually is injected into the gastrocnemius-soleus complex, and for femoral lengthening, it is injected into the hamstring complex. The maximum amount of botulinum toxin that can be administered is 8 units per kilogram of body weight, and repeat injections cannot be administered more frequently than every 3 months. A dynamic hinged brace can help stretch joint contractures and is most frequently used across the femur and tibia. Careful wire placement also is important to avoid causing contractures. Any wire that transfixes the pes anserinus insertion will result in painful knee extension, leading to knee flexion contracture.

With tibial lengthening, the fibula also must be transfixed at both ends to prevent fibular subluxation. This can be accomplished with a transfixation pin or wire (**Figure 6**).

Axial Deviation and Residual LLD

Tjernström et al[13] reported that angular deviation occurred during lengthening and was corrected in 18 of 28 cases. García-Cimbrelo et al[6] reported that axial deviation occurred in 8 of 100 cases and attributed the deviation to unstable frame assembly. Because a spatial frame is used for most tibial lengthening procedures, any axial deviation can be corrected during treatment with the external fixator. The regenerate bone is much less likely to deform after the frame is removed if it is not removed prematurely. Occasionally, bending of the regenerate bone does occur. It is important to monitor the regenerate bone for several months after frame removal. Bending of the regenerate bone is painless, and patients often are unaware that it is occurring. When detected early, regenerate bone bending can be treated with the insertion of an interlocking rod or Rush rod and cast. If the bone bending is detected later, application of an external fixator might be required to correct the axial deviation.

Residual LLD can occur for a variety of reasons. The most common reason is flexion contracture of the knee

FIGURE 6

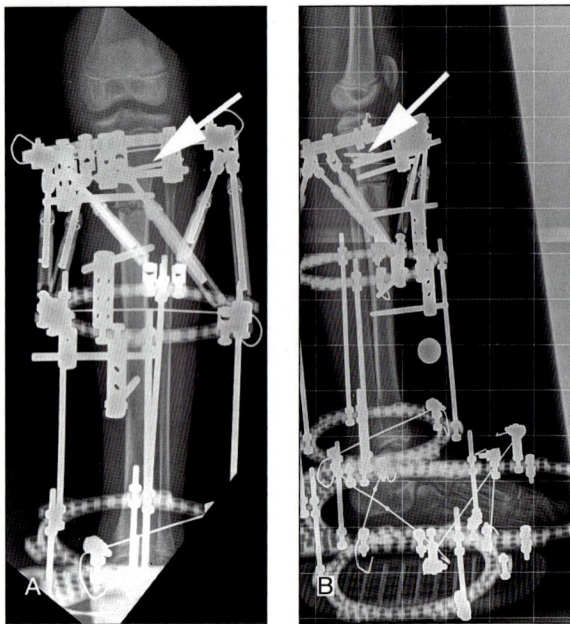

AP (**A**) and lateral (**B**) radiographs of an 11-year-old patient with hemiatrophy who underwent tibial lengthening. Note the proximal tibiofibular screw (arrow) to prevent subluxation of the proximal tibiofibular joint during lengthening. The distal tibiofibular joint is transfixed with a wire. (© 2009, Rubin Institute for Advanced Orthopaedics, Sinai Hospital of Baltimore, Baltimore, MD.)

that prevents the surgeon from obtaining true measurements of the limb with a weight-bearing radiograph. Until the knee flexion contracture resolves, the best way to accurately measure limb length is to obtain a lateral radiograph and use magnification markers. Residual LLD also can occur if the patient undergoes lengthening before skeletal maturity. In addition, the methods used to predict LLD are not 100% accurate, and occasionally, lengthening will cause a slowing of the normal growth of the tibia.[18] When the knee contracture resolves or the patient reaches skeletal maturity, the patient may have an LLD of 2 cm or greater.

Nerve and Vascular Injuries

Nerve injuries and palsies occur as the nerve becomes stretched or lengthened during deformity correction.

Tjernström et al[13] reported five cases of nerve palsy. Maffulli et al[10] reported that 149 patients developed nerve symptoms. The patients were treated by reducing the rate of lengthening; 17 patients, however, were still symptomatic at the time of fixator removal. Velazquez et al[5] reviewed their first 40 patients treated with Ilizarov fixation at the Hospital for Sick Children in Toronto and reported that four transient nerve palsies occurred.

Preoperative planning is required for a procedure such as correction of proximal tibial alignment from valgus to neutral, which will stretch the peroneal nerve at several tethering points as it enters the anterior compartment of the calf. When nerve stretching is anticipated, prophylactic nerve decompression is performed before symptoms occur.

Pin-Tract and Wire-Tract Infections

Pin-tract infections are common complications of distraction osteogenesis because the frame needs to be worn for several months. Several authors report the incidence of pin-tract infections to be approximately 50%.[17,19,20] Maffulli et al[10] treated 240 patients with LLD using distraction osteogenesis with various types of pins and wires. Of the 267 Orthofix pins (Orthofix Orthopaedics North America, McKinney, TX) used, 146 pin sites developed infections: 125 were managed with local care and orally administered antibiotics, 13 developed deep infections that were treated with pin exchange, and eight developed infections that were treated with pin removal only. Hydroxyapatite-coated pins have helped tremendously in decreasing the rate of pin-tract infection because of the ability of bone to grow into the hydroxyapatite coating. This dramatically decreases loosening of the pin, which promotes infection of the soft tissue and bone.[21] Most pin-tract infections are treated with local wound care and orally administered antibiotics. **Table 1** lists the three types of pin-tract problems and their treatment. A pin culture is obtained in the surgeon's office to make sure the proper antibiotic is administered.

Careful handling of the surrounding soft tissue helps to avoid pin and wire complications. Pins and wires should be placed into the skin without any skin tension. If skin tension occurs around the pin or wire, it should be released. Also, pins in the femur traverse a large amount of soft tissue. The soft tissue pistons on the

T A B L E 1 **Classification and Treatment of Pin-Tract Problems**

Grade	Description	Treatment
1	Soft-tissue inflammation	Pin care; apply local antiseptic or antibiotics; ensure proper wire tension
2	Soft-tissue infection	Administer oral antibiotics (typically, a 10-day course); pin care
3	Bone infection	Remove pin; curettage of the pin tract and bone; if necessary, antibiotic delivery using bone cement

(© 2009, Rubin Institute for Advanced Orthopaedics, Sinai Hospital of Baltimore, Baltimore, MD.)

pins with knee range of motion, causing inflammation and soft-tissue trauma, which lead to infection. Tightly wrapping the pins with Kerlix gauze (Covidien, Mansfield, MA) keeps the pistoning to a minimum and helps eliminate some of the femoral pin-tract problems (**Figure 7**). García-Cimbrelo et al[6] reported that wires that were tensioned using a dynamometric tensioner incurred a 7.8% rate of grade 1 problems versus 24.5% for wires tensioned manually.

Systemic and Life-Threatening Complications
Toxic Shock Syndrome
Maffulli et al[10] reported that one patient who underwent femoral lengthening for sequelae of multifocal osteomyelitis developed a pin-tract infection that initially was treated with orally administered antibiotics. The infection recurred, however, with accompanying symptoms of malaise, fever, and vomiting. *Staphylococcus aureus* toxin was identified in the blood. The symptoms resolved with removal of the fixator. Other cases of toxic shock syndrome have been reported.[22] Quick recognition of the symptoms is very important because the hypotension and resulting septic shock can be fatal.

Hypertension
Idiopathic hypertension developed in five of 240 patients in a series presented by Maffulli et al.[10] The hypertension resolved by discontinuing distraction for 2 to 3 days and resuming the rate at 0.5 mm/d for 1 week. The 1 mm/d rate was then resumed, and no additional hypertension occurred.

Soft-Tissue Envelope Compromise
When using distraction osteogenesis for bone transport, the soft-tissue envelope at the transporting end often is scarred. During transport, the bone end can start to protrude through the soft tissue, or the soft tissue can invaginate, preventing good bone contact. El-Alfy et al[23] reported 11 cases of bone transport for bone and soft-tissue defects. In their series, one patient had bone protruding through the wound during transport that was treated with resection, which restored good soft-tissue coverage. Transport was then continued successfully. Three patients experienced docking-site soft-tissue invagination during transport. The cases were treated with elevation of the skin and soft tissue, and no additional problems occurred.

Rare Complications
Rare complications from distraction osteogenesis include case reports of osteogenic sarcoma after a femoral lengthening through fibrous dysplasia,[24] pseudoaneurysms following corticotomy and lengthenings,[25] and arteriovenous fistulas.[26,27]

Compartment syndrome is a complication that occurs very rarely after osteotomy and external fixator application for lengthening. Velazquez et al[5] reported two cases that required fasciotomy and secondary wound closure.

METABOLIC BONE DISEASE AND POLIOMYELITIS
The rate of complications in patients with metabolically abnormal bone (eg, enchondromatosis, melorheostosis, hypophosphatemic rickets, monostotic fibrous dysplasia, and irradiated bone) is higher than in patients

FIGURE 7

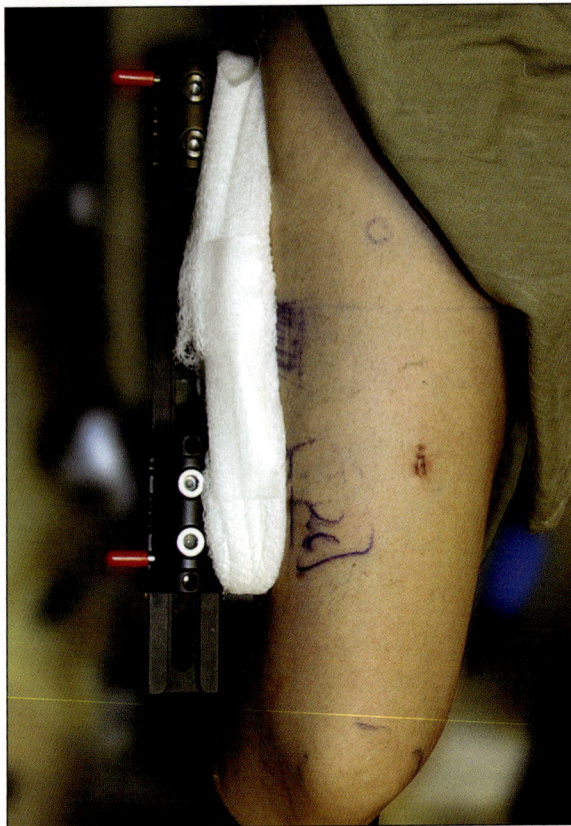

Photograph shows proper wrapping technique used during monolateral external fixation to prevent the skin from pistoning on femoral pins. Tightly wrapping the Kerlix gauze (Covidien, Mansfield, MA) decreases the soft-tissue trauma around the pins and helps prevent infection. (© 2009, Rubin Institute for Advanced Orthopaedics, Sinai Hospital of Baltimore, Baltimore, MD.)

with healthy bone, as documented by Naudie et al.[28] The worst complication occurred in a patient who had melorheostosis. Ischemia developed in the leg, accompanied by nerve palsy, flexion contracture of the knee, and pressure sores that required a transfemoral amputation. Younge et al[29] also had difficulty performing a lengthening in a patient with melorheostosis and the onset of distal ischemia. The abnormal bone characteristics of such conditions make the results of limb-lengthening procedures unpredictable. Stanitski[30] showed that

distraction osteogenesis can be safely performed in patients with metabolic bone disease, but the healing index is slower than in unaffected patients. In Stanitski's series, the rate of distraction was 0.5 mm/d and the healing index was 1.6 months per centimeter, as opposed to the average 1.0 month per centimeter. No regenerate bone complications secondary to the slower rate were reported in the series.

Ring et al[31] described six cases of limb lengthening in patients with osteogenesis imperfecta. A slower rate of distraction was used, the frame was left in place for a longer period of consolidation, and all limbs were protected with a cast or brace after removal. In addition to the standard problems encountered with lengthening, one patient experienced a fracture that occurred in the nonsurgical extremity during the rehabilitation phase, one patient experienced a fracture that occurred through a previous pin site in the surgical extremity, and one patient experienced intraoperative hemorrhage, which has previously been reported as a problem in patients with osteogenesis imperfecta.[32] Even with the reported complications, four of the six patients achieved good functional improvement.

Patients with poliomyelitis also have difficulty regenerating bone and need to be treated with caution. In my experience, the rate of lengthening must be slower in these patients; however, this has not been documented in the literature.

Ollier disease, or enchondromatosis, is a dyschondroplasia that seems to be the exception with regard to slower regenerate healing. Jesus-Garcia et al[33] documented 10 patients who were treated with distraction osteogenesis at a rate of 1 mm/d and did not incur regenerate bone complications. Price et al[34] and Paley[2] documented increased risk for premature consolidation in cases of Ollier disease.

COMPLICATIONS SPECIFIC TO ANATOMIC REGIONS
The Hand

Heo et al[35] documented complications in 16 of 51 distraction osteogenesis procedures performed in the hand (31%). Major complications included premature consolidation, nonunion, fracture, angular deformity, and pin loosening. Minor complications included delayed healing and joint stiffness. The rate of distraction was

0.25 mm/d for the phalanges and 0.5 mm/d for the metacarpals. Distraction of the phalanges was associated with more complications than was distraction of the metacarpals. A safe distraction rate for the metacarpals is 0.25 mm twice per day. It is important to avoid damaging the periosteum and to avoid lengthening by more than 40% of the initial bone length. Lengthening greater than 40% is associated with nonunion, joint stiffness, and subluxation.[36]

The Foot

Numerous articles have documented metatarsal lengthening for brachymetatarsia.[37-40] The most common indication for metatarsal lengthening is for a congenitally short fourth metatarsal. Oh et al,[37] in one of the largest published series, reported on 47 metatarsals that were lengthened in 33 patients at a distraction rate of 0.25 mm twice per day. The average increase in metatarsal length was 35% in children and 30% in adults. The most common complications were metatarsophalangeal joint subluxation and stiffness, especially with the more extensive lengthenings. This joint subluxation can be minimized by pinning the metatarsophalangeal joint during lengthening.

ACKNOWLEDGMENTS

The author thanks John E. Herzenberg, MD, FRCSC, for contributing the case shown in **Figure 3**.

REFERENCES

1. Krishnan A, Pamecha C, Patwa JJ: Modified Ilizarov technique for infected nonunion of the femur: The principle of distraction-compression osteogenesis. *J Orthop Surg (Hong Kong)* 2006;14(3):265-272.

2. Paley D: Problems, obstacles, and complications of limb lengthening by the Ilizarov technique. *Clin Orthop Relat Res* 1990(250)81-104.

3. Paley D: Current techniques of limb lengthening. *J Pediatr Orthop* 1988;8(1):73-92.

4. Dahl MT, Gulli B, Berg T: Complications of limb lengthening: A learning curve. *Clin Orthop Relat Res* 1994(301):10-18.

5. Velazquez RJ, Bell DF, Armstrong PF, Babyn P, Tibshirani R: Complications of use of the Ilizarov technique in the correction of limb deformities in children. *J Bone Joint Surg Am* 1993;75(8):1148-1156.

6. García-Cimbrelo E, Olsen B, Ruiz-Yagüe M, Fernandez-Baíllo N, Munuera-Martínez L: Ilizarov technique: Results and difficulties. *Clin Orthop Relat Res* 1992(283)-:116-123.

7. Ilizarov GA, Deviatov AA: Surgical lengthening of the shin with simultaneous correction of deformities. *Ortop Travmatol Protez* 1969;30(3):32-37.

8. Fischgrund J, Paley D, Suter C: Variables affecting time to bone healing during limb lengthening. *Clin Orthop Relat Res* 1994(301):31-37.

9. Niemelä BJ, Tjernström B, Andersson G, Wahlsten VS: Does leg lengthening pose a threat to a child's mental health? An interim report one year after surgery. *J Pediatr Orthop* 2007;27(6):611-617.

10. Maffulli N, Lombari C, Matarazzo L, Nele U, Pagnotta G, Fixsen JA: A review of 240 patients undergoing distraction osteogenesis for congenital post-traumatic or postinfective lower limb length discrepancy. *J Am Coll Surg* 1996;182(5):394-402.

11. Simpson AH, Cole AS, Kenwright J: Leg lengthening over an intramedullary nail. *J Bone Joint Surg Br* 1999;81(6):1041-1045.

12. Paley D, Herzenberg JE, Paremain G, Bhave A: Femoral lengthening over an intramedullary nail: A matched-case comparison with Ilizarov femoral lengthening. *J Bone Joint Surg Am* 1997;79(10):1464-1480.

13. Tjernström B, Olerud S, Rehnberg L: Limb lengthening by callus distraction: Complications in 53 cases operated 1980-1991. *Acta Orthop Scand* 1994;65(4):447-455.

14. Paley D, Tetsworth K: Percutaneous osteotomies: Osteotome and Gigli saw techniques. *Orthop Clin North Am* 1991;22(4):613-624.

15. Jochymek J, Gal P: Evaluation of bone healing in femurs lengthened via the gradual distraction method. *Biomed Pap Med Fac Univ Palacky Olomouc Czech Repub* 2007;151(1):137-141.

16. Herzenberg JE, Scheufele LL, Paley D, Bechtel R, Tepper S: Knee range of motion in isolated femoral lengthening. *Clin Orthop Relat Res* 1994(301):49-54.

17. Zhang X, Liu T, Li Z, Peng W: Reconstruction with callus distraction for nonunion with bone loss and leg shortening caused by suppurative osteomyelitis of the femur. *J Bone Joint Surg Br* 2007;89(11):1509-1514.

18. Sharma M, MacKenzie WG, Bowen JR: Severe tibial growth retardation in total fibular hemimelia after limb lengthening. *J Pediatr Orthop* 1996;16(4):438-444.

19. Magyar G, Toksvig-Larsen S, Lindstrand A: Hemical-lotasis open-wedge osteotomy for osteoarthritis of the knee: Complications in 308 operations. *J Bone Joint Surg Br* 1999;81(3):449-451.

20. Fowler JL, Gie GA, Maceachern AG: Upper tibial valgus osteotomy using a dynamic external fixator. *J Bone Joint Surg Br* 1991;73(4):690-691.

21. Moroni A, Vannini F, Mosca M, Giannini S: State of the art review: Techniques to avoid pin loosening and infection in external fixation. *J Orthop Trauma* 2002;16(3):189-195.

22. Turker R, Lubicky JP, Vogel LC: Toxic shock syndrome in patients with external fixators. *J Pediatr Orthop* 1992;12(5):658-662.

23. El-Alfy B, El-Mowafi H, El-Moghazy N: Distraction osteogenesis in management of composite bone and soft tissue defects. *Int Orthop* 2010;34(1):115-118.

24. Harris NL, Eilert RE, Davino N, Ruyle S, Edwardson M, Wilson V: Osteogenic sarcoma arising from bony regenerate following Ilizarov femoral lengthening through fibrous dysplasia. *J Pediatr Orthop* 1994; 14(1):123-129.

25. Bowman JN, Ellozy SH, Ting J, Ghiassi S: Successful repair of popliteal artery pseudoaneurysm after tibial lengthening osteotomy in a 7-year-old boy. *Vasc Endovascular Surg* 2008;42(6):610-614.

26. Spinelli F, Spinelli R, Stilo F, De Caridi G, Mirenda F: Vascular lesions secondary to osteotomy by cortico-tomy. *Chir Ital* 2007;59(4):575-579.

27. Lang W, Ott R, Haas P, Schweiger H: Popliteal arteri-ovenous fistula after corrective upper tibial osteotomy. *Arch Orthop Trauma Surg* 1993;112(2):99-100.

28. Naudie D, Hamdy RC, Fassier F, Duhaime M: Compli-cations of limb-lengthening in children who have an underlying bone disorder. *J Bone Joint Surg Am* 1998;80(1):18-24.

29. Younge D, Drummond D, Herring J, Cruess RL: Melorheostosis in children: Clinical features and natu-ral history. *J Bone Joint Surg Br* 1979;61-B(4):415-418.

30. Stanitski DF: Treatment of deformity secondary to metabolic bone disease with the Ilizarov technique. *Clin Orthop Relat Res* 1994(301):38-41.

31. Ring D, Jupiter JB, Labropoulos PK, Guggenheim JJ, Stanitsky DF, Spencer DM: Treatment of deformity of the lower limb in adults who have osteogenesis imper-fecta. *J Bone Joint Surg Am* 1996;78(2):220-225.

32. Yong-Hing K, MacEwen GD: Scoliosis associated with osteogenesis imperfecta. *J Bone Joint Surg Br* 1982; 64(1):36-43.

33. Jesus-Garcia R, Bongiovanni JC, Korukian M, Boatto H, Seixas MT, Laredo J: Use of the Ilizarov external fix-ator in the treatment of patients with Ollier's disease. *Clin Orthop Relat Res* 2001(382):82-86.

34. Price CT, Bright RW, Wang L: Limb lengthening after immediate correction of deformity using the Orthofix unilateral fixator. *American Academy of Orthopaedic Surgeons 58th Annual Meeting, Final Program.* Ana-heim, CA, 1991, p 80.

35. Heo CY, Kwon S, Back GH, Chung MS: Complications of distraction lengthening in the hand. *J Hand Surg Eur Vol* 2008;33(5):609-615.

36. Erdem M, Sen C, Eralp L, Kocaoğlu M, Ozden V: Lengthening of short bones by distraction osteogenesis: Results and complications. *Int Orthop* 2009;33(3): 807-813.

37. Oh CW, Sharma R, Song HR, Koo KH, Kyung HS, Park BC: Complications of distraction osteogenesis in short fourth metatarsals. *J Pediatr Orthop* 2003;23(4): 484-487.

38. Oh CW, Satish BR, Lee ST, Song HR: Complications of distraction osteogenesis in short first metatarsals. *J Pediatr Orthop* 2004;24(6):711-715.

39. Masada K, Fujita S, Fuji T, Ohno H: Complications fol-lowing metatarsal lengthening by callus distraction for brachymetatarsia. *J Pediatr Orthop* 1999;19(3):394-397.

40. Levine SE, Davidson RS, Dormans JP, Drummond DS: Distraction osteogenesis for congenitally short lesser metatarsals. *Foot Ankle Int* 1995;16(4):196-200.

CHAPTER 11

VAN NES ROTATIONPLASTY

JOSEPH IVAN KRAJBICH, MD, FRCSC

INTRODUCTION

Van Nes rotationplasty,[1] also known as tibial rotation-plasty, Borggreve operation,[2] or simply as rotationplasty, is neither clearly an amputation nor a limb-sparing procedure. Most orthopaedic surgeons are relatively unfamiliar with the Van Nes rotationplasty, and most orthopaedic trainees have never examined a patient who has undergone the procedure, much less seen it performed. Even among surgeons familiar with the procedure, few perform it on a routine basis. If performed well, however, and for the right indications, it is an excellent alternative to more conventional procedures. Some may not consider Van Nes rotationplasty to be a true limb salvage procedure, yet its capability to preserve function is generally not disputed.[3-5]

The basic principle of rotationplasty in all of its modifications is to substitute a turned-around ankle and foot for an absent or nonfunctional knee joint, with the foot acting as the proximal tibia. The rotation is a full 180°, so normal ankle extension (dorsiflexion) becomes knee flexion, and ankle flexion (plantar flexion) becomes knee extension (**Figure 1**). The foot fits into a prosthetic socket, enabling function similar to that of a below-knee (transtibial) amputation[6-10] (**Figure 2**).

Although the principle is the same, there is enough difference in the technique and potential complications in the procedure performed for congenital limb deficiency

(proximal femoral focal deficiency [PFFD]) and malignant tumor resections[11-14] to warrant separate description and discussion. The procedure used for PFFD and related congenital abnormalities is the subject of this review.

VAN NES ROTATIONPLASTY AND PFFD

PFFD is the congenital deficiency most commonly treated with Van Nes rotationplasty. PFFD is one of the greatest challenges to extremity restoration. In addition to a complete absence (Aitken type C and D, Krajbich class II/Alman class II deformities) or significant abnormality (Aitken type A and B, Krajbich class I/Alman class I deformities) of the hip joint, a significant defect also is centered in the subtrochanteric area of the femur. In an extreme situation, this includes virtually all of the femur, as well as a significant abnormality of the knee joint with associated ligamentous deficiencies and soft-tissue contractures.[15-18] Associated fibular hemimelia (longitudinal fibular deficiency) also is present in most cases. All these factors lead to marked longitudinal deficiency in the affected extremity compared with the opposite, unaffected limb. In virtually all cases, the foot of the affected extremity is at a level somewhere between the mid tibia and the knee of the opposite extremity. Before Van Nes developed the rotationplasty procedure, this complex deformity

---

FIGURE 1

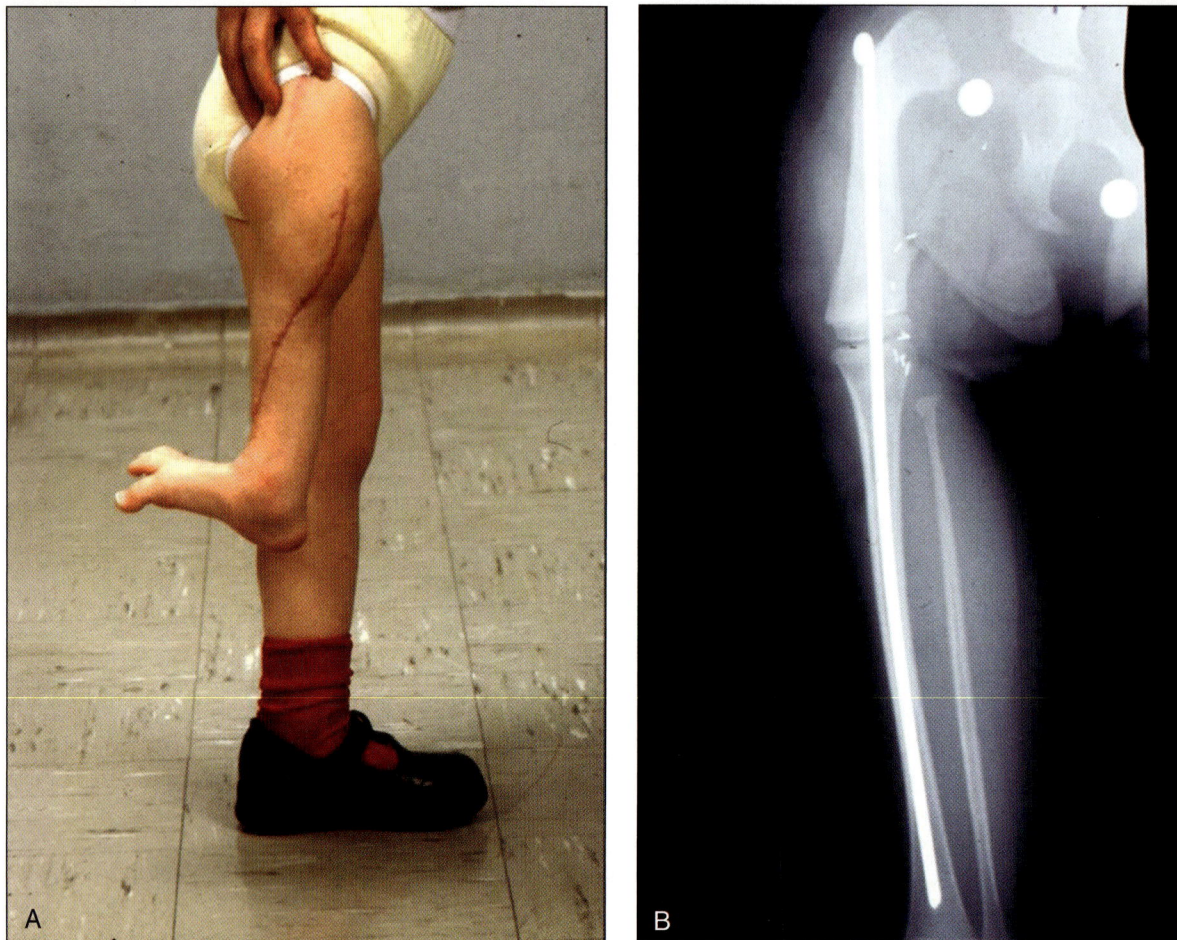

Photograph (**A**) and AP radiograph (**B**) of a child who underwent a Van Nes rotationplasty procedure for proximal femoral focal deficiency. The new ankle/knee is slightly below the level of the opposite knee in anticipation of ongoing growth difference in the thighs. The knees are expected to be at equal heights at skeletal maturity.

was treated using an extension prosthesis with a prosthetic knee joint located below the foot or with no joint at all. These patients functioned either in the manner of above-knee (transfemoral) amputees with a thigh-length discrepancy or knee arthrodesis patients, with neither solution being very functional.

Van Nes described performing an osteotomy of the tibia and fibula and turning the distal fragment 180°, allowing function in the anatomic range of the knee joint. The final limb length was adjusted to be approximately at the level of the opposite knee. Independently, a significant advance in the surgical treatment of PFFD was proposed by King,[19] who described a combined knee arthrodesis, Syme disarticulation, and above-knee prosthetic fitting. This procedure had the advantage of giving the patient a solid "one-bone" thigh with an excellent residual limb for prosthetic fitting, and a prosthetic knee at the level of the opposite knee joint. Torode and Gillespie[20] combined the knee fusion with the rotationplasty, achieving at least partial rotation through the knee fusion and the rest through the

FIGURE 2

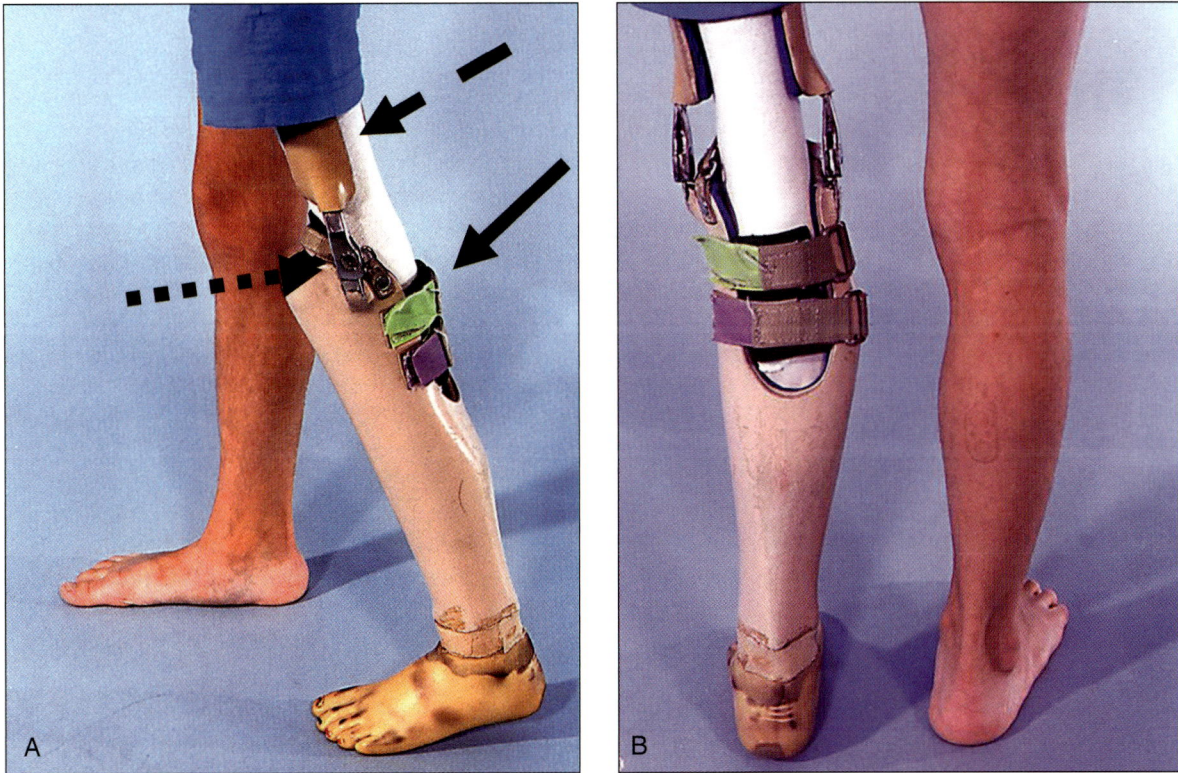

Lateral (**A**) and posterior (**B**) photographs show a Van Nes rotationplasty patient wearing her prosthesis. The main components of the prosthesis are the foot socket (solid arrow), the external hinges that provide coronal plane stability (dotted arrow), and the thigh cuff (dashed arrow).

traditional tibial osteotomy. This procedure decreased the tendency for postoperative derotation. I further modified the procedure, to achieve all the rotation through the knee arthrodesis. In this technique, all the muscles and tendons crossing the knee joint are detached and then reattached so they are anatomically aligned. This modification allows for a better retention of the muscle biomechanics and alleviates the tendency for derotation of the distal fragment with growth. The resulting extremity is then fitted with Van Nes rotationplasty prostheses, which have functionality similar to that of a transtibial amputation. The one-bone thigh also provides a good platform for hip reconstructive surgery for the Aitken type A and B and Krajbich class I and Alman class I deficiencies. My colleagues and I have successfully used this modification for the past 20 years.

INITIAL EVALUATION AND TREATMENT

The rotationplasty is usually performed when the patient is between 2.5 and 3.5 years of age, although it can be performed at almost any age. In older age groups, the procedure may be technically easier; however, the rehabilitation potential is greatest at a younger age.[21] Careful physical examination helps assess the presence of additional deficiencies involving other limbs, particularly of the surgical limb. If a fibular deficiency exists, it is carefully evaluated, particularly with respect to abnormality of the ankle joint and the foot. Complete absence of the fibula with stiff equinovalgus ankle deformity and a foot with fewer than three rays usually are contraindications to rotationplasty. Radiologic examination sometimes is supplemented by MRI of the hip area and is used to correctly classify the deformity so that the optimal treatment plan can be determined and outlined for the caregivers.

When the child starts to stand, at 9 to 12 months of age, a simple extension prosthesis is provided to facilitate the child's ability to learn to walk independently. He or she is then followed up in the clinic at 6- to 8-month intervals. If the child is a candidate for rotationplasty and the parents prefer it as a treatment, the procedure is then performed at 2.5 to 3.5 years of age, leaving enough time for the child to be fully rehabilitated in time to begin school, even if additional surgery for hip reconstruction (for Aitken type A or B and Krajbich grade I or Alman grade I deformities) is planned at 4 or 5 years of age.

INDICATIONS
Any condition resulting in a severe shortening of the affected extremity can be salvaged by rotationplasty, usually with significant functional improvement, as long as the foot/ankle complex is present and has a combined active range of motion of at least 50° to 60°. The status of the hip and the knee is of only secondary importance. All children with unilateral PFFD of the Krajbich/Alman class I or II; Aitken A, B, C, or D; or Gillespie type II deformities are potential candidates for Van Nes rotationplasty, provided that they have a functional foot/ankle complex. Other conditions that are significantly less common also can fulfill the criteria for the surgery, such as a rare variant of tibial hemimelia with absent proximal tibia, severe congenital knee dislocation with significant overlap of the femur and tibia, and some acquired conditions such as neonatal osteomyelitis of the distal femur.

CONTRAINDICATIONS
In children born with PFFD, the only absolute contraindication to rotationplasty is the absence of a functional ankle/foot unit. If the ankle and foot do not meet the minimum requirements of at least three rays and a range of motion of the combined ankle–subtalar joint complex of at least 50°, the procedure is contraindicated and some variant of the procedure described by King or prosthetic fitting without surgery should be considered. The most common relative contraindication is the cos-

metic and social unacceptability of having the foot rotated backward, which happens only very rarely in my experience.

A competent prosthetist familiar with the pediatric population and the design of rotationplasty prostheses is required.[22] Gaining access to such an expert may be an issue in some countries. On the other hand, the prosthetic components are relatively simple and inexpensive. The simple SACH foot, socket for the foot, and external knee hinges are the minimum required components.

Multiple congenital limb deficiencies such as bilateral PFFD also can be relative contraindications. Most patients with this condition spend a fair amount of time ambulating directly on their feet. Having both feet rotated 180° makes for both a more awkward gait and an unusual appearance. If a child has significant bilateral upper extremity deficiencies, the feet may become the child's main prehensile extremity used for typing, writing, feeding, and other activities of daily living. Rotationplasty would clearly lead to functional loss for the child and is therefore contraindicated.

Unfortunately, a significant reason why rotationplasty is still rejected as a treatment option is surgeons' unfamiliarity with the procedure and misconceptions about it. The procedure requires specific technical skills and is best performed by a pediatric surgeon familiar with the procedure.

SURGICAL TECHNIQUE
General anesthesia is administered and all monitoring lines are inserted per the anesthesia service. The child is typed and screened for blood but not cross-typed because blood product replacement is almost never needed. The patient is positioned supine with a slight prop under the surgical side. The surgical extremity is then prepared and draped from the toes to the side of the pelvis and lower abdominal quadrant, in a manner similar to that as for any major hip procedure, allowing easy access to the greater trochanter. Using a sterile Doppler ultrasonographic probe, the locations of the posterior tibial artery and the anterior tibial artery are noted at the ankle level. The incision is then marked on the skin. I prefer to use a lazy S–shape incision, starting proximally on the lateral side of the thigh about 2 to 3 inches above the knee, and extending distally toward the knee. The incision curves medially across the knee joint

FIGURE 3

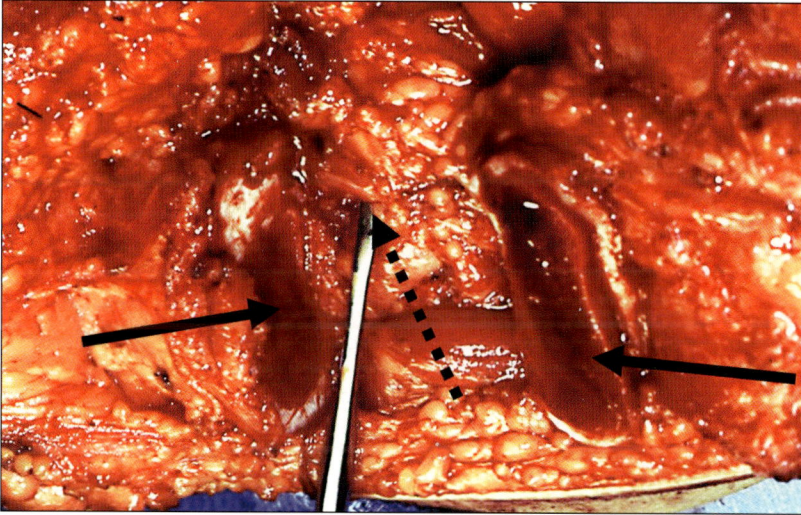

Intraoperative photograph of the technique. Note the osteotomized bony surfaces of the distal femur and proximal tibia (solid arrows) and the main neurovascular bundle (dotted arrow).

at the level of the distal femur and then curves distally along the anteromedial border of the tibia. The advantages of this incision are twofold. First, it facilitates distal fragment external rotation, which allows the peroneal nerve and the femoral-popliteal artery to assume a "straight" course rather than winding around the leg. Second, it places the incision scar more or less on the lateral side of the extremity, with no neurovascular structures immediately deep to it, which is important if any further surgery, such as hip realignment osteotomy, is needed.

After the incision is completed and skin flaps are developed, I prefer to first identify the peroneal nerve on the lateral side. Cases of significant fibular deficiency have abnormal anatomy, making this slightly less straightforward than usual. In such a case, locating the nerve more proximally (at the sciatic nerve division) may be safer and more advisable. Once the nerve is identified, isolated, and protected, the tendons crossing the knee anteriorly, laterally, and medially can all be divided. The patellar tendon, biceps femoris, and pes anserinus tendons are all divided approximately 1 inch from their insertions. A knee capsulotomy is then performed. The capsule is divided completely circumferentially, which allows visualization of the posterior neurovascular structures.

At this point, the femoral condyles and metaphysis are dissected free of the residual soft tissue, including detachment of the gastrocnemius heads at their origin on the femoral condyles, taking care not to disrupt the neurovascular supply. Approximately 2 inches of the distal femur is then osteotomized and removed from the surgical field. Next, the proximal tibia is dissected free and transected just distal to the epiphyseal plate. On rare occasions, with a very short femoral fragment, the epiphyseal plate is preserved by doing the osteotomy through the epiphysis (**Figure 3**). Good visualization of the remaining posterior structures is now possible. The remaining popliteus and semimembranosus tendons and muscles are divided. The popliteal vessels are carefully dissected past the adductor hiatus to allow free mobilization into the anterior aspect of the thigh. The distal fragment is then checked for ease of rotation, checking carefully for a good vascular supply of the rotated fragment. If needed, additional freeing of soft tissues or even further femoral shortening is performed.

Next, under fluoroscopic guidance, a Rush rod or a heavy Kirschner wire (K-wire) is introduced into the medullary cavity of the femur in retrograde fashion, exiting the bone proximally in the region of the greater trochanter. The leg is then rotated the desired 180° and the rod is advanced antegrade into the tibia. The tibia

FIGURE 4

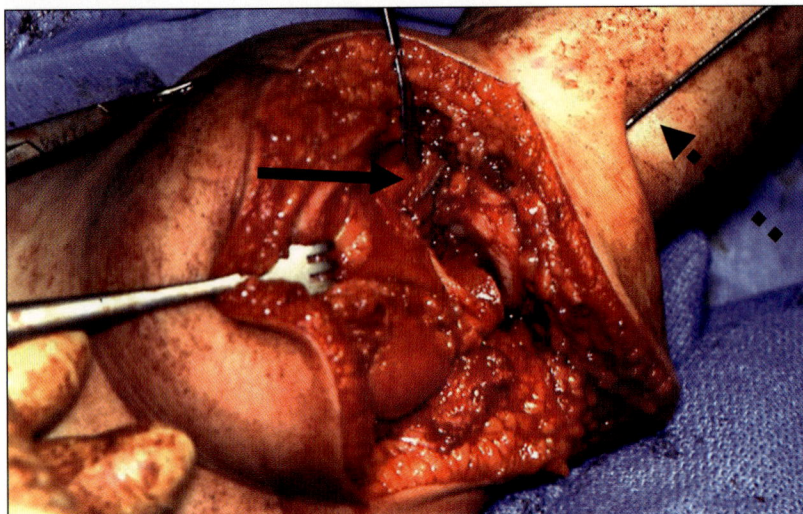

Intraoperative photograph of the technique. The final position is held by the cross K-wire (dotted arrow). Note the unobstructed position of the neurovascular bundle on the anterior surface (solid arrow).

is held in close apposition to the femur, and care is taken not to trap any of the soft-tissue structures in the osteotomy site.

The final adjustment of the desired rotation is now performed. The leg and foot are carefully checked for adequate circulation by assessing perfusion, palpating distal pulses, and checking them with a Doppler probe if needed. Any inadequate circulation can be addressed at this time by derotation and further freeing of the vessels.

Once the final position is achieved, the K-wire across the osteotomy site is used to hold the position (**Figure 4**). The desired rotation has to be evaluated carefully. Many cases of so-called derotation are simply cases of inadequate rotation during the index procedure. In a child with a significant degree of fibular deficiency, the motion of the ankle joint alone may not be adequate, and the motion of the final Van Nes knee will be a combination of ankle and subtalar motion. The amount of rotation achieved during surgery as well as the construction of the prosthesis must account for this motion. Next, the heads of the gastrocnemius muscle (now anterior) are attached to the quadriceps after excising the patella and the very distal portion of the quadriceps muscle. The skin flaps are then closed, trimming any obvious dog-ear edges. The dressing is applied, and the child is placed in a half hip spica splint (**Figure 5**). An opening is left over the posterior tibial artery behind the

medial malleolus to allow vascular monitoring. At 7 to 10 days after surgery, the splint is changed to a solid half hip spica cast under anesthesia. The cast is worn for 6 to 8 weeks, by which time union will have occurred and the child will be ready for removal of the cross K-wire, the start of physical therapy with both gentle passive and active range-of-motion exercises, and prosthetic fittings.

POTENTIAL COMPLICATIONS

The most immediate and potentially devastating complication of rotationplasty is a loss of adequate circulation in the affected extremity. This must be promptly recognized and circulation must be restored by derotating the extremity and freeing the vessels with or without further shortening of the femoral fragment. Good pulse and perfusion must be established before applying a dressing and waking the child from the anesthesia. Circulation is then carefully monitored for the following 48 hours, and the child is kept well hydrated with intravenous fluids.

Postoperative derotation is thought to be a frequent complication of rotationplasty. In my experience, when the technique discussed above is used, derotation is quite rare and most cases of inadequate rotation are likely present at the time of the index operation. It is therefore of paramount importance to pay adequate atten-

FIGURE 5

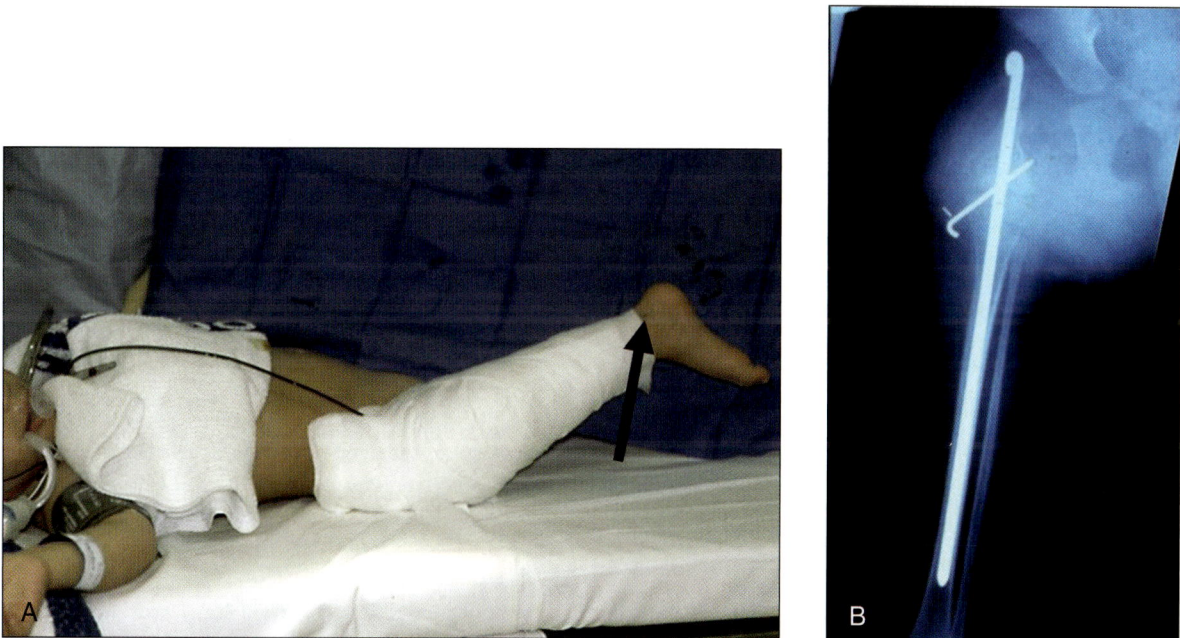

Images of a patient obtained after Van Nes rotationplasty. **A,** Immediate postoperative photograph shows the patient supine, before final spica-like splint application. The posterior tibial artery pulse site (arrow) is marked for ease of postoperative monitoring. **B,** AP radiograph shows intramedullary rod and cross K-wire used for internal fixation.

tion to the degree of rotation achieved. When additional hip reconstruction surgery is planned, final adjustment of both the rotation and length can be potentially addressed at that time.

The most common complication (if one can call it such) is an extremity that is too long. Ideally, the level of the heel on the rotationplasty side should be approximately at the level of the contralateral knee (ie, the thighs should be the same length) at skeletal maturity. Clearly, overall leg length can be manipulated by the length of the prosthesis, but symmetry of gait and cosmetic effect when sitting is best served by having the knees at the same level. In a young child, the optimal length can be achieved by good planning, taking into account the length of the femoral and tibial fragments and the growth potential in the tibial growth plates (both distal and proximal) and in the hindfoot. If the thigh is left too long, additional equalization can be performed during the hip reconstruction surgery if planned or by appropriately timed epiphysiodesis of the remaining growth plates.

PROCEDURE MODIFICATIONS

When the femur is completely absent or comprises only a small cartilaginous fragment that is frequently fused to the proximal tibial epiphysis, achieving a complete 180° rotation through the knee can be a challenge. In these situations, I modify the procedure, sometimes delaying surgery 1 to 2 years to allow a little extra growth; I modify the procedure similar to the way described by Torode and Gillespie.[20] As much rotation as possible is done proximally through the cartilage anlage of the fused knee, and any remaining rotation is then achieved with a mid tibial osteotomy. In this situation, it is sometimes helpful to delay the surgery for 1 to 2 years to allow for extra growth.

The rotationplasty procedure has been modified by Brown[23] to allow stabilization of the femoropelvic junction in Aitken type C and D and Krajbich/Alman class 2 cases and to substitute a rotated knee joint for a uniplanar hip joint, similar to the procedure described by Winkelmann[13] for malignant lesions of the proximal femur. Even greater attention must be given to protecting an adequate blood supply to the distal part of the extremity because the neurovascular structures are the only tissues left undivided.

DISCUSSION

Over time, the Van Nes rotationplasty has undergone several modifications from its first description in the literature by Van Nes.[1] The procedures most commonly performed are the technique described by Torode and Gillespie and my technique, with the rotation attained primarily through the knee, combined with knee fusion. This variant largely eliminates the issue of late derotation and gives the patient a solid one-bone thigh and functional, biologic knee joint. A solid normal-length thigh allows stretching of associated contractures around the hip, improves the range of motion, and makes any planned hip reconstruction easier.

Several gait studies have demonstrated appropriate in-phase muscle function in the thigh after rotationplasty, making the patient's gait highly functional.[5,21,24] Psychologic testing of these patients failed to demonstrate any adverse effect of the procedure.

I consider rotationplasty to be the treatment of choice in children who have been diagnosed with unilateral PFFD and whose overall limb-length discrepancy and associated hip and knee deficiencies make them less than ideal candidates for leg-lengthening procedures. A single procedure with a short hospital stay, minimal risk of complications, and a predictably good functional outcome offers many advantages over current alternatives. Rotationplasty should be part of the armamentarium of any pediatric orthopaedic surgeon with significant interest in limb deficiency treatment.

REFERENCES

1. Van Nes CP: Rotation-plasty for congenital defects of the femur. *J Bone Joint Surg Br* 1950;32:12.
2. Borggreve J: Kniegelenksersatz durch das in der Beinlängsachse um 180 Grad gedrehte Fussgelenk. *Arch Orthop Chir* 1930;28:175-178.
3. Steenhoff JR, Daanen HA, Taminiau AH: Functional analysis of patients who have had a modified Van Nes rotationplasty. *J Bone Joint Surg Am* 1993;75(10): 1451-1456.
4. Murray MP, Jacobs PA, Gore DR, Gardner GM, Mollinger LA: Functional performance after tibial rotationplasty. *J Bone Joint Surg Am* 1985;67(3):392-399.
5. McClenaghan BA, Krajbich JI, Pirone AM, Koheil R, Longmuir P: Comparative assessment of gait after limb-salvage procedures. *J Bone Joint Surg Am* 1989;71(8):1178-1182.
6. Hall JE: Rotation of hypoplastic lower limbs to use the ankle joint as a knee. *Intern Clin Inform Bull* 1966;6(2):3.
7. Hall JE, Bochman D: The surgical and prosthetic management of proximal femoral focal deficiency, in *A Symposium on Proximal Femoral Focal Deficiency: A Congenital Anomaly*. National Academy of Sciences, 1969.
8. Kostuik JP, Gillespie R, Hall JE, Hubbard S: Van Nes rotational osteotomy for treatment of proximal femoral focal deficiency and congenital short femur. *J Bone Joint Surg Am* 1975;57(8):1039-1046.
9. Kritter AE: Tibial rotation-plasty for proximal femoral focal deficiency. *J Bone Joint Surg Am* 1977;59(7):927-934.
10. Kotz R, Salzer M: Rotation-plasty for childhood osteosarcoma of the distal part of the femur. *J Bone Joint Surg Am* 1982;64(7):959-969.
11. Krajbich JI, Carroll NC: Van Nes rotationplasty with segmental limb resection. *Clin Orthop Relat Res* 1990(256):7-13.
12. Krajbich JI: Modified Van Nes rotationplasty in the treatment of malignant neoplasms in the lower extremities of children. *Clin Orthop Relat Res* 1991(262): 74-77.
13. Winkelmann WW: Hip rotationplasty for malignant tumors of the proximal part of the femur. *J Bone Joint Surg Am* 1986;68(3):362-369.
14. de Bari A, Krajbich JI, Langer F, Hamilton EL, Hubbard S: Modified Van Nes rotationplasty for osteosarcoma of the proximal tibia in children. *J Bone Joint Surg Br* 1990;72(6):1065-1069.
15. Aitken GT: Proximal femoral deficiency: Definition, classification and management, in *A Symposium on Proximal Femoral Focal Deficiency: A Congenital Anomaly*. National Academy of Sciences, 1969.

16. Alman BA, Krajbich JI, Hubbard S: Proximal femoral focal deficiency: Results of rotationplasty and Syme amputation. *J Bone Joint Surg Am* 1995;77(12):1876-1882.

17. Gillespie R, Torode IP: Classification and management of congenital abnormalities of the femur. *J Bone Joint Surg Br* 1983;65(5):557-568.

18. Krajbich I: Proximal femoral focal deficiency, in Kalamchi A, ed: *Congenital Lower Limb Deficiencies*. New York, NY, Springer-Verlag, 1989, pp 108-127.

19. King RE: Providing a single skeletal lever in proximal femoral focal deficiency. *Inter Clin Inform Ball* 1966;6(2):23.

20. Torode IP, Gillespie R: Rotationplasty of the lower limb for congenital defects of the femur. *J Bone Joint Surg Br* 1983;65(1):569-573.

21. Hillmann A, Rosenbaum D, Schröter J, Gosheger G, Hoffmann C, Winkelmann W: Electromyographic and gait analysis of forty-three patients after rotationplasty. *J Bone Joint Surg Am* 2000;82(2):187-196.

22. Bochman D: Prosthetic devices for the management of proximal femoral focal deficiency. *Orthop Prosthet* 1980;12(4):4-85.

23. Brown KL: Resection, rotationplasty, and femoropelvic arthrodesis in severe congenital femoral deficiency: A report of the surgical technique and three cases. *J Bone Joint Surg Am* 2001;83-A(1):78-85.

24. Roux N, Pieters S: Prosthetic management 56 years after rotationplasty due to proximal femoral focal deficiency (PFFD). *Prosthet Orthot Int* 2007;31(3):313-320.

CHAPTER 12

AMPUTATION AND PROSTHETIC FITTING

ANTHONY A. SCADUTO, MD
NORMAN Y. OTSUKA, MD

INTRODUCTION

Most limb-length discrepancies (LLDs) that are large enough to require prosthetic fitting arise from congenital limb anomalies.[1] Amputations in children require special attention because of continued growth and ongoing psychologic and motor development.

ASSESSMENT OF CONGENITAL LLD

Many congenital limb deficiencies have both a true and an apparent LLD. Apparent discrepancies can result from angular deformities as well as hip and knee contractures. In a typical patient with proximal femoral focal deficiency (PFFD) [also called proximal longitudinal deficiency of the femur], the flexed-hip position will lead to an underestimation of the total femoral length on a standard AP scanogram or teleoradiograph. A simple way to measure the true femoral or tibial length when the hip or knee cannot be fully extended is to obtain a lateral radiograph, placing a ruler parallel to the femur or tibia (**Figure 1**).

PSYCHOSOCIAL CONSIDERATIONS

Although significant gains in the outcome of lengthening have occurred over the last 25 years, it is important to discuss realistic expectations and possible future advances with the patient's family. Often, it is preferable to perform a single amputation rather than a prolonged and staged surgical reconstruction that precludes normal childhood activities.[2-4] A higher incidence of complications has been reported when amputation is performed as a salvage procedure in a multiply operated limb rather than as a primary procedure.[5]

Many families are concerned with the future psychologic impact of an amputation on their child. Birch et al[6] examined the long-term psychologic impact of a Syme disarticulation in cases of fibular deficiency. When patients who were treated with a Syme disarticulation as a child underwent psychologic testing as adults, they did not differ from the norm with regard to occupational satisfaction, personal growth, relationships with peers, or self-reported quality of life and self-esteem.

Cultural norms can heavily influence a family's priorities regarding appearance and function. Clinics that provide psychologic, social, and pediatric support are more likely to identify these cultural influences and better assist parents in making an informed decision. The importance of being able to sit or kneel on the floor or wear regular shoes or of preserving the anatomic foot can vary greatly among families. Even with this variability, we have always

Dr. Scaduto or an immediate family member is a member of a speakers' bureau or has made paid presentations on behalf of Abbott; serves as a paid consultant to or is an employee of Abbott; and has received research or institutional support from DePuy, a Johnson & Johnson company. Dr. Otskua or an immediate family member serves as a board member, owner, officer, or committee member of the American Academy of Orthopaedic Surgeons, the California Orthopaedic Association, and the Pediatric Orthopaedic Society of North America; and has received research or institutional support from the National Institutes of Health (NIAMS & NICHD) and Shriners Hospitals for Children.

FIGURE 1

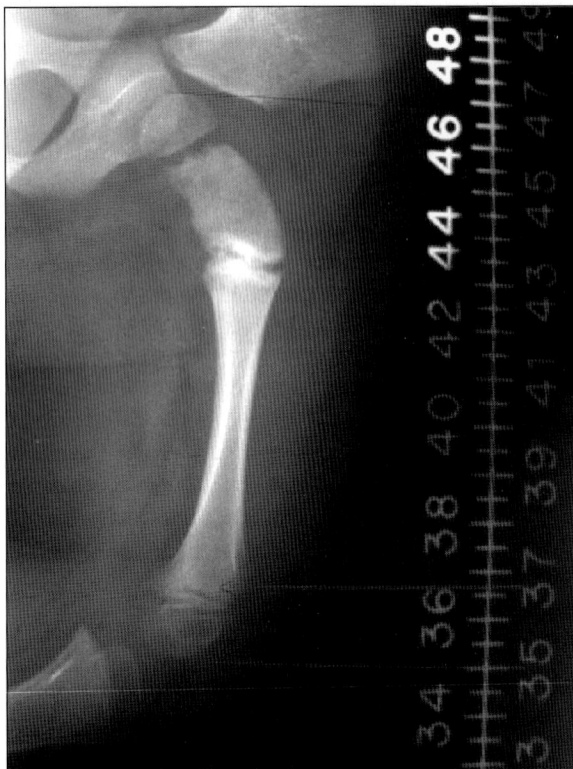

AP radiograph shows the best method to measure bone length when hip or knee contractures are present: the child should be in the lateral position, with the ruler lying parallel to the femur or tibia.

found it especially helpful to provide families considering amputation an opportunity to meet other families who have faced similar difficult treatment decisions.

FUNCTION AFTER AMPUTATION

Nearly all children with congenital lower extremity anomalies gain functional mobility, attend regular school, and lead quality lives;[5] many participate in competitive sports.[6] Amputations performed to address significant LLDs rarely lead to a loss in baseline function, and in some cases, they may enhance function. In a series comparing lengthening and amputation for fibular hemimelia (also called longitudinal fibular deficiency), children who underwent amputation were more active than those who underwent lengthening.[7] Recent suc-

cesses by Olympic-level athletes with lower extremity amputations who competed with and without prostheses underscore the remarkable abilities of amputees and the recent advances in prosthetic design.[8,9]

TIMING OF AMPUTATION

Families with a limb-deficient child may wish to postpone treatment until their child is able to participate in the decision, but this must be weighed against the psychologic drawbacks of waiting. Parents should never feel pressured into amputation for their child, but they also should be aware of the optimal age to amputate.

Most children begin to walk around 12 months of age. Ideally, amputation surgery and any recovery from it are completed just before walking age. Fibular deficiency is a common diagnosis in which amputation, when indicated, is optimally performed around 10 months of age because there is usually no delay in motor development when performed at this age. Parents also seem to have an easier time adjusting to an amputation performed before their child begins walking, as opposed to one that interrupts early walking.

The ideal timing of an amputation for a child with tibial deficiency or PFFD depends on the anatomy present, but it is usually a bit older than the age for fibular deficiency. For example, in some cases of partial tibial deficiency, it may be helpful to delay the amputation until the child is 3 to 4 years old. Part of the definitive surgery is fusing the fibula to the upper tibia, and this is much easier after the tibial anlage has ossified.

Postponing amputation and prosthetic fitting in toddlers because they lack the balance or skills needed to use advanced prosthetic components is ill advised. Rather, the amputation should be performed early and the child should be provided with a prosthesis that is simple in design. Limiting components and simplifying the suspension will help ensure rapid acceptance of the prosthesis. After knee disarticulation or knee fusion, toddlers using an above-knee prosthesis are initially fitted with a nonarticulated prosthesis. Usually, articulated prostheses can be used skillfully by 4 years of age, and they become essential at school age, to allow the child to sit comfortably at a school desk. Advanced prosthetic knee components and energy-storing feet can be added as a child grows to deal with athletic demands or challenging walking environments.

FIGURE 2

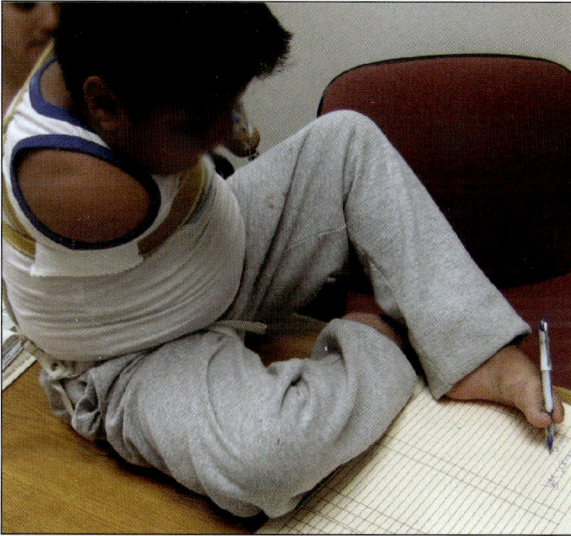

Photograph of a child with a limb-length discrepancy and bilateral upper extremity deficiencies. His dexterity with his feet for manual activities requires special consideration when selecting treatment options.

FIGURE 3

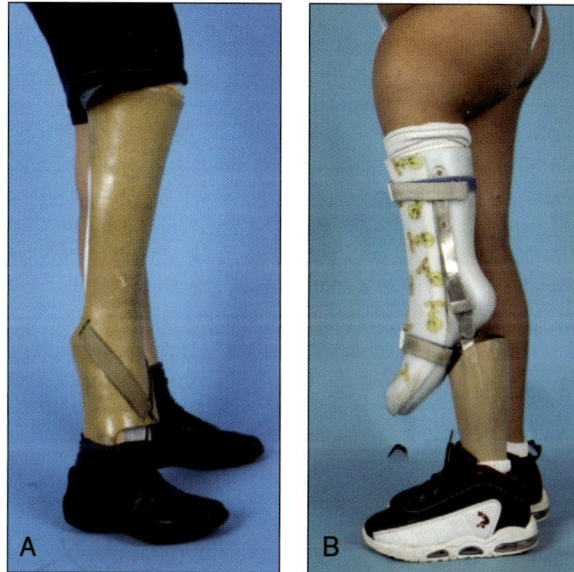

Photographs show an extension prosthesis (**A**) and an extension orthosis (**B**).

CONTRAINDICATIONS TO AMPUTATION

Occasionally, patients with lower extremity defects have concurrent hand and upper extremity deficiencies. In such cases, it is important to postpone any decisions regarding lower extremity amputation or lengthening until the child has established preferences for manual activities. Many children with bilateral upper extremity deficiencies develop excellent dexterity with their toes and feet, allowing them to feed and dress themselves. Children born with significant bilateral upper extremity deficiencies are usually more skilled with their feet at complex tasks, such as writing, than are children who use functional prostheses (**Figure 2**). Early amputation or lengthening in such children should be avoided.

Toe-to-hand transfers are now well-established procedures.[10] A surgeon performing a lower extremity amputation for a limb anomaly should always search for possible uses for the "spare parts" for the reconstruction of the upper extremity. We have, on occasion, postponed an amputation to allow parts of the lower extremity to become large enough to facilitate the vessel and nerve repair needed for a toe-to-hand transfer.[11]

AWAITING DEFINITIVE TREATMENT: ORTHOTIC MANAGEMENT

Regardless of the ultimate treatment decision, many children with an LLD require nonsurgical management for large discrepancies. A shoe lift is indicated when a child is toe-walking to compensate for the LLD. Internal shoe lifts should not exceed 1.5 cm because larger internal lifts make it difficult to keep the shoe on. Discrepancies of 5 cm or less are usually well corrected with a shoe lift applied to the sole of the shoe. Lifts larger than 5 cm can lead to ankle sprains, but adding an ankle-foot orthosis can be helpful in these circumstances.

When a discrepancy is larger than 8 cm, a special ankle-foot orthosis can be useful. These devices come in many styles and have been given a variety of names, including extension orthosis, extension prosthesis, equinus prosthesis, and prosthesis (**Figure 3**). They consist of a suspension component with the foot set in some

T A B L E 1 Differences Between Child and Adult Amputees

Parameter	Adults	Children
Peripheral vascular disease and diabetes	Common	Rare
Phantom pain and neuromas	Common	Rare
Terminal overgrowth	None	Common
Residual limb shape and length changes	Unlikely	Common
Surgical priorities	Wound healing more important than length	Length more important than wound healing
Gait training	Intensive training needed	Less training needed

equinus and a shank component attached to a prosthetic foot. Nearly any discrepancy can be corrected with this type of orthosis. An extension orthosis allows the child to wear a normal shoe and will significantly improve gait in a child with a large discrepancy. Occasionally, a family and patient will elect to use an extension orthosis as definitive treatment of a severe discrepancy. Patient satisfaction and mobility may be comparable to surgical conversion in some cases.[12] The most common complaints with this device relate to the foot location, which can lead to poor cosmesis from the distal flare in the prosthesis, as well as difficulty when wearing pants.

PRINCIPLES OF AMPUTATION IN CHILDREN

Amputation surgery in children differs from that in adults, as summarized in **Table 1**. To avoid terminal overgrowth problems in growing children, one should always attempt an ankle disarticulation as opposed to a below-knee (transtibial) amputation. Likewise, knee disarticulation is preferred over transfemoral amputation. In pediatric patients, the residual limb often becomes conical or tapered with growth. This leads to difficulties with prosthetic suspension and rotation control. Techniques that reduce distal bony architecture (eg, cutting the malleoli or condyles, as is often done for disarticulation surgeries in adults) should be avoided.

RESIDUAL LIMB LENGTH

A common and important error to avoid when devising a surgical plan for an amputation in a child is the failure to consider what the ideal residual limb length will be to maximize prosthetic function or appearance. Problems can arise from either excess or insufficient length of the residual limb. For a prosthetic knee joint to be level with the opposite knee, the residual limb must be 7 to 10 cm shorter than the opposite side. Excess length also can hinder prosthetic function in patients with transtibial amputations and Syme disarticulations. Standard energy-storing feet require a minimum of 7 cm of distance from the residual limb to the floor, whereas the latest dynamic feet used by high-performance amputees require more than 15 cm.[13]

Many surgeons are reluctant to resect either the distal femoral or proximal tibial physis when performing a knee arthrodesis and Syme disarticulation for PFFD; in our experience, however, failure to do so leads to problems with excessive length. We recently reviewed a series of 62 patients with PFFD and found that residual limb lengths would be excessive 94% of the time when both the femoral and tibial physes were preserved at the time of knee arthrodesis, whereas no patients would have too short a residual limb if the femoral physis was resected.[14]

The minimum residual limb length needed to ensure maximum prosthetic function is not well established. Excessively short residual limbs make load transfer and suspension difficult. A short residual limb often requires extending the prosthesis to the next proximal joint, such as an above-knee prosthesis for a very short transtibial amputation. This problem is more likely to occur with acute traumatic amputations, as opposed to carefully planned elective amputations performed for LLDs. Our goal for the minimum length of an above-knee residual limb is 20 cm and for a below-knee residual limb is 10 cm. In a series of 22 residual limb lengthening procedures, Bowen et al[15] reported an average increase in femoral length of 8.7 cm and a tibial increase of 6.9 cm; 85% of their patients were able to wear a standard prosthesis after lengthening, whereas none could before.

T A B L E 2 Treatment Guidelines Based on Jones Classification of Tibial Deficiency

Type	Radiographic Findings	Treatment
1a	Tibia not seen during infancy or later; hypoplastic distal femoral epiphysis	Knee disarticulation
1b	Tibia not seen during infancy but appears with growth; normal-size lower femoral epiphysis	Syme disarticulation or Boyd amputation; tibiofibular synostosis
2	Proximal tibia anlage seen early	Syme disarticulation or Boyd amputation
3	Distal tibia present; proximal tibia absent	Syme disarticulation
4	Distal tibia diastasis	Syme disarticulation vs ankle reconstruction/lengthening

FIBULAR DEFICIENCY

Previously, many factors were considered critical in the decision to treat fibular deficiency with either lengthening or amputation, including the extent of the fibular deficiency and the number of deficient rays. Currently, the issues considered most important are function of the foot and the percentage of inequality.[16] Amputation should be considered when the tibial discrepancy is greater than 30% (>12 cm at maturity) or when the foot is nonfunctional, as defined by severe ankle instability and foot deficiency (two or fewer rays). Lengthening procedures are best suited for patients with lesser discrepancies and a functional foot defined by a stable, plantigrade position with four or more rays. A few studies directly compare the outcomes of lengthening and amputation for fibular deficiency.[3,7] Choi et al[3] reported 88% satisfactory results after amputation compared with 55% after lengthening. McCarthy et al[7] found that at a mean of 7 years postoperatively, children who had undergone amputation had less pain and were more satisfied than children who had undergone lengthening, although both groups were highly functional and satisfied. More recently, Walker et al[17] compared 36 patients who underwent amputation with 26 patients who underwent lengthening at an average age of 33 years. No significant differences existed in 16 of 17 quality-of-life measures; both groups had average to above-average quality of life compared with an unaffected adult population.

SYME DISARTICULATION VERSUS BOYD AMPUTATION

The goal of early amputation for fibular deficiency is to create an end-bearing residual limb with a shape and length that maximizes suspension and cosmesis. Both the Syme (ankle disarticulation) and Boyd (retention of the calcaneus with fusion to the distal tibia) techniques have been used effectively to treat fibular deficiency. The Syme procedure is simpler, requires less healing time, and results in a tapered end that is cosmetically appealing, but it also leads to greater need for supplemental supracondylar suspension.[18] By retaining the calcaneus, the Boyd amputation enables supramalleolar suspension and keeps the heel pad on the end of the residual limb; however, it is less cosmetically appealing when the residual limb is long because the prosthesis cannot be tapered distally to match the opposite leg. We prefer the Boyd amputation over the Syme disarticulation and strongly recommend resecting the distal tibial physis at the time of calcaneal-tibial fusion to create room for a dynamic energy-storing foot and to help avoid the cosmetic problems of a long residual limb.

TIBIAL DEFICIENCY

The treatment of congenital tibial deficiencies is determined by which segment of the tibia is present and whether there is a functional quadriceps mechanism (**Table 2**). This is not always easily discerned during infancy. Motor examinations are limited in this age group and the proximal tibia may consist of only a cartilaginous anlage not visible on radiographs. When a child has no active knee extension and no palpable or radiographic evidence of a tibia, a knee disarticulation is the treatment of choice. Brown[19] described an alternate treatment method of centralizing the fibula under the femur to enable use of a modified below-knee prosthesis. Most reported long-term outcomes of the Brown procedure have been disappointing because of flexion

FIGURE 4

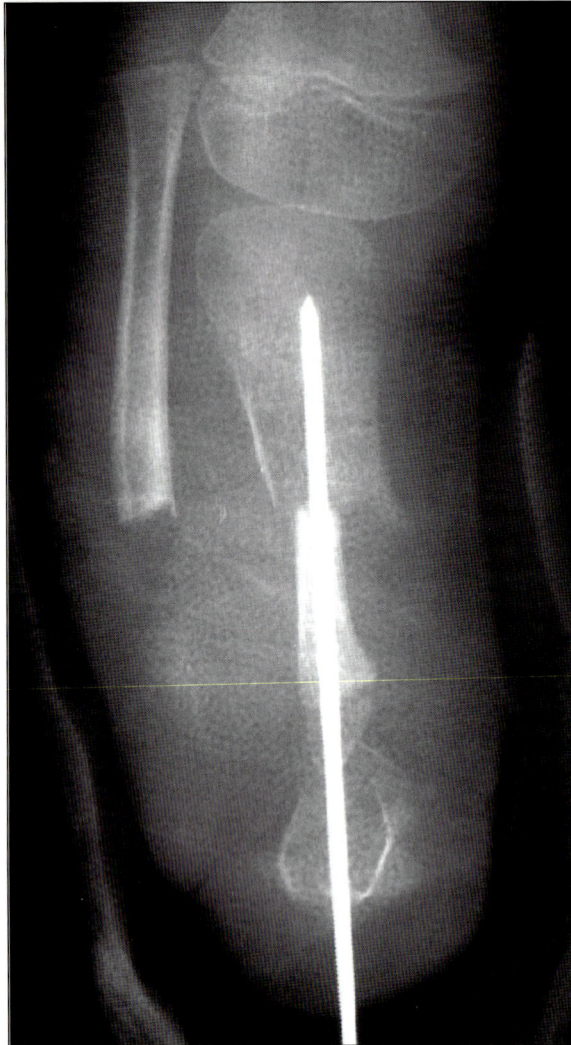

Postoperative AP radiograph shows end-to-end tibiofibular synostosis and modified Boyd amputation.

contractures, weak quadriceps function, and ligamentous instability.[20,21]

When the proximal tibia segment is present and powered, the child can function as a transtibial amputee after a side-to-side or end-to-end tibiofibular synostosis (**Figure 4**). Unlike the results of the Brown procedure, the results are good when the biologic knee joint is preserved with a tibiofibular synostosis and Syme disarticulation.[22,23] We prefer to perform a Syme or Boyd procedure at 10 to 12 months of age and then perform the tibiofibular synostosis when most of the proximal tibia anlage is ossified, at 2 to 7 years of age (**Table 2**).

The Jones type 4 tibial deficiency (distal diastasis) can be treated with either amputation or ankle reconstruction and lengthening. Functional results after early amputation are usually excellent.[24] A few series have reported good short-term outcomes after ankle fusion/reconstruction and lengthening;[25,26] therefore, treatment should be individualized based on the family's preferences and the anatomy present.

CONGENITAL DEFICIENCY OF THE FEMUR

The treatment options for a marked LLD resulting from a femoral deficiency are as follows: (1) provide an extension orthosis only; (2) remove the foot and fit as a transtibial amputee; (3) remove the foot, shorten the limb, fuse the knee, and fit as an above-knee (transfemoral) amputee; (4) perform a Van Nes rotationplasty; or (5) perform multiple lengthening procedures, with hip and knee stabilization procedures as needed.

Although the parents and the medical team must consider many factors when selecting a treatment plan, the most important factor is the predicted discrepancy at maturity. If the final predicted discrepancy is less than 20 cm (or the affected femur is >50% of the contralateral side) the child may be a suitable candidate for lengthening. A rotationplasty improves gait efficiency in comparison with foot ablation options but may be cosmetically unacceptable to some families. Both lengthening and Van Nes rotationplasty are reviewed elsewhere in this monograph.

Removing the foot by means of a Syme or Boyd procedure and using an extra-long below-knee prosthesis is one treatment for marked discrepancies in children with PFFD. It is preferable over the Van Nes rotationplasty when ankle instability or poor foot function exists. Preserving the knee joint at the time of the Syme disarticulation can lead to cosmetic and functional problems if the femoral segment is short. The long segment below the knee is obvious when the child sits and is especially problematic when sitting at a desk or low table. The knee flexion that occurs at the prosthetic brim contributes to gait abnormalities as well. During weight bearing, the prosthesis moves anteriorly and superiorly relative to the pelvis. To compensate, the child lurches forward and to the side. If the femoral segment is extremely short, the child can be fitted with an above-knee prosthesis that controls knee flexion, which does little to improve gait or cosmesis. The prosthesis still must accommodate the flexed, abducted, and externally rotated hip (**Figure 5**).

Fusing the knee joint creates a single lever and improves hip alignment. The prosthesis can then be positioned under the pelvis and is more in line with the center of gravity of the body, which reduces the child's forward and lateral trunk lurch and improves distal loading. Opinions vary on when to convert the affected limb to a functional transfemoral amputation. Ideally, after a Syme disarticulation and knee arthrodesis, the distal end of the residual limb will be at least 7 cm higher than the contralateral limb. In most cases of PFFD, the tibia on the affected side is nearly normal in length (mean, 92% of contralateral side).[14] The tibia alone would be of sufficient length for the residual limb; therefore, preserving the femoral physis at the time of arthrodesis is likely to lead to excess residual limb length. We prefer to resect the femoral physis at the time of the knee arthrodesis and combine it with the foot ablation surgery when the child is 2 to 3 years old.

FIGURE 5

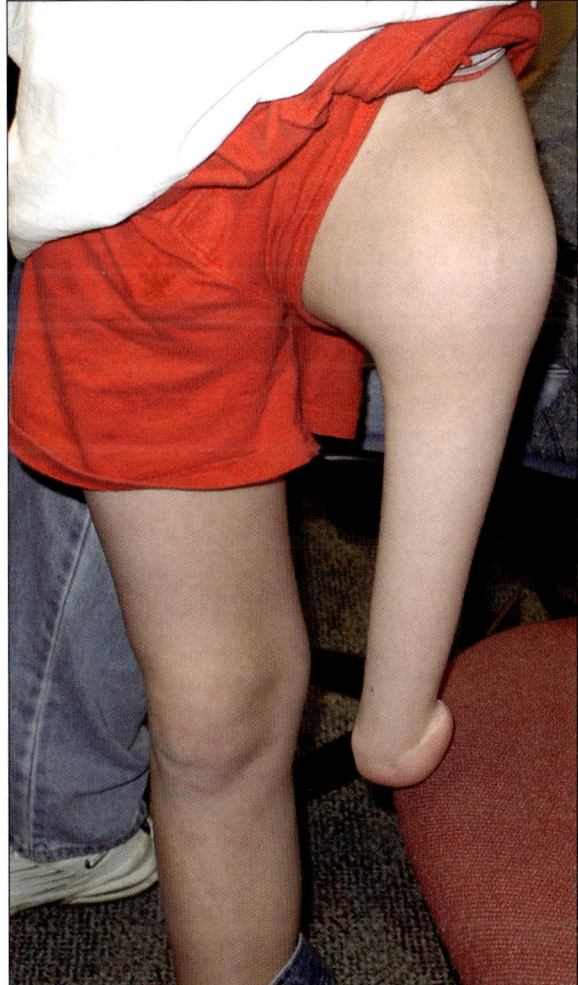

Photograph of a child with proximal femoral focal deficiency shows typical flexion, abduction, and external rotation deformity with a short femoral segment and an unfused knee.

REFERENCES

1. Amstutz HC: The morphology, natural history, and treatment of proximal femoral focal deficiencies, in Aitken GT, ed: *Proximal Femoral Focal Deficiency, A Congenital Anomaly.* Washington, D.C., National Academy of Sciences, 1969, pp 50-76.
2. Kruger LM, Talbott RD: Amputation and prosthesis as definitive treatment in congenital absence of the fibula. *J Bone Joint Surg Am* 1961;43-A:625-642.
3. Choi IH, Kumar SJ, Bowen JR: Amputation or limb-lengthening for partial or total absence of the fibula. *J Bone Joint Surg Am* 1990;72(9):1391-1399.
4. Naudie D, Hamdy RC, Fassier F, Morin B, Duhaime M: Management of fibular hemimelia: Amputation or limb lengthening. *J Bone Joint Surg Br* 1997;79(1):58-65.
5. Anderson L, Westin GW, Oppenheim WL: Syme amputation in children: Indications, results, and long-term follow-up. *J Pediatr Orthop* 1984;4(5):550-554.
6. Birch JG, Walsh SJ, Small JM, et al: Syme amputation for the treatment of fibular deficiency: An evaluation of long-term physical and psychologic functional status. *J Bone Joint Surg Am* 1999;81(11):1511-1518.
7. McCarthy JJ, Glancy GL, Chnag FM, Eilert RE: Fibular hemimelia: Comparison of outcome measurements after amputation and lengthening. *J Bone Joint Surg Am* 2000;82-A(12):1732-1735.

8. Robinson J: Amputee ineligible for Olympic events. *The New York Times.* January 14, 2008.

9. Whiteside K: Open water swimmer overcomes disability. *USA Today.* August 20, 2008.

10. Jones NF, Hansen SL, Bates SJ: Toe-to-hand transfers for congenital anomalies of the hand. *Hand Clin* 2007;23(1):129-136.

11. Chang J, Jones NF: Simultaneous toe-to-hand transfer and lower extremity amputations for severe upper and lower limb defects: The use of spare parts. *J Hand Surg Br* 2002;27(3):219-223.

12. Kant P, Koh SH, Neumann V, Elliot C, Cotter D: Treatment of longitudinal deficiency affecting the femur: Comparing patient mobility and satisfaction outcomes of Syme amputation against extension prosthesis. *J Pediatr Orthop* 2003;23(2):236-242.

13. Osebold WR, Lester EL, Christenson DM: Problems with excessive residual lower leg length in pediatric amputees. *Iowa Orthop J* 2001;21:58-67.

14. Farng E, Longrace M, Bowen RE, Scaduto AA: Limb length discrepency in proximal femoral focal deficiency. *Pediatric Orthopaedic Society of North America Annual Meeting.* Boston, MA, 2009.

15. Bowen RE, Struble SG, Setoguchi Y, Watts HG: Outcomes of lengthening short lower-extremity amputation stumps with planar fixators. *J Pediatr Orthop* 2005;25(4):543-547.

16. Birch JG, Lincoln TL, Mack PW: Functional classification of fibular deficiency, in Herring JA, ed: *The Child with a Limb Deficiency.* Rosemont, IL, American Academy of Orthopaedic Surgeons, 1998, p 161.

17. Walker JL, Knapp D, Minter C, et al: Adult outcomes following amputation or lengthening for fibular deficiency. *J Bone Joint Surg Am* 2009;91(4):797-804.

18. Fulp T, Davids JR, Meyer LC, Blackhurst DW: Longitudinal deficiency of the fibula: Operative treatment. *J Bone Joint Surg Am* 1996;78(5):674-682.

19. Brown FW: Construction of a knee joint in congenital total absence of the tibia (paraxial hemimelia tibia): A preliminary report. *J Bone Joint Surg Am* 1965;47:695-704.

20. Epps CH Jr, Tooms RE, Edholm CD, Kruger LM, Bryant DD III: Failure of centralization of the fibula for congenital longitudinal deficiency of the tibia. *J Bone Joint Surg Am* 1991;73(6):858-867.

21. Loder RT, Herring JA: Fibula transfer for congenital absence of the tibia: A reassessment. *J Pediatr Orthop* 1987;7(1):8-13.

22. Davids JR, Meyer LC: Proximal tibiofibular bifurcation synostosis for the management of longitudinal deficiency of the tibia. *J Pediatr Orthop* 1998;18(1):110-117.

23. Spiegel DA, Loder RT, Crandall RC: Congenital longitudinal deficiency of the tibia. *Int Orthop* 2003;27(6):338-342.

24. Jones D, Barnes J, Lloyd-Roberts GC: Congenital aplasia and dysplasia of the tibia with intact fibula: Classification and management. *J Bone Joint Surg Br* 1978;60(1):31-39.

25. Tokmakova K, Riddle EC, Kumar SJ: Type IV congenital deficiency of the tibia. *J Pediatr Orthop* 2003;23(5):649-653.

26. Schoenecker PL, Capelli AM, Millar EA, et al: Congenital longitudinal deficiency of the tibia. *J Bone Joint Surg Am* 1989;71(2):278-287.

LENGTHENING FOR CONGENITAL LOWER LIMB DEFICIENCIES

JOHN G. BIRCH, MD

INTRODUCTION

In the pediatric population, the most common (and most challenging) indications for limb lengthening are for the management of congenital limb deficiencies. The morphologic categories of congenital lower extremity deficiencies include congenital femoral, tibial, and fibular deficiencies. Almost all published authors and active clinicians involved with limb-lengthening procedures will caution the novice surgeon (and the patient) that limb lengthening for congenital deficiencies is more difficult and has a higher complication rate than limb lengthening for acquired limb-length discrepancy (LLD) secondary to physeal disruption due to trauma, infection, tumor destruction, other traumatic causes, and perhaps even skeletal dysplasias characterized by primary physeal disturbance (such as achondroplasia). Although that belief is widespread, most literature does not clearly support that impression.[1-7]

The increased challenges of managing LLD by means of a lengthening procedure include the need for prolonged cooperation from a young patient and the presence of associated joint distortion, restricted motion, or instability, which increases the risk of joint complications resulting from lengthening. Also of concern are the increased soft-tissue resistance to lengthening, particularly skeletal muscle, which likely increases the potential for increased pain and functional disturbance during lengthening, joint contracture and subluxation, and

regenerate bone bending after apparatus removal. This chapter reviews some aspects of patient assessment specific to limb lengthening for congenital limb deficiency, treatment strategies for limb reconstruction, and considerations specific to the type of congenital deficiency.

ASSESSMENT OF CONGENITAL LIMB DEFICIENCY

Although treatment of any patient with LLD by means of limb lengthening requires comprehensive assessment by a physician, it is particularly important in pediatric patients with a congenital limb deficiency. In assessing a family unit's ability to endure prolonged, stressful, and frequently painful treatment, the physician must be able to develop a comprehensive plan using all available information to maximize the patient's function. The physician must take into account the current and the expected final discrepancy in skeletally immature patients, associated joint and soft-tissue abnormalities, the expectations of the patient and family, and psychosocial factors

Predicting Limb-Length Discrepancy at Skeletal Maturity

The surgeon must be able to make an etiology-specific diagnosis and, as is the most common case, extrapolate in the skeletally immature patient the predicted discrepancy at the end of growth. The most useful methods of

Dr. Birch or an immediate family member has received royalties from Orthofix, and WB Saunders.

predicting ultimate LLD in patients with congenital limb deficiencies include Moseley straight-line graphs,[8] the Green-Anderson method,[9] and the Paley multiplier method.[10] All of these methods assume a constant rate of growth inhibition relative to the long (normal) leg. As Shapiro[11] has elegantly pointed out, however, this assumption is frequently inaccurate in limb growth disturbance of any cause, including congenital deficiencies, except for those resulting from complete physeal growth arrest. Thus, surgeons must be cautious in their estimation of ultimate LLD and must reevaluate existing and projected discrepancies on a regular basis during growth.

Associated Deformities

Major (most severe) congenital limb deficiencies typically have associated deformities that are less dramatic than shortening and may not significantly affect function until limb lengthening is considered. As part of the assessment of the lower extremities, however, the surgeon must document the angular and rotational states of both limbs and note potential upper extremity deficiencies as well.

Joint Abnormalities

Congenital LLD rarely occurs without associated joint distortion. The surgeon must determine range of motion, clinical instability, and radiographic distortion for each lower extremity joint as part of the overall assessment of the limb. These abnormalities may increase the risk of damage to the affected joint by limb lengthening and so must be taken into account when planning major limb-lengthening reconstruction.

Other Functional Deformities

Perhaps the most functionally important abnormality is associated upper extremity deficiency. This can make rehabilitation difficult (for example, if the patient cannot use standard crutches or a walker for assisted ambulation during use of an external fixator for lower extremity lengthening) or require the child to use a deformed lower extremity as a substitution for upper extremity prehension. The surgeon should also screen for rare pelvic or spinal congenital anomalies.

Patient Assessment

Limb-lengthening procedures are prolonged, painful, intrusive procedures that tax the patient, parents, and entire family unit.[12-14] The ability and willingness to comply with pin care and physical therapy regimens are crucial to a satisfactory treatment outcome. Parents of a child with a visible deformity, whether or not that deformity interferes with comfort or function, are eager to have that deformity resolved and often harbor unrealistic expectations regarding the degree of correction and the complexity of treatment. The physician must exercise caution not to respond to the natural intense desire to start treatment too early in an unwilling, noncomprehending child who bears the primary burden of limb-lengthening treatments. Participation in specific patient/parent educational programs to inform all parties of what to expect postoperatively should be mandatory if such programs are available. Preoperative psychologic counseling also helps identify unspoken child/parent concerns and expectations as well as provides strategies to address pain, sleep disturbance, loss of appetite, and academic disruptions. Nonnuclear (single-parent, divorced, remarried) families and those with a history of alcohol or other drug abuse or psychiatric illness are at higher risk for inability to comply with the rigors and stresses created by limb-lengthening procedures.

Treatment Strategies

The physician must develop and keep in mind a "big picture" of current and future functional effects of the child's limb deformity, as well as strategies to maximize function in both the short and long term. Techniques available to manage LLD in the growing child include shoe lifts, extension orthoses, appropriately timed contralateral epiphysiodeses, and ipsilateral limb lengthening. These options should be considered and offered to the family at the appropriate time. Shoe lifts and extension orthoses are rarely accepted by patients or families as permanent solutions to LLD, but they can temporarily improve function before or between limb-lengthening sessions in more complex cases.

First, the physician must establish a baseline assessment of the nature of the deformity, specifically, the existing LLD; axial (mal)alignment; joint flexibility, deformity, and instability; and overall functional impair-

TABLE 1   **Assessment Checklist for Congenital Limb Deficiency**

Diagnosis
Current and predicted final limb-length discrepancy
   Joint assessment
      Range of motion
      Instability
      Radiographic abnormality
      Associated deformity
         Axial
         Rotational
   Neuromuscular assessment
Patient/parent assessment/education
Staged treatment strategy for management of limb-
   length discrepancy and associated deformities

ment (**Table 1**). An estimation of LLD at skeletal maturity should be determined as soon as considered feasible, and family expectations and goals should be identified. Using this information, the surgeon should try to develop an overall treatment strategy with the family.

I prefer to consider lengthening for congenital limb deficiency when the functional status of the limb will be improved only by means of a lengthening procedure. Typical relative indications are a patient with an LLD associated with an angular deformity that exceeds 5% (approximately 4 cm at skeletal maturity in a patient in the 50th percentile). An absolute indication is an LLD greater than 10% (8 cm at skeletal maturity). No patient, however, should be encouraged to undergo a lengthening procedure that requires a postoperative treatment program he or she is unable or unwilling to comply with.

Most surgeons identify an increased risk of complications when limb lengthening exceeds 15% to 20% of the initial length of the bone segment, which translates to 4 to 6 cm of lengthening in average deformities.[2,3,7,15,16] I use the following method to outline the general strategy:

First, if the estimated discrepancy at skeletal maturity is between 4 and 6 cm and treatment by lengthening has been agreed to by all parties, I try to delay lengthening until after skeletal maturity. This allows accurate determination of the lengthening required and avoids the potential growth deceleration sometimes noted in skeletally immature patients after a lengthening procedure.

Second, if the projected discrepancy is between 6 and 10 cm at skeletal maturity, I attempt the first lengthening at a time when the anticipated residual discrepancy can be managed by means of contralateral epiphysiodesis. In general, this corresponds to the preadolescent to early teenage years. Females achieve lower extremity skeletal maturation at a mean age of 14.25 years; males achieve it at a mean age of 16.25 years (the White-Menelaus method[17]). The surgeon and patient then have the option of a second lengthening at skeletal maturity, or contralateral epiphysiodesis.

Third, if the discrepancy is anticipated to exceed 10 cm, I encourage an initial lengthening procedure when the child (with the assistance of preoperative family psychologic counseling) is able to understand, effectively agree to, and comply with postoperative treatment regimens. This typically is between the ages of 7 and 10 years but varies with the individual. I do not set specific lengthening goals at that initial lengthening procedure. Although I anticipate a 15% to 20% increase in bone length, the actual amount achieved depends on the patient's psychologic and physical response. A vigorous effort to achieve an additional centimeter of length in this age group is unwarranted because it risks a significant aversion to a second lengthening procedure, has a higher risk of joint and regenerate complications, and may have a higher risk of secondary physeal growth deceleration.[18-20]

LENGTHENING FOR CONGENITAL FEMORAL DEFICIENCY

A discussion of management of congenital femoral deficiency is immediately impeded by confusion regarding terminology. This is a result of the enormous clinical spectrum of severity of deformity, not only with respect to length, but also in the nature and severity of hip dysplasia, knee abnormalities, and associated lower-leg congenital abnormalities (tibial shortening, fibular deficiency, or tibial deficiency). Specifically, the extent of femoral deficiency can vary from only a few centimeters at maturity to complete absence of the femur. Radiographically, hips can be normal, have upper femoral varus or valgus (with or without associated acetabular dysplasia), or, in the most severe cases, associated upper

TABLE 2 Gillespie Classification of Congenital Femoral Deficiency

Group	Description	Feature	General Treatment
A	Femur long enough	Foot can be pulled to level of opposite mid tibia	Lengthening/shortening strategies to equalize limb lengths
B	Femur too short	Foot above level of opposite mid tibia; flexed, abducted externally rotated funnel-shaped thigh	Individualized limb reconstruction to maximize prosthetic function
C	Femur too short	Similar to B, but absent femur results in less hip positional deformity	Similar to B, but hip deformity less problematic to weight bearing in prosthesis

(Data from Gillespie R, Torode IP: Classification and management of congenital abnormalities of the femur. *J Bone Joint Surg Br* 1983;65[5]:557-568.)

FIGURE 1

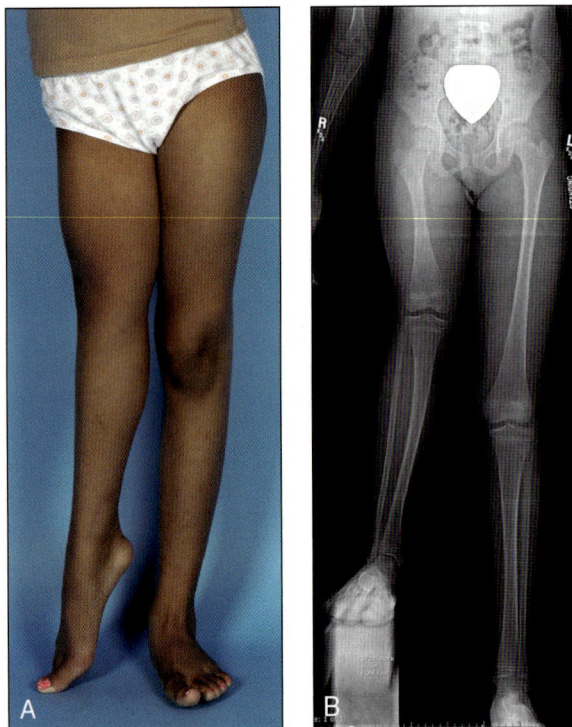

Gillespie group A ("femur long enough") patient. **A,** Clinical photograph shows the limb is short but the foot is beyond the level of the contralateral mid tibia. Note the associated external rotation and distal femoral valgus deformity. **B,** AP radiograph shows mild upper femoral dysplasia and distal femoral valgus associated with hypoplastic lateral condyles and tibial spines, in addition to femoral shortening.

femoral pseudarthrosis, stiffness, or complete absence of the upper femur. Knees typically have hypoplastic or absent anterior cruciate ligaments, multiplanar instability, and hypoplastic lateral femoral condyles, resulting in valgus deformity and potential patellar instability; knees can be stiff as well. The most common associated lower leg deformity is congenital fibular deficiency, which aggravates total limb shortening and axial deformity and may limit rotationplasty reconstructive options because of associated foot weakness, reduction, or stiffness. The deformity can be bilateral, resulting in a short-stature syndrome, but usually causes little functional deficit.

Coincident with this morphologic spectrum is the existence of multiple classification systems (eg, Aitken,[21] Gillespie,[22] Pappas[23]). I find that the Gillespie system[22] provides the best guidelines for management of LLD for congenital femoral deficiency syndromes (**Table 2**). In Gillespie group A patients (described as "femur long enough"), the foot can be drawn to the level of the opposite mid tibia (**Figure 1**). This implies a projected discrepancy of as much as 17 to 20 cm at skeletal maturity, assuming relatively constant growth inhibition; management of this extreme amount of shortening will typically require up to three stages of lengthening, as well as contralateral epiphysiodesis. In addition, complications requiring surgical intervention almost certainly will occur. A significant commitment to the treatment strategy, therefore, is required from all parties. Also, an assumption that the hip, knee, and foot are sufficiently stable and functional to withstand this aggressive length-

FIGURE 2

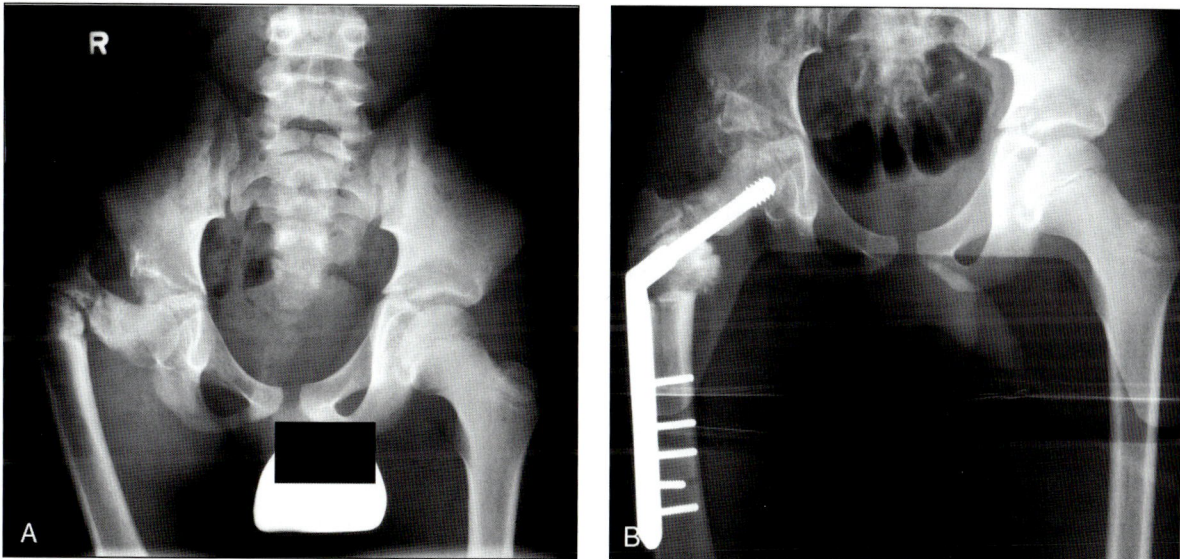

Patient with congenital femoral deficiency. **A,** Preoperative AP pelvic radiograph shows significant proximal femoral varus deformity and associated acetabular dysplasia. Femoral lengthening performed without correcting this deformity has significant risk for hip subluxation. **B,** Postoperative AP pelvic radiograph after upper femoral valgus osteotomy and Dega pelvic osteotomy.

ening protocol is inherent in qualifying the limb as "femur long enough" for lengthening.

Group B (described as "femur too short") patients have more severe shortening. Group C patients are similar to group B patients but have no femur (also referred to as Aitken D) and do not have the severe flexion/valgus/external rotation deformity of the thigh that makes prosthesis fitting in group B patients so challenging. Gillespie group B and C patients in my care are most often treated by means of reconstructive options that maximize prosthetic function without striving to achieve total limb preservation and limb-length equality. These options, which include rotationplasty, foot ablation with or without knee fusion, and hip stabilization procedures, obligate the patient to use a prosthesis or extension orthosis.[22,24] Highly experienced centers committed to limb preservation may recommend lengthening reconstruction in Gillespie group B patients. Such lengthening strategies require significantly more procedures to stabilize the hip or knee and involve substantially greater and more frequent lengthening stages.

In patients with congenital femoral deficiency deemed appropriate for femoral lengthening (Gillespie group A), the surgeon must assess for associated hip dysplasia, knee flexion deformity and/or instability, and associated lower leg deformity and shortening. In addition to shortening, virtually all of these patients demonstrate distal femoral valgus (often masked in stance or not detected by cursory examination, owing to increased external and decreased internal rotation of the hip). The first decision is whether to treat associated hip dysplasia with a stabilizing pelvic osteotomy (Salter, Dega, or equivalent procedure) with or without upper femoral realignment (usually for associated upper femoral varus deformity) (**Figure 2**). Although no universally accepted guidelines exist as to when such intervention is required, the surgeon must recognize that femoral lengthening risks subluxation, even when the hip is radiographically normal, and that risk is increased when associated acetabular dysplasia is present. The surgeon must proceed accordingly because subluxation will result in hip stiffness and almost certainly in early degenerative

FIGURE 3

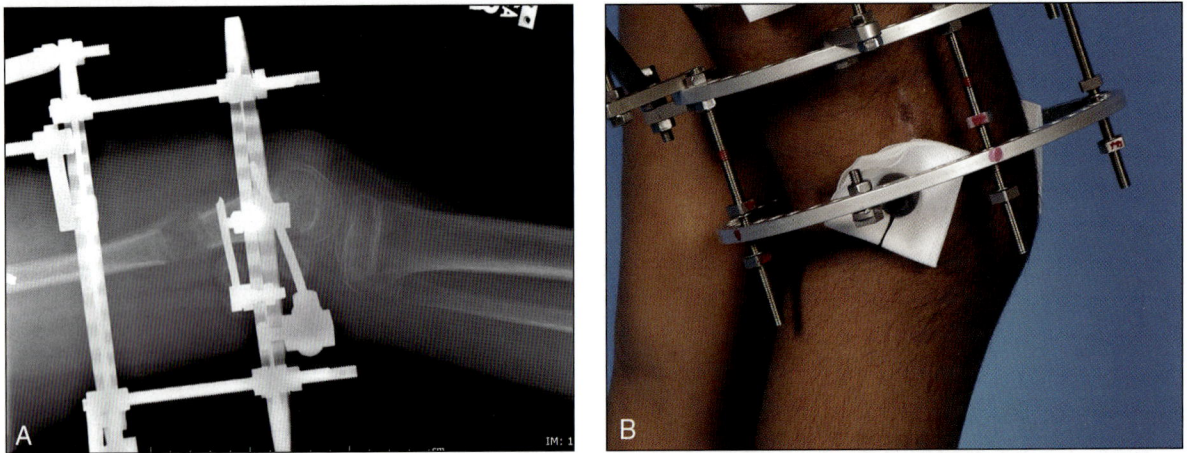

Patient whose knee subluxated during limb lengthening. **A,** Lateral radiograph shows posterior translation of the tibia relative to the femur, with lack of full knee extension. **B,** Clinical photograph shows lack of full knee extension and posterior sag of the tibia relative to the femur.

arthritis. Similarly, whereas untreated patients rarely report knee instability before lengthening, cruciate hypoplasia and multiplanar instability increase, at least theoretically, the risk of knee subluxation during lengthening, which has the same undesirable outcome as hip subluxation. The patient, therefore, must commit to undergoing vigorous and continual physical therapy and the surgeon must be vigilant in confirming that the patient maintains full (baseline) hip extension and abduction and knee extension (**Figure 3**). Typically, there will be little motion of the knee, and the patient will report pain localized to the patellar ligament. Some authors recommend prophylactic extension of external fixation across the knee to protect the articular cartilage from compression and/or knee subluxation.

The choice of lengthening method depends on the surgeon's preference. Four options are available.

Monolateral Fixation

This option has the advantages of relative simplicity of application and being less cumbersome for the patient. Monolateral fixators, however, generally also have limited angular and rotational adjustability and less capability for extension across joints, specifically the knee and the ankle.

Circular External Fixation

This option is more complicated to apply and care is more difficult than with monolateral fixation. Circular external fixation also is particularly cumbersome for femoral lengthening. On the other hand, that complexity offers the theoretical and often real advantages of flexibility and adaptability to specific cases: specifically, multilevel osteotomies performed to correct deformity at one level and lengthen at another are easier to execute. In addition, angular and rotational deformities, either primary or developing during a course of lengthening, often can be corrected by revision of the apparatus without a need to return to surgery, and extension across the knee or ankle is relatively easily accomplished.

Intramedullary Rods and Locking Plates

The third option is lengthening by means of supplemental internal fixation of the distraction gap using an intramedullary rod or locking plate.[25-29] Lengthening for congenital femoral deficiency has a reported rate of regenerate bone bending or fracture as high as 40% after removal of the external fixator. To prevent this complication, some authors have reported using internal fixation to supplement external fixation for lengthening,

FIGURE 4

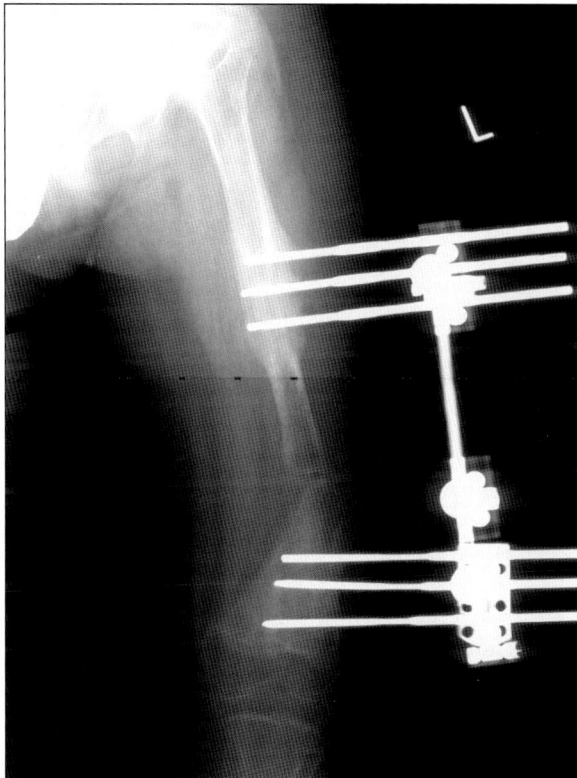

AP radiograph shows varus deformity that occurred during distal femoral lengthening. The linear half-pin construct of the distal femoral segment has become unstable, with resultant varus deformity of the limb. Note the associated hypoplastic regenerate bone.

using either locked intramedullary rods or locking plates. These internal devices may be implanted at the index procedure and locked at the time of external fixator removal, or inserted simultaneously with removal of the fixator.

Intramedullary Lengthening Device

Soft-tissue resistance to lower limb lengthening can result in typical secondary deformity; specifically, varus deformity of the femur (**Figure 4**) or apex anteromedial deformity (procurvatum) of the tibia (**Figure 5**). Any fixation device used must have adequate inherent stability to prevent the development of these deformities, or the surgeon must have a strategy to correct them

FIGURE 5

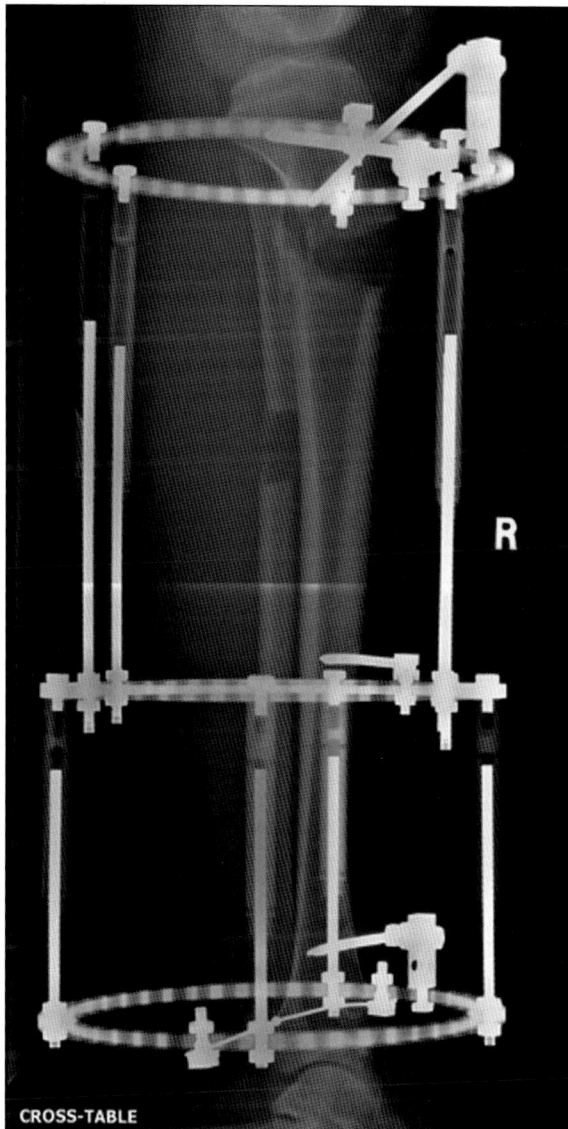

Lateral radiograph of typical procurvatum/flexion deformity of the tibia that occurred during tibial lengthening.

subsequently. Inadequate proximal or distal segmental fixation yields to posterolateral muscle compartment resistance to lengthening. During clinical examination, the deformity may be inappropriately attributed to loss of knee extension.

T A B L E 3 Birch Classification of Congenital Fibular Deficiency

Type	Features	General Treatment Guidelines
IA	Functional foot; limb-length discrepancy 0%–5%	None, orthosis, or contralateral epiphysiodesis
IB	Functional foot, limb-length discrepancy 6%–10%	Epiphysiodesis or single-stage lengthening at skeletal maturity
IC	Functional foot, limb-length discrepancy 11%–30%	Up to three staged lengthenings with or without contralateral epiphysiodesis
ID	Functional foot, limb-length discrepancy >30%	Same as IC, or consider Syme disarticulation or Boyd amputation
IIA	Nonfunctional foot, effective upper extremity function	Syme disarticulation or Boyd amputation at walking age
IIB	Nonfunctional foot with ineffective or uncertain upper extremity function	Defer amputation until substitution patterns for lack of upper extremity function established

(Adapted with permission from Birch JG, Lincoln TL, Mack PW: Functional classification of fibular deficiency, in Herring JA, Birch JG, eds: *The Child With a Limb Deficiency.* Rosemont, IL, American Academy of Orthopaedic Surgeons, 1998, pp 161-170.)

All currently available intramedullary devices have the same limitation of only one function (telescopic distraction), with no opportunity to correct deformity subsequent to lengthening or to manage joint contracture problems, so patients must therefore be chosen and monitored carefully with this method.

LENGTHENING FOR CONGENITAL FIBULAR DEFICIENCY

As with congenital femoral deficiency, congenital fibular deficiency is characterized by a broad spectrum of severity of limb shortening, lower limb deformity, and foot reduction. The mildest cases may escape detection until adolescence, presenting as a mild LLD, with the radiographic identification of a ball-and-socket ankle and subtle femoral abnormalities. The most severe cases have marked tibial shortening and only a remnant of an appendage passing as a foot. As with congenital femoral deficiency, multiple classification systems have been published, most notably those of Coventry and Johnson,[30] Achterman and Kalamchi,[31] and Letts and Vincent.[32] Although most publications and treatment centers recommend Syme disarticulation or Boyd amputation for patients with severe LLD and/or foot deformity and reduction,[6,31,33-35] extensive surgical reconstructive options are increasingly requested by

families that are aware of such opportunities. Positive, functional long-term results for reconstructive management of the more severe cases are lacking in the literature; published reports favor foot ablation at walking age in the more severe cases.[33-36]

The most effective approach at my institution involves a functional classification,[37] whereby we assess the severity of the foot deformity first (generally, the presence of three or fewer rays or severe ankle/foot deformity), and the total limb shortening, with an estimation of ultimate discrepancy at skeletal maturity. If the foot is deemed salvageable, the strategy for management of the associated LLD is the same as outlined previously and summarized in **Table 3.**

Several characteristics unique to congenital fibular deficiency must be taken into account when planning reconstructive strategies; most important is the near-universal prevalence of associated, usually milder, congenital femoral deficiency (**Figure 6**). Consequently, not only must variable femoral shortening be considered when estimating ultimate LLD, but also the risk of associated hip dysplasia and knee instability, which may require intervention. Most importantly, the patients usually have increased external rotation/valgus deformity of the femur, which usually requires surgical correction by means of osteotomy, lengthening, and

FIGURE 6

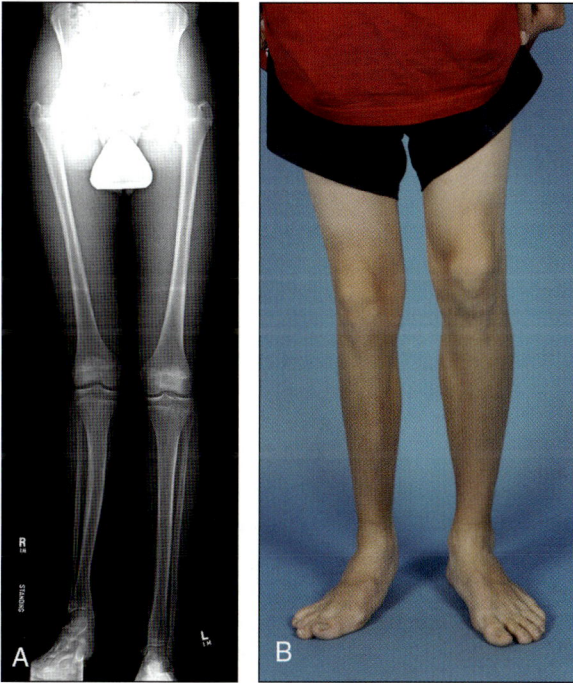

Patient with a moderately severe fibular deficiency. **A,** Weight-bearing 6-ft AP radiograph shows patient with 7 cm of tibial shortening and planar ankle, as well as associated mild femoral shortening, valgus deformity, and external rotational deformity. **B,** Clinical appearance of patient.

FIGURE 7

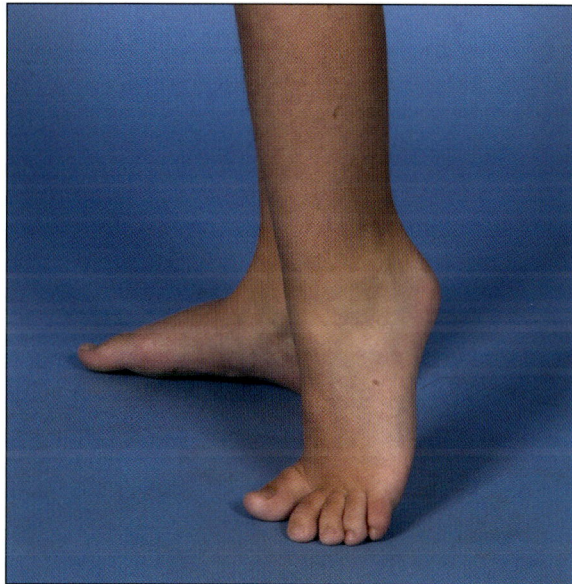

Clinical photograph of a patient with severe fibular deficiency. This patient may function very well with the foot in rigid equinus.

angular deformity correction, or by appropriately timed medial distal femoral growth modulation. The method depends on the surgeon's preference, the overall reconstructive strategy, and the extent of associated shortening.

A second important consideration is the presence of inherent ankle and foot stiffness and deformity. The ankle may be planar (more common when the fibula is rudimentary or absent) or ball-and-socket, and the hindfoot usually will demonstrate tarsal coalition, which is sometimes massive. Consequently, patients with moderately severe shortening may function well during childhood by walking on the ball of the foot or by using an extension orthosis, using a stiff plantar flexed foot as an extension of the leg (**Figure 7**). After the ankle and foot have been subjected to lengthening procedures,

however, and the stiff foot and ankle have been rendered plantigrade by means of successful lengthening, the foot may become painful, have atypical excessive weight-bearing characteristics, and function as an obstruction to ambulation. Ankle joint fusion and/or tarsal osteotomies may be necessary to ameliorate these symptoms or functional deficit.

Fibular deficiency, more than any other pediatric limb deficiency, requires the development of a long-term strategy developed in conjunction with the child's family. Full assessment of the limb, including hip dysplasia, associated femoral shortening and deformity, knee instability, severity of tibial shortening, and nature and severity of foot and ankle deformity all must be taken into account when planning a reconstructive strategy. At my institution, we find that providing the families of an affected infant the opportunity to visit with the families of other patients who elected multistage reconstructive procedures or primary amputation helps clarify the expectations and goals of the treatments they select for their children.

T A B L E 4 Classification of Congenital Tibial Deficiency

Type	Features	General Treatment Recommendations
Ia	No proximal tibia	Knee disarticulation
Ib	Proximal tibia present but unossified at birth	Syme disarticulation or Boyd amputation and fibular transfer to upper tibial remnant
II	Proximal tibia present, ossified at birth; no distal tibia	Syme disarticulation or Boyd amputation and fibular transfer to upper tibial remnant
III	Distal tibia preserved, proximal tibia absent	Knee disarticulation
IV	Tibiofibular diastasis with severe lower-leg shortening and equinovarus foot deformity	Staged reconstruction (tibiotalar fusion and tibial lengthening) or Syme disarticulation or Boyd amputation

(Data from Jones D, Barnes J, Lloyd-Roberts GC: Congenital aplasia and dysplasia of the tibia with intact fibula: Classification and management. *J Bone Joint Surg Br* 1978;60[1]:31-39.)

LENGTHENING FOR CONGENITAL TIBIAL DEFICIENCY

Congenital tibial deficiency is extremely rare. The Jones classification[38] provides an excellent overview of the nature and spectrum of this deficiency. Table 4 summarizes the major deficiency types and standard treatments currently recommended. This is the only congenital deficiency that is most commonly bilateral and that may be hereditary; both autosomal dominant and autosomal recessive forms have been reported. Abnormalities of the upper extremities frequently occur with severe bilateral congenital fibular deficiency. Whenever primary amputation of the lower extremities is being seriously considered for patients with severe fibular or tibial deficiencies, the nature and severity of associated upper extremity deficiency must be assessed. Patients are rarely dependent on their deformed feet to substitute for absent effective upper extremity function, but in those circumstances the feet must be preserved.

Type Ia congenital tibial deficiency is characterized by severe tibial shortening, no true knee articulation or function, no ankle, and a foot in severe varus (with or without medial ray duplication). Brown[39] described knee reconstruction involving transfer of the fibular remnant to the femoral notch with quadriceps reconstruction, typically accompanied by foot ablation; however, studies have demonstrated relatively poor results (stiffness, flexion deformity, and pain) with this reconstruction.[40-43] Consequently, type Ia tibial deficiency is usually best managed by means of primary knee disarticulation, which I typically perform at "cruising" age (after the child has achieved good sitting balance and is attempting to pull to stand).

Congenital tibial deficiency types Ib and II are distinct from type Ia in that there is preservation of a proximal tibial remnant (distinguished by the absence or presence, respectively, of ossification of that remnant at birth), usually resulting in a functional knee (adequate arc of motion and quadriceps function). Reconstructive efforts to preserve knee function are usually warranted in such cases. Transfer of the fibula to the proximal tibial remnant (combined with foot ablation) provides the patient with a functional below-knee (transtibial) amputation without the concerns of diaphyseal overgrowth that can complicate diaphyseal or metaphyseal amputations in children. Anecdotal reports of limb preservation by means of combining knee reconstructive procedures with subsequent staged lengthenings of the tibia/fibula have been described,[44] but these approaches are subject to the same controversies as discussed with severe congenital femoral and fibular deficiencies.

Type III tibial deficiency is an exceptionally rare form, characterized by absence of a proximal tibia, preservation of the distal tibia, and severe leg shortening. This type is not amenable to limb lengthening, to my knowledge or experience.

Type IV congenital tibial deficiency (tibiofibular diastasis) is a unique deformity characterized by moderately severe tibial shortening, absent ankle articulation, and

FIGURE 8

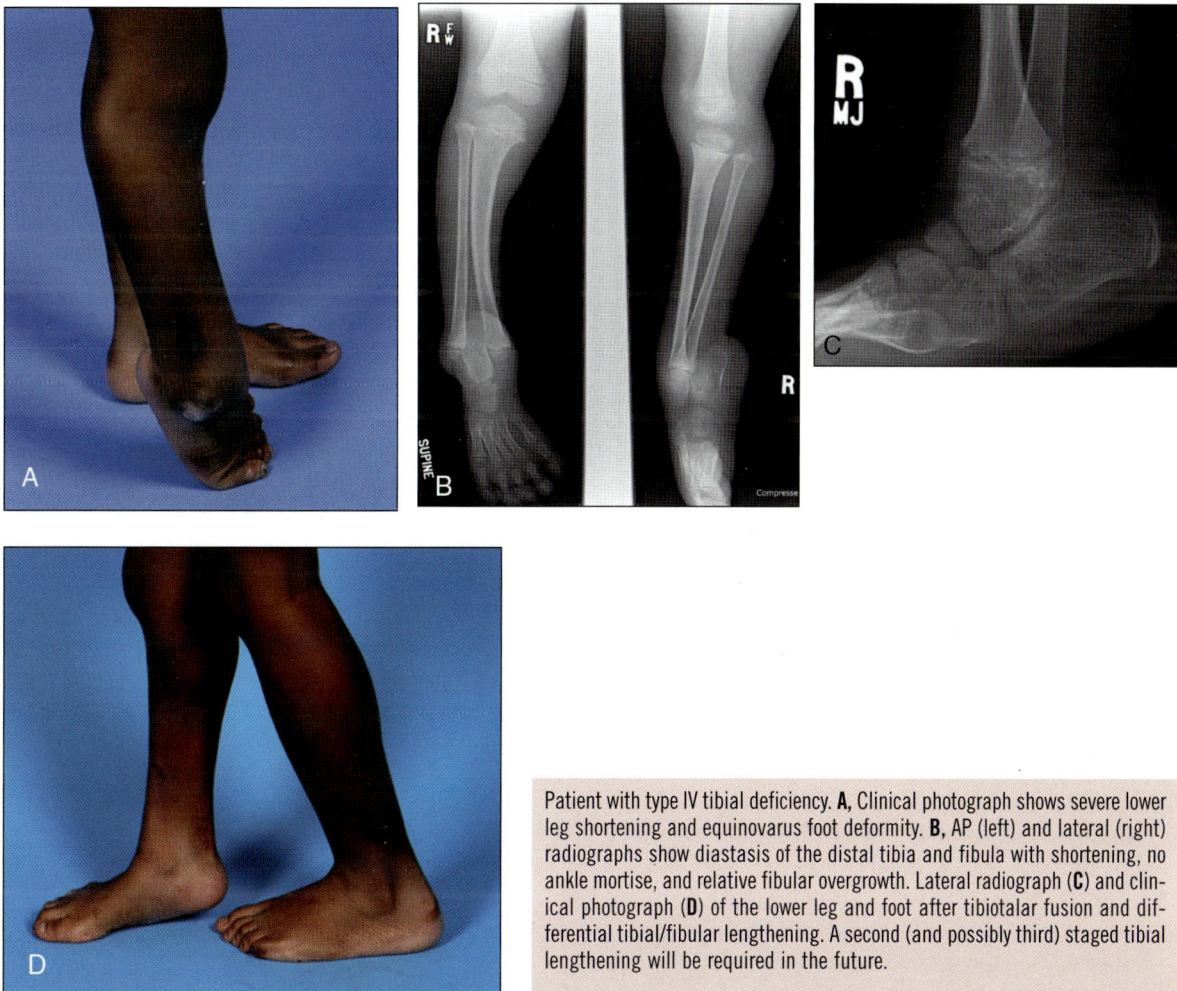

Patient with type IV tibial deficiency. **A,** Clinical photograph shows severe lower leg shortening and equinovarus foot deformity. **B,** AP (left) and lateral (right) radiographs show diastasis of the distal tibia and fibula with shortening, no ankle mortise, and relative fibular overgrowth. Lateral radiograph (**C**) and clinical photograph (**D**) of the lower leg and foot after tibiotalar fusion and differential tibial/fibular lengthening. A second (and possibly third) staged tibial lengthening will be required in the future.

severe foot equinus and internal rotation (**Figure 8,** *A* and *B*). Two reconstructive options exist: primary foot ablation and staged surgical reconstruction. When primary foot ablation is chosen, because the fibula is often hypertrophic relative to the tibia distally, revision may be required to allow comfortable prosthetic fit and end bearing. Staged surgical reconstruction consists of tibiotalar fusion and staged tibial lengthenings and typically involves up to three tibial lengthening procedures, with or without contralateral epiphysiodesis.[41,45] Significant deformity of the foot with soft-tissue shortening is char-

acteristic of this deficiency; therefore, rendering the foot in a stable, plantigrade position can be accomplished only with fairly extensive shortening and soft-tissue release, or by means of external fixator–assisted gradual distraction of the foot to the end of the tibia, with second-stage tibiotalar fusion (**Figure 8,** *C* and *D*). I approach type IV tibial deficiency like severe fibular deficiency, by providing families the opportunity to visit with families of patients that have been treated using both methods. Most families at my institution subsequently elect primary amputation to treat their child's limb deformity.

REFERENCES

1. Aldegheri R: Distraction osteogenesis for lengthening of the tibia in patients who have limb-length discrepancy or short stature. *J Bone Joint Surg Am* 1999; 81(5):624-634.

2. Dahl MT, Gulli B, Berg T: Complications of limb lengthening: A learning curve. *Clin Orthop Relat Res* 1994(301):10-18.

3. Karger C, Guille JT, Bowen JR: Lengthening of congenital lower limb deficiencies. *Clin Orthop Relat Res* 1993(291):236-245.

4. Miller LS, Bell DF: Management of congenital fibular deficiency by Ilizarov technique. *J Pediatr Orthop* 1992;12(5):651-657.

5. Fixsen JA: Major lower limb congenital shortening: A mini review. *J Pediatr Orthop B* 2003;12(1):1-12.

6. Griffith SI, McCarthy JJ, Davidson RS: Comparison of the complication rates between first and second (repeated) lengthening in the same limb segment. *J Pediatr Orthop* 2006;26(4):534-536.

7. Antoci V, Ono CM, Antoci V Jr, Raney EM: Bone lengthening in children: How to predict the complications rate and complexity? *J Pediatr Orthop* 2006; 26(5):634-640.

8. Moseley CF: A straight-line graph for leg-length discrepancies. *J Bone Joint Surg Am* 1977;59(2):174-179.

9. Anderson M, Green WT, Messner MB: Growth and predictions of growth in the lower extremities. *J Bone Joint Surg Am* 1963;45-A:1-14.

10. Paley D, Bhave A, Herzenberg JE, Bowen JR: Multiplier method for predicting limb-length discrepancy. *J Bone Joint Surg Am* 2000;82-A(10):1432-1446.

11. Shapiro F: Developmental patterns in lower-extremity length discrepancies. *J Bone Joint Surg Am* 1982;64(5):639-651.

12. Ghoneem HF, Wright JG, Cole WG, Rang M: The Ilizarov method for correction of complex deformities: Psychological and functional outcomes. *J Bone Joint Surg Am* 1996;78(10):1480-1485.

13. Hrutkay JM, Eilert RE: Operative lengthening of the lower extremity and associated psychological aspects: The Children's Hospital experience. *J Pediatr Orthop* 1990;10(3):373-377.

14. Ramaker RR, Lagro SW, van Roermund PM, Sinnema G: The psychological and social functioning of 14 children and 12 adolescents after Ilizarov leg lengthening. *Acta Orthop Scand* 2000;71(1):55-59.

15. Sakurakichi K, Tsuchiya H, Uehara K, Kabata T, Tomita K: The relationship between distraction length and treatment indices during distraction osteogenesis. *J Orthop Sci* 2002;7(3):298-303.

16. Yun AG, Severino R, Reinker K: Attempted limb lengthenings beyond twenty percent of the initial bone length: Results and complications. *J Pediatr Orthop* 2000;20(2):151-159.

17. Westh RN, Menelaus MB: A simple calculation for the timing of epiphysial arrest: A further report. *J Bone Joint Surg Br* 1981;63-B(1):117-119.

18. Lee SH, Szöke G, Simpson H: Response of the physis to leg lengthening. *J Pediatr Orthop B* 2001;10(4):339-343.

19. Sabharwal S, Paley D, Bhave A, Herzenberg JE: Growth patterns after lengthening of congenitally short lower limbs in young children. *J Pediatr Orthop* 2000; 20(2):137-145.

20. Sharma M, MacKenzie WG, Bowen JR: Severe tibial growth retardation in total fibular hemimelia after limb lengthening. *J Pediatr Orthop* 1996;16(4):438-444.

21. Aitken GT: Proximal femoral focal deficiency: Definition, classification, and management, in Aitken GT, ed: *Proximal Femoral Focal Deficiency: A Congenital Anomaly.* Washington, DC, National Academy of Sciences, 1969, pp 1-22.

22. Gillespie R, Torode IP: Classification and management of congenital abnormalities of the femur. *J Bone Joint Surg Br* 1983;65(5):557-568.

23. Pappas AM: Congenital abnormalities of the femur and related lower extremity malformations: Classification and treatment. *J Pediatr Orthop* 1983;3(1):45-60.

24. Alman BA, Krajbich JI, Hubbard S: Proximal femoral focal deficiency: Results of rotationplasty and Syme amputation. *J Bone Joint Surg Am* 1995;77(12):1876-1882.

25. Gordon JE, Goldfarb CA, Luhmann SJ, Lyons D, Schoenecker PL: Femoral lengthening over a humeral intramedullary nail in preadolescent children. *J Bone Joint Surg Am* 2002;84-A(6):930-937.

26. Kocaoglu M, Eralp L, Kilicoglu O, Burc H, Cakmak M: Complications encountered during lengthening over an intramedullary nail. *J Bone Joint Surg Am* 2004; 86-A(11):2406-2411.

27. Kristiansen LP, Steen H: Lengthening of the tibia over an intramedullary nail, using the Ilizarov external fixator: Major complications and slow consolidation in 9 lengthenings. *Acta Orthop Scand* 1999;70(3):271-274.

28. Lai KA, Lin CJ, Chen JH: Application of locked intramedullary nails in the treatment of complications after distraction osteogenesis. *J Bone Joint Surg Br* 2002;84(8):1145-1149.

29. Paley D, Herzenberg JE, Paremain G, Bhave A: Femoral lengthening over an intramedullary nail: A matched-case comparison with Ilizarov femoral lengthening. *J Bone Joint Surg Am* 1997;79(10):1464-1480.

30. Coventry MB, Johnson EW Jr: Congenital absence of the fibula. *J Bone Joint Surg Am* 1952;34-A(4):941-955.

31. Achterman C, Kalamchi A: Congenital deficiency of the fibula. *J Bone Joint Surg Br* 1979;61-B(2):133-137.

32. Letts M, Vincent N: Congenital longitudinal deficiency of the fibula (fibular hemimelia): Parental refusal of amputation. *Clin Orthop Relat Res* 1993(287):160-166.

33. Choi IH, Kumar SJ, Bowen JR: Amputation or limb-lengthening for partial or total absence of the fibula. *J Bone Joint Surg Am* 1990;72(9):1391-1399.

34. McCarthy JJ, Glancy GL, Chnag FM, Eilert RE: Fibular hemimelia: Comparison of outcome measurments after amputation and lengthening. *J Bone Joint Surg Am* 2000;82-A(12):1732-1735.

35. Naudie D, Hamdy RC, Fassier F, Morin B, Duhaime M: Management of fibular hemimelia: Amputation or limb lengthening. *J Bone Joint Surg Br* 1997;79(1):58-65.

36. Birch JG, Walsh SJ, Small JM, et al: Syme amputation for the treatment of fibular deficiency: An evaluation of long-term physical and psychological functional status. *J Bone Joint Surg Am* 1999;81(11):1511-1518.

37. Birch JG, Lincoln TL, Mack PW: Functional classification of fibular deficiency, in Herring JA, Birch JG, eds: *The Child with a Limb Deficiency.* Rosemont, IL, American Academy of Orthopaedic Surgeons, 1998, pp 161-170.

38. Jones D, Barnes J, Lloyd-Roberts GC: Congenital aplasia and dysplasia of the tibia with intact fibula: Classification and management. *J Bone Joint Surg Br* 1978;60(1):31-39.

39. Brown FW: Construction of a knee joint in congenital total absence of the tibia (paraxial hemimelia tibia): A preliminary report. *J Bone Joint Surg Am* 1965;47: 695-704.

40. Loder RT, Herring JA: Fibular transfer for congenital absence of the tibia: A reassessment. *J Pediatr Orthop* 1987;7(1):8-13.

41. Schoenecker PL, Capelli AM, Millar EA, et al: Congenital longitudinal deficiency of the tibia. *J Bone Joint Surg Am* 1989;71(2):278-287.

42. Epps CH Jr, Schneider PL: Treatment of hemimelias of the lower extremity: Long-term results. *J Bone Joint Surg Am* 1989;71(2):273-277.

43. Wada A, Fujii T, Takamura K, Yanagida H, Urano N, Yamaguchi T: Limb salvage treatment for congenital deficiency of the tibia. *J Pediatr Orthop* 2006;26(2): 226-232.

44. Hosny GA: Treatment of tibial hemimelia without amputation: Preliminary report. *J Pediatr Orthop B* 2005;14(4):250-255.

45. Tokmakova K, Riddle EC, Kumar SJ: Type IV congenital deficiency of the tibia. *J Pediatr Orthop* 2003;23(5):649-653.

CHAPTER 14

LIMB LENGTHENING FOR UPPER LIMB DEFICIENCIES

DROR PALEY, MD, FRCSC

INTRODUCTION

A limb-length discrepancy (LLD) of the upper limb is much better tolerated than a lower limb discrepancy because humans do not need to walk on the hands. Patients rarely report small LLDs (<3 cm) unless there is an associated discrepancy between the forearm bones. Length issues for the upper limb can be categorized by limb segment affected (humerus, forearm, metacarpals, phalanges) and whether they are unilateral or bilateral.

HUMERAL DEFICIENCIES

Growth disturbance of the humerus may be unilateral or bilateral. Unilateral cases are usually the result of birth palsy, congenital conditions, or damage to the proximal or distal humeral physis due to trauma, infection, or tumor. Bilateral deficiencies are usually congenital or caused by dysplasias.

The proximal humeral physis contributes 80% of humeral growth.[1,2] Damage to this physis leads to significant loss of growth remaining at all ages and can lead to physeal growth arrest. Extension, varus, and internal rotation deformities often are associated with physeal injury because of the patterns of displacement and physeal damage. Unicameral bone cysts, Ollier disease, and multiple hereditary exostoses (MHEs, also known as multiple osteochondromatosis) are benign tumors that are known to cause growth disturbance or arrest of the proximal humerus. Osteomyelitis of the proximal humerus and infection of the shoulder joint also are well-recognized causes of proximal humeral growth arrest. The varus extension pattern of deformity is common to all these causes of physeal injury, suggesting that the capital part of the physis is the part that is most susceptible to premature closure, whereas the greater tuberosity is less likely to close early. The varus deformity and the prominence of the greater tuberosity lead to loss of active abduction and flexion of the shoulder and shoulder impingement. In some patients, subluxation and dislocation of the shoulder will develop. Birth palsy, poliomyelitis, cerebral palsy, and other neurologic conditions lead to atrophic deficiency of the humerus and forearm of the affected side. Birth palsy also leads to forward subluxation of the scapula on the thorax.[3] Finally, congenital deficiency often is associated with limited motion of the shoulder and inferior subluxation of the humeral head.

Unilateral Humeral Deficiency

Most patients or their parents will report a humeral deficiency of 5 cm or more, usually because of concerns about cosmesis. If one arm is more than 5 cm shorter than the other, the deformity is obvious and sometimes

Dr. Paley or an immediate family member has received royalties from Smith & Nephew and Pega Medical; serves as a paid consultant to or is an employee of Biomet, Orthofix, and Smith & Nephew; and has received research or institutional support from Biomet, Orthofix, and Smith & Nephew.

unsightly. Adults with such a deficiency reported problems with appearance, inability to sit comfortably with the arm on an armrest, tailoring issues for clothes with one shorter sleeve, and limited shoulder and elbow motion because of associated deformities. Atrophy or hypoplasia of the shoulder girdle is another common symptom.

In the young, growing child, the first step is to measure the length discrepancy on radiographs of both humeri and forearms. Prediction of the final LLD at maturity is the next step. The Pritchett growth remaining method,[1] the Bortel and Pritchett straight-line graph method,[2] or the Paley multiplier method[4] can be used. With the Paley method, the formula used for the prediction depends on whether the cause is congenital or developmental.[4,5]

After the predicted LLD is calculated, the strategy for treatment can be determined. Epiphysiodesis of the long limb is not as reasonable an option in the upper limb as it is in the lower limb, for both functional and cosmetic reasons. The main role of epiphysiodesis in the upper limb is to complete closure of a partially closed physis to prevent recurrence of deformity.

Lengthening of the humerus is the preferred treatment of discrepancy (**Figure 1**). For predicted discrepancies greater than 8 cm, two smaller lengthenings are preferred to one large one. In the young child, one lengthening can be performed between the ages of 7 and 10 years and the second between the ages of 12 and 16 years. The ideal level at which to perform a lengthening osteotomy is just below and/or through the deltoid tuberosity. Lengthening at this level avoids stretching the deltoid muscle and avoids applying pressure to the shoulder joint. In cases in which inferior subluxation of the glenohumeral joint is present, a lengthening osteotomy performed at a level proximal to the deltoid tuberosity is preferred to help reduce the humeral head.

When an associated deformity exists in the proximal humerus, the lengthening osteotomy can be performed at the same level as the deformity correction. Alternately, the deformity can be corrected acutely with an osteotomy at the surgical neck of the humerus and the lengthening can be performed through a second osteotomy below the deltoid tuberosity.

The type of external fixation used for lengthening depends on the complexity of the case, the need for gradual versus acute correction of the deformity, and the number of osteotomies required. My preferences in different situations are summarized in **Table 1**.

Currently, I prefer to use all hydroxyapatite-coated half pins instead of wires.[6] It is important to avoid lateral half pins anywhere in the third quarter of the humerus to avoid damaging the radial nerve.

Bilateral Humeral Deficiency

Achondroplasia and hypochondroplasia are the two most common dysplasias treated with lengthening. Patients with these dysplasias have both a limb-trunk disproportion and a rhizomelic disproportion. Lengthening is performed on both sides at the same time to normalize both of these disproportions. Most patients require approximately 10 cm of lengthening performed at 14 years of age. The benefit of lengthening both arms is not only cosmetic. Arm lengthening greatly improves the reach of these little people, which aids in all activities of daily living (eg, reaching across the sink or stove and reaching light switches, closet hangers, and automatic teller machines). When combined with lower limb lengthening, humeral lengthening also helps the patient reach high objects, sit farther back from the steering wheel of a car so the airbag does not need to be disabled, comfortably use the armrest of a chair, etcetera. One of the biggest benefits relates to perineal care. Patients with achondroplasia are very flexible when young but develop spinal stiffness and stenosis as adults. Although they can compensate for their short arm reach for perineal hygiene when they are young, they often cannot when they are older. Longer arms help with ease of perineal hygiene all through life.

Bilateral short upper extremities of congenital origin often are not an indication for arm lengthening unless the elbow has full range of motion and the shoulder has good motion. Many of these patients also have short forearms (eg, bilateral radial clubhand). In such cases, it is more functionally beneficial to lengthen both forearms than the humeri.

Complications of Humeral Lengthening

Lengthening of one or both humeri is very well tolerated.[7-9] Often, little pain is involved and little functional disability is caused by the lengthening process. Patients are able to use their arms nearly normally during the

FIGURE 1

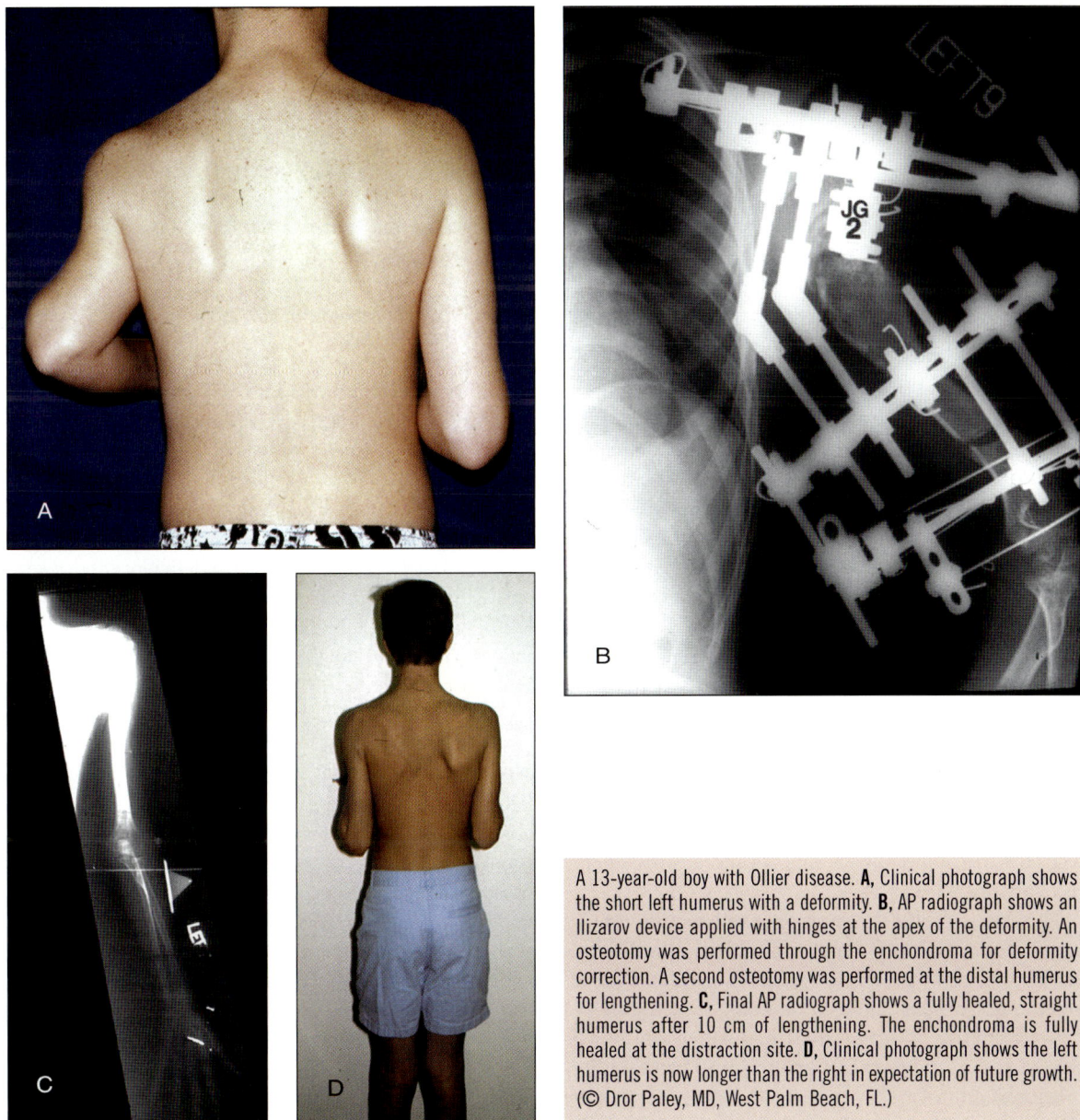

A 13-year-old boy with Ollier disease. **A**, Clinical photograph shows the short left humerus with a deformity. **B**, AP radiograph shows an Ilizarov device applied with hinges at the apex of the deformity. An osteotomy was performed through the enchondroma for deformity correction. A second osteotomy was performed at the distal humerus for lengthening. **C**, Final AP radiograph shows a fully healed, straight humerus after 10 cm of lengthening. The enchondroma is fully healed at the distraction site. **D**, Clinical photograph shows the left humerus is now longer than the right in expectation of future growth. (© Dror Paley, MD, West Palm Beach, FL.)

lengthening process. Pain during lengthening most often is due to pin infection or loosening pin sites, which are the most common complications of humeral lengthening.[7,10] This is especially common with monolateral external fixation, in which all the pins are in one plane.

Hydroxyapatite-coated pins have reduced but not eliminated the loosening associated with the fixator being in place for long periods of time.[6]

Failure of or delay in bone formation is uncommon. The humerus usually heals quickly and at a faster rate

TABLE 1 Author's Preferred Fixation for Upper Limb Lengthening

Surgical Treatment	Type of Fixator
Straight lengthening of the humerus below the tuberosity without deformity correction	Monolateral external fixator
Straight lengthening of the humerus below the tuberosity with a second osteotomy performed to acutely correct proximal deformity	Ilizarov external fixator
Lengthening with gradual deformity correction at the same osteotomy level	Ilizarov device[a] or Taylor Spatial Frame[a]

[a]Manufactured by Smith & Nephew, Memphis, TN.

than the tibia and femur for similar amounts of lengthening.[9] Prophylactic Rush rods (Zimmer, Warsaw, IN) can be used to prevent fracture after removal. Failure of bone formation requires resection of the interposing fibrous tissue and autologous bone grafting while fixation is maintained. Care should be taken to avoid injury to the radial nerve, which is under tension.

Nerve injury can occur at the time of fixator application or during distraction. Any time the radial nerve is injured at the time of fixator application, it should be explored early to identify the cause of the injury and to avoid secondary nerve injury due to entrapment from swelling into a tight fascial space. Most of the time, the nerve is intact and tethered by surrounding fascia or an adjacent pin. Decompression and replacement of offending pins improves the likelihood of an earlier recovery and allows distraction to proceed while nerve recovery occurs.[11]

The dorsal first web sensation and extensor pollicis longus function and strength should be assessed frequently during lengthening. Problems will alert the surgeon to early radial nerve entrapment. If symptoms of entrapment are observed, the lengthening rate can be slowed. If the symptoms or signs abate, no further intervention is required. If symptoms and signs worsen, the radial nerve should be decompressed, after which the lengthening may continue.

Flexion or extension contractures of the elbow may occur. Daily physical therapy to stretch the elbow and shoulders through their passive range of motion is important to prevent contractures. If the lengthening is performed distal to the deltoid tuberosity, shoulder con-

tracture and stiffness are rarely an issue. Elbow contracture can be treated with dynamic splinting.

FOREARM DEFICIENCIES
Forearm deficiencies have been classified generically by Paley[8,12,13] (**Figure 2**). In addition, there are disease-specific classifications for forearm deficiency (eg, Bayne and Klug radial clubhand,[14] Bayne ulnar clubhand,[15] Masada multiple hereditary exostoses[16]). The treatment strategy depends on the combined knowledge of the Paley generic deficiency type and the degree of dysplasia of the disease-specific deficiency type.

Radial Clubhand
Patients with this condition have instability of the hand, absent or hypoplastic thumb, contractures, limitation of motion of the fingers and elbow, and deficiency of one or both forearms. My treatment algorithm depends on the degree of radial aplasia. For complete radial aplasia, treatment starts with correction and stabilization of the hand, pollicization if needed, and staged lengthening of one or both forearms.

Complete Radial Aplasia
Since 1999, I have used a technique I developed and call ulnarization of the carpus (**Figure 3**) to treat complete radial aplasia. This is a modified version of the Buck-Gramcko radialization technique performed through a volar approach and combined with transfer of the flexor carpi ulnaris tendon to the dorsum of the hand.[17,18] Recurrence and growth arrest have thus far not occurred in any of my patients and stability, active dorsiflexion,

and grip strength are improved. I perform this procedure on patients as young as 12 months.

As early as 3 months after the ulnarization, I perform the Buck-Gramcko pollicization of the index finger using the method described by Manske.[19,20] In cases with thrombocytopenia-absent radius (TAR) syndrome, in which the thumb is present but hypoplastic, I widen the first web space and perform an extensor indicis proprius tendon transfer when indicated.

Lengthening is performed between the ages of 8 and 10 years (**Figure 3**). In bilateral cases, both sides are lengthened at the same time. A proximal ulnar osteotomy is performed for lengthening using circular external fixation that extends to the hand with wire fixation. Half pins are used for fixation of the ulna. Proximally, two divergent pins are used to prevent flexion deviation during lengthening. Distally, two half pins are used in the ulna and two wires are used in the metacarpals. The lengthening rate should not exceed 0.8 mm/d. The goal of lengthening should be no more than 6 cm at this age. A second lengthening of up to 8 cm can be performed between the ages of 12 and 14 years. When external fixation is removed, a prophylactic wire or rod can be inserted to prevent fracture (**Figure 3**). This is augmented by a cast. Daily physical and/or occupational therapy of the hand and elbow should be performed to maintain range of motion. If the range of motion starts to decrease because of elbow and/or finger flexion contractures, the lengthening should be slowed or stopped. Nerve problems are rarely an issue with forearm lengthening, but bone healing and flexion deformity of the regenerate bone should be prevented, recognized, and treated.

Incomplete Radial Aplasia

When 50% or more of the radius is present, and especially if the distal radial physis exists, the preferred strategy is different than the one used to treat complete radial aplasia. With patients as young as 1 year, the hand should be distracted on the ulna with circular external fixation to correct the radial deviation contracture. The hypoplastic radius should be simultaneously lengthened with a mini monolateral external fixator. The hand distraction moves the carpus away from the radius, creating a space for it to be lengthened into. The radius should be overlengthened as much as possible to create a bone block to prevent recurrent deformity.

FIGURE 2

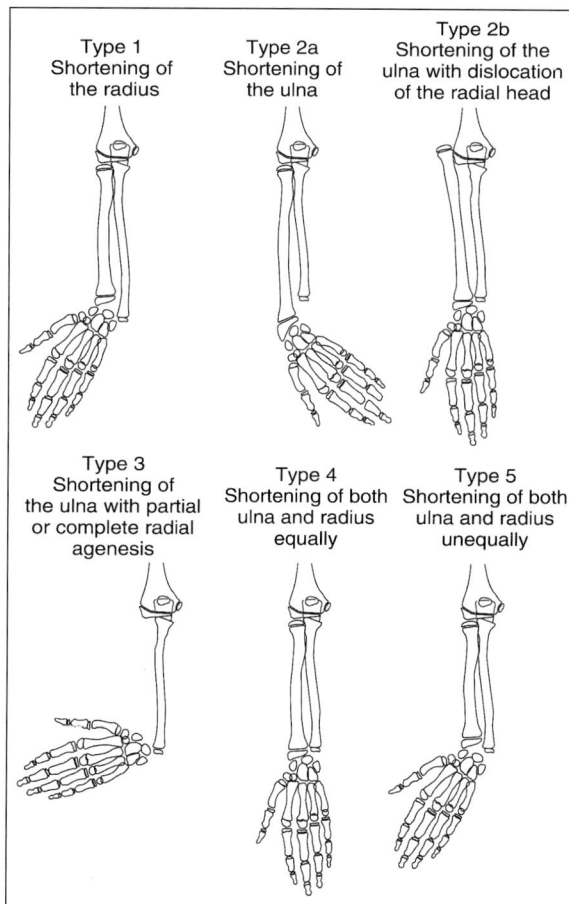

The Paley classification of forearm deficiency. (© 2009, Rubin Institute for Advanced Orthopaedics, Sinai Hospital of Baltimore, Baltimore, MD.)

As early as 3 months after the correction of the hand, the thumb should be treated as described above for complete radial aplasia. If the patient has weak wrist extension, a flexor carpi ulnaris transfer can be performed at the same time.

The forearm should be lengthened again between the ages of 6 and 8 years, depending on the rate of recurrence of radial deviation deformity. This deformity recurs because of the differential undergrowth of the radius relative to the ulna. During the second lengthening, both the ulna and radius are lengthened, albeit differentially.

FIGURE 3

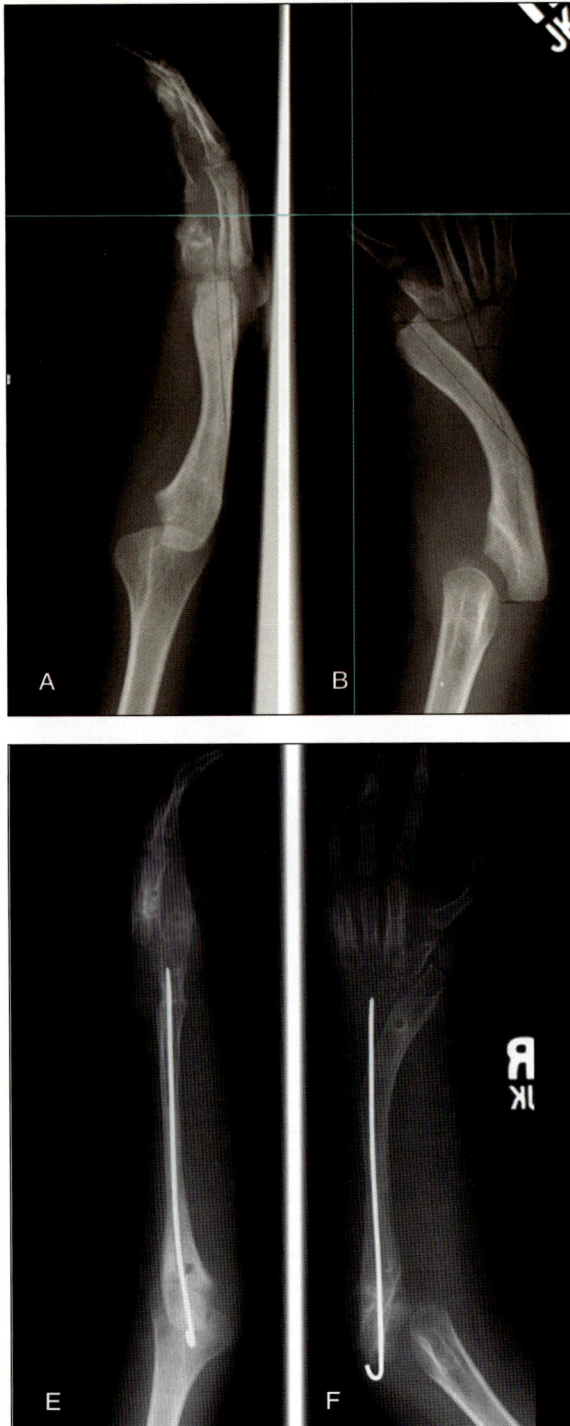

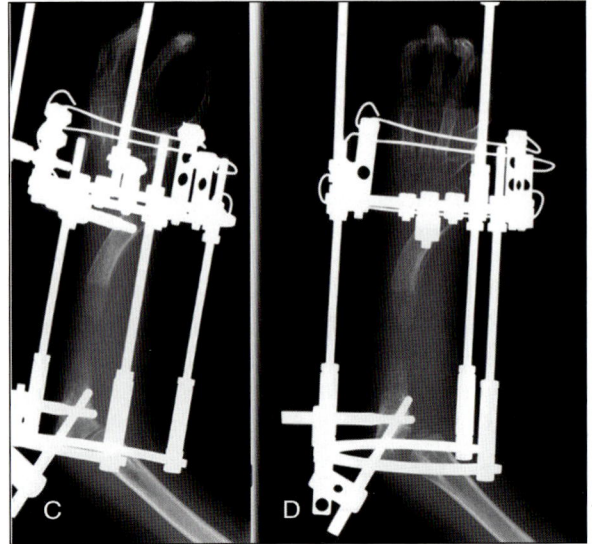

Lateral (**A**) and PA (**B**) radiographs of a child's forearm and hand obtained at age 8 years. Lateral (**C**) and PA (**D**) radiographs obtained during forearm lengthening with an Ilizarov device (7 cm of lengthening). Lateral (**E**) and PA (**F**) radiographs obtained after removal of the external fixator and pinning of the ulna to prevent fracture. (© Dror Paley, MD, West Palm Beach, FL.)

Ulnar Clubhand

Ulnar dysplasia ranges from differential deficiency of the ulna compared with the radius, to partial absence of the distal ulna, to complete absence of the entire ulna, to radiohumeral synostosis.[15] The spectrum of deformities with ulnar dysplasia is much larger than with radial aplasia.

Hypoplasia (Bayne Type I)

In Bayne type I ulnar hypoplasia, the ulna is shortened relative to the radius and the wrist and elbow are present.[15] The distal radius may increase its tilt and bow around the shortened ulna. The radial head may dislocate over time. Bayne type I dysplasia can be described as either Paley type 2a or 2b. For Paley type 2a dysplasia, lengthening of the ulna is performed relative to the radius with correction of distal radial deformity if needed. The latter can be performed gradually or acutely while the ulna is gradually overlengthened relative to the radius. For cases of Paley type 2b dysplasia, in which the

FIGURE 4

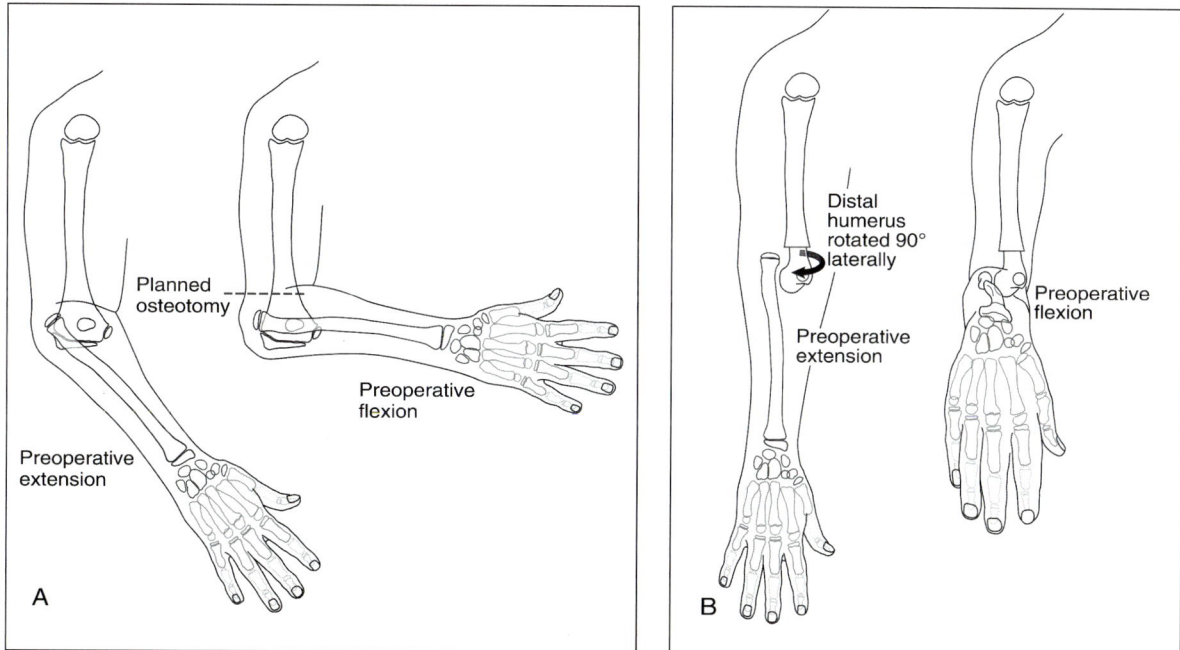

Drawings of Bayne type III complete ulnar aplasia. **A,** With this condition, the radius tends to rotate internally around the humerus so that the flat surface of the humerus is articulating with the shaft of the radius. **B,** The Paley technique of distal humeral external rotation osteotomy to reorient the forearm. The elbow flexion contracture can be treated by gradual distraction with an external fixator that extends from the humerus to the forearm and is hinged at the elbow. (© 2009, Rubin Institute for Advanced Orthopaedics, Sinai Hospital of Baltimore, Baltimore, MD.)

radial head is subluxated or dislocated, the radius should be distracted simultaneously with the ulnar lengthening until it reduces in the joint. I prefer to apply external fixation to the ulna only and allow the radius to passively reduce as a result of the pull of the interosseous membrane. Once the radius reduces, it can be fixed in place with a proximal wire while the ulnar lengthening continues.

Distal Absence (Bayne Type II Ulnar Dysplasia)

With an absent distal ulnar physis (Bayne type II ulnar dysplasia),[15] the degree of deficiency is greater. Although lengthening of the ulna may still be considered in some cases of lesser deficiency, usually the radial head is dislocated and forearm rotation is compromised or limited. The preferred option is a one-bone forearm procedure.

If the forearm is still short, lengthening at a later age can be considered. Resection of the radial head can be performed during the same surgical procedure.

Absent Ulna and Dislocated, Unstable Radius (Bayne Type III)

When the ulna is absent and the radius is dislocated and unstable (Bayne type III complete ulnar aplasia),[15] the radius rotates internally around the humerus until it rests against its flat, broad, distal surface (**Figure 4,** *A*). Instability of flexion and extension of the elbow as well as limited rotation of the forearm with malrotation of the wrist position are the biggest problems in addition to a shortened forearm.

I developed a new method to treat this rare dysplasia by performing a ~90° distal humeral external rotation osteotomy such that the flat side of the distal humerus is in an anterior-posterior orientation rather than a medial-lateral orientation (**Figure 4,** *B*). The radius remains dislocated and is not rotated but now is oriented anterior-posteriorly so that it scissors up and down against the flat surface of the humerus. This gives improved range in a more functional orientation with greatly improved stability. The humeral rotational osteotomy is combined with a forearm rotational osteotomy to reorient the rotation of the wrist and to lengthen the forearm.

Radiohumeral Synostosis (Bayne Type IV)

Radiohumeral synostosis (Bayne type IV ulnar dysplasia)[15] is the most functionally debilitating of all the ulnar dysplasias, especially when it is bilateral. In some cases, a vestigial ulnohumeral joint is present. Resection of the radiohumeral synostosis liberates the elbow and permits some limited motion. Separating the synostosis also restores some forearm rotation and may restore some elbow motion. Most recently, I have restored elbow function by invaginating the humerus between the radius and ulna after surgically separating the two bones. This required a rotational osteotomy of the humerus similar to Bayne type III. Lengthening has a small role in unilateral cases for aesthetic and functional reasons. If the elbow is fused in too flexed a position, an osteotomy can be used both to lengthen the short humerus or forearm and to extend the elbow to 135°, which is a more optimal functional position for unilateral elbow function.

Multiple Hereditary Exostoses

Masada et al[16] classified forearm deficiency due to MHE into three types. These types correspond to Paley generic deficiency types 2a, 2b, and 4.

Osteochondromas of the forearm bones usually lead to differential deficiency of the ulna relative to the radius (Masada types 1 and 2) and, less commonly, to deficiency of the radius relative to the ulna (Masada type 3).[16] Associated deformities include loss of interosseous space between the radius and ulna, with bowing of the ulnar apex toward the radius; subluxation and dislocation of the radial head; increased tilt of the distal radius toward the ulna; and carpal slip toward the ulna.

Significant controversy exists regarding the benefit of osteochondroma resection and reduction of the radial

head. Inconsistent improvement of forearm rotation has been reported with these procedures. Most of these reports did not combine lengthening of the ulna or restoration of the interosseous space between the bones.[21,22]

My method is a five-step approach (**Figure 5**): (1) Resect osteochondromas from the distal radius and ulna. (2) Correct distal radial tilt with a closing wedge osteotomy of the distal radius (staple fixation). (3) Widen the interosseous space by diaphyseal ulnar osteotomy and acute correction (half pins perpendicular to proximal and distal ulna). (4) Lengthen the short ulna at a rate of 0.75 mm/day. (5) Gradually reduce the radial head by distal transport of the radius with lengthening of the ulna (transfixation wire or half pin through the distal radius and ulna). If the radial head does not spontaneously reduce due to proximal interosseous osteochondromas or radial neck valgus, open reduction with osteochondroma resection and/or valgus neck osteotomy should be performed.

Short-term results of this approach include removal of obstructing and tethering exostoses, equalization of the radial and ulnar lengths, reduction of the radial head in the joint, restoration of the interosseous space, reduction of the radial tilt, reduction of the carpal slip, and restoration of forearm rotation.

Growth Arrest of Distal Radius

The distal radius contributes 75% of the radial growth.[1,2] Growth arrest of the distal radius is usually posttraumatic and leads to a short radius relative to the ulna (Paley type 1). If the growth arrest is associated with a malunion or is partial, the orientation of the distal radius also is altered. Ulnar deficiency or radial lengthening can be used to treat this condition. In most cases, the discrepancy between the radius and ulna is too great for ulnar deficiency. Radial lengthening is therefore the preferred option.

In most cases, it is safest to include the hand in the fixation to prevent wrist contracture. Because deformity correction is part of the treatment of most cases of distal growth arrest of the radius, circular external fixation is preferable (Ilizarov device or TSF). It is best to fix the hand in the deformed position and then correct the deformity gradually with lengthening, which brings the hand to a neutral position. If the patient is near the end of growth according to either the Paley multiplier[4,5] or

FIGURE 5

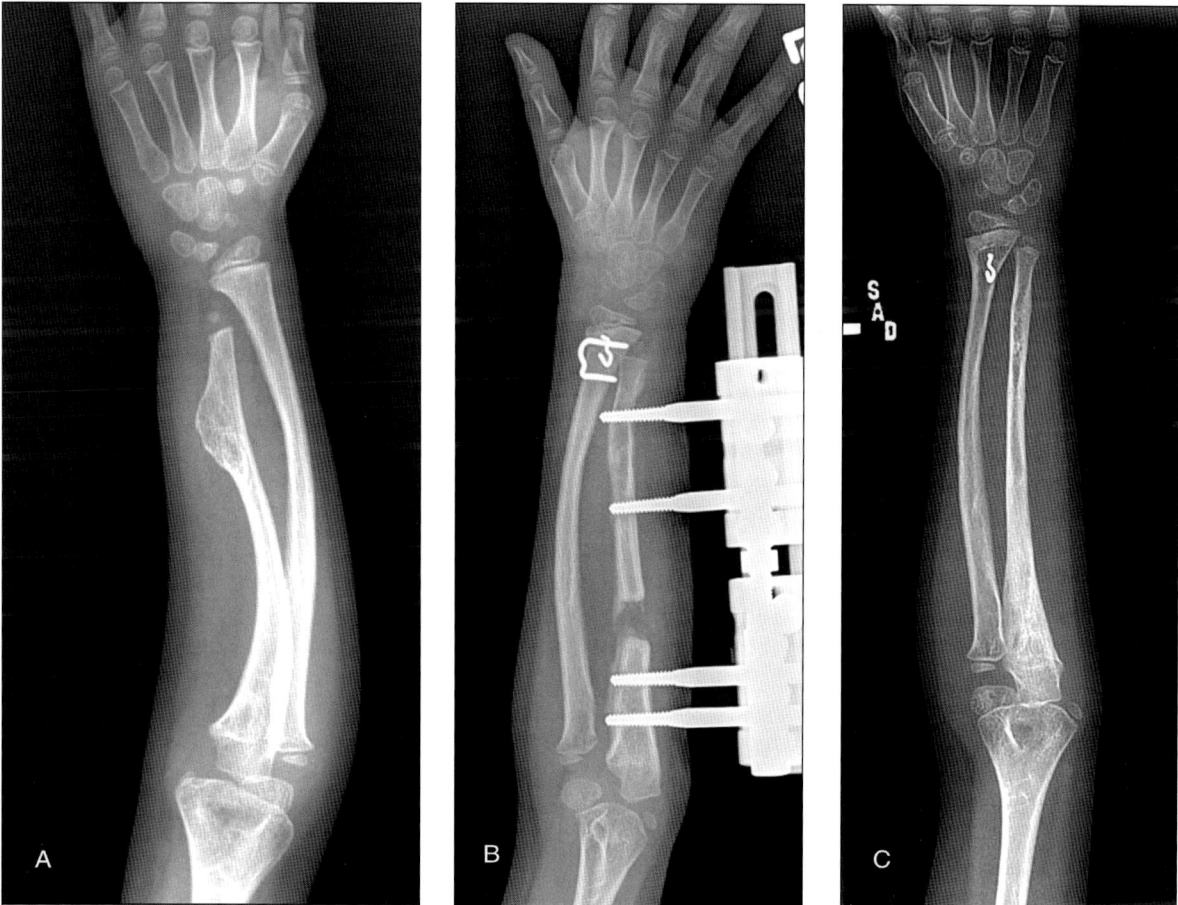

Surgical treatment of multiple hereditary exostoses (multiple osteochondromatosis). **A,** PA radiograph of the forearm (Paley type 2b) in a patient with a large osteochondroma of the distal ulna. The ulnar diaphysis is bowed toward the bow in the radius, narrowing the interosseous space. The radial head is subluxated and the ulna is short compared with the radius as evidenced by the position of the ulnar head proximal to the joint line of the distal radius. **B,** PA radiograph of the forearm obtained after acute correction of ulnar bowing to widen the interosseous space, lengthening of the ulna using monolateral external fixation with distal transport of the radius to reduce the radial head subluxation, and a closing wedge osteotomy of the distal radius to correct increased radial tilt. Fixation of the osteotomy is with memory staples. **C,** PA radiograph of the forearm obtained after removal of external fixator. The interosseous space is restored to normal, the ulnar diaphysis is straight, the length of the ulna is restored to the length of the radius, the radial head is fully reduced, and the distal radial tilt is normal. (© Dror Paley, MD, West Palm Beach, FL.)

Pritchett[1] and the Bortel and Pritchett[2] growth remaining methods, the radius can be overlengthened up to 3 cm relative to the ulna according to the predicted ulnar length at skeletal maturity. The goal of treatment is for the radius and ulna to be the same length at skeletal maturity.

Madelung Deformity

A Madelung deformity is Blount disease of the wrist. The lunate facet is hypoplastic with tethering of the physis adjacent to it, and the carpus herniates in both volar and proximal directions. The distal radioulnar joint is dissociated and dislocated. In most cases, the dislocation is ulna-dorsal, but sometimes it is ulna-volar, which is more symptomatic.

I use a volar approach to expose the lunate facet and perform a hemifacet elevation to the level of the lunate facet with the scaphoid facet. I then perform a complete extra-articular osteotomy to reorient the entire distal radius. The osteotomies are fixed with a plate. The distal radioulnar joint dislocation is repaired with autologous palmaris longus tendon using the Brian Adams technique.[23] Lengthening for Madelung deformity is performed only if the radius is significantly shorter than the ulna.

Growth Arrest of the Distal Ulna

The distal ulna represents 85% of ulnar growth.[1,2] Posttraumatic growth arrest can produce a Paley 2a or 2b deformity, depending on whether the radial head subluxates. The tethering ulna causes the distal radius to increase its tilt. Therefore, as with patients with MHE, in patients with growth arrest of the distal ulna, correction of the distal radius is combined with lengthening of the ulna. These patients also undergo reduction of radial head subluxation, much like patients with MHE.

Lengthening of both bones of the forearm at the same time (for Paley types 4 and 5) has a high risk of permanent loss of forearm rotation. It is reasonable to do this if the forearm has limited rotation to begin with and if this situation is not expected to change. If the forearm has normal rotation, or if the rotation can be restored by resection of blocking osteochondromas or by widening the interosseous space, it is not advisable to lengthen both forearm bones.

DEFICIENCIES IN THE HAND

Isolated metacarpal deficiency (brachymetacarpia) is not as commonly seen as equivalent deficiency in the foot. When it is seen, it is most common in the fourth metacarpal. Lengthening of an isolated short metacarpal is easily accomplished with a miniature distraction device. Lengthening rates should not exceed 0.5 mm/d. Acromelia should not be treated by multiple metacarpal lengthenings.

The main indication for finger lengthening is congenital or posttraumatic amputation of the tip of the finger or thumb. This can be accomplished with a miniature distraction device.

REFERENCES

1. Pritchett JW: Growth in the upper extremity, in Pritchett JW, ed: *Practical Bone Growth.* Seattle, WA, JW Pritchett, 1993, pp 49-63.

2. Bortel DT, Pritchett JW: Straight-line graphs for the prediction of growth of the upper extremities. *J Bone Joint Surg Am* 1993;75(6):885-892.

3. Nath RK: *Obstetric Brachial Plexus Injuries: The Nath Method of Diagnosis and Treatment.* College Station, TX, Virtualbookworm.com Publishing, 2007.

4. Paley D, Gelman A, Shualy MB, Herzenberg JE: Multiplier method for limb-length prediction in the upper extremity. *J Hand Surg Am* 2008;33(3):385-391.

5. Paley D, Bhave A, Herzenberg JE, Bowen JR: Multiplier method for predicting limb-length discrepancy. *J Bone Joint Surg Am* 2000;82-A(10):1432-1446.

6. Pizà G, Caja VL, González-Viejo MA, Navarro A: Hydroxyapatite-coated external-fixation pins: The effect on pin loosening and pin-track infection in leg lengthening for short stature. *J Bone Joint Surg Br* 2004;86(6):892-897.

7. Kashiwagi N, Suzuki S, Seto Y, Futami T: Bilateral humeral lengthening in achondroplasia. *Clin Orthop Relat Res* 2001(391):251-257.

8. Tetsworth K, Krome J, Paley D: Lengthening and deformity correction of the upper extremity by the Ilizarov technique. *Orthop Clin North Am* 1991;22(4):689-713.

9. Cattaneo R, Villa A, Catagni MA, Bell D: Lengthening of the humerus using the Ilizarov technique: Description of the method and report of 43 cases. *Clin Orthop Relat Res* 1990(250):117-124.

10. Hosny GA: Unilateral humeral lengthening in children and adolescents. *J Pediatr Orthop B* 2005;14(6):439-443.

11. Nogueira MP, Paley D, Bhave A, Herbert A, Nocente C, Herzenberg JE: Nerve lesions associated with limb-lengthening. *J Bone Joint Surg Am* 2003;85-A(8):1502-1510.

12. Villa A, Paley D, Catagni MA, Bell D, Cattaneo R: Lengthening of the forearm by the Ilizarov technique. *Clin Orthop Relat Res* 1990(250):125-137.

13. Paley D, Kelly D: Lengthening and deformity correction in the upper extremities, in Raskin K, ed: *Atlas of the Hand Clinics.* Philadelphia, PA, WB Saunders, 2000, vol 5, pp 117-172.

14. Bayne LG, Klug MS: Long-term review of the surgical treatment of radial deficiencies. *J Hand Surg Am* 1987;12(2):169-179.

15. Bayne LG: Ulnar club hand (ulnar deficiencies), in Green DP, ed: *Operative Hand Surgery,* ed 3. New York, NY, Churchill Livingstone, 1993, pp 288-303.

16. Masada K, Tsuyuguchi Y, Kawai H, Kawabata H, Noguchi K, Ono K: Operations for forearm deformity caused by multiple osteochondromas. *J Bone Joint Surg Br* 1989;71(1):24-29.

17. Buck-Gramcko D: Radialization as a new treatment for radial club hand. *J Hand Surg Am* 1985;10(6 Pt 2): 964-968.

18. Buck-Gramcko D: Radialization for radial club hand. *Tech Hand Up Extrem Surg* 1999;3(1):2-12.

19. Manske PR, McCaroll HR Jr: Index finger pollicization for a congenitally absent or nonfunctioning thumb. *J Hand Surg Am* 1985;10(5):606-613.

20. Manske PR, Rotman MB, Dailey LA: Long-term functional results after pollicization for the congenitally deficient thumb. *J Hand Surg Am* 1992;17(6): 1064-1072.

21. Peterson HA: Multiple hereditary osteochondromata. *Clin Orthop Relat Res* 1989(239):222-230.

22. Peterson HA: Deformities and problems of the forearm in children with multiple hereditary osteochondromata. *J Pediatr Orthop* 1994;14(1):92-100.

23. Adams BD, Berger RA: An anatomic reconstruction of the distal radioulnar ligaments for posttraumatic distal radioulnar joint instability. *J Hand Surg Am* 2002;27(2): 243-251.

CHAPTER 15

LOWER LIMB LENGTHENING IN SKELETAL DYSPLASIAS

WILLIAM G. MACKENZIE, MD, FRCSC, FACS

MARIA JULIA CORNES, MD

INTRODUCTION

Skeletal dysplasias are a heterogeneous group of disorders characterized by abnormalities of articular cartilage and bone growth, affecting between 2 and 4.7 per 10,000 individuals.[1] The modes of inheritance are heterogeneous: autosomal recessive, autosomal dominant, X-linked recessive, or X-linked dominant. To date, more than 300 distinct genetic disorders of bone growth and articular cartilage have been identified.[2]

Skeletal dysplasias have two major classification systems; one was developed by Sir Thomas Fairbank in 1951 in *An Atlas of General Affections of the Skeleton*,[3] and the other was described in 1964 by the Rubin Institute.[4,5] Both systems group skeletal dysplasias according to the anatomic distribution of bone changes at the epiphyseal, physeal, metaphyseal, and diaphyseal regions.

When planning limb lengthening and realignment, the clinician should be aware of the different skeletal dysplasias and associated concomitant bone or cartilage morphology, as the results of limb lengthening in a patient with skeletal dysplasia are not the same as in those with other types of discrepancies. Skeletal dysplasias may result in short stature, limb-length discrepancy (LLD), angular deformity, and/or joint abnormalities. Patients with achondroplasia have well-formed joints with normal cartilage. Extended limb lengthening for stature in these individuals is less complex than in patients with other diagnoses such as pseudoachondroplasia and spondyloepiphyseal dysplasia, who have abnormal cartilage and significant joint laxity.

LIMB LENGTHENING AND REALIGNMENT FOR SKELETAL DYSPLASIA

Indications for limb lengthening include short stature, LLD, and angular and/or rotational deformity. The assessment of the patient starts with a thorough history and physical examination, including an evaluation of current function and any limitation of daily activities. Evaluation of the proportion of the trunk to the upper and lower extremities should ensure that the planned procedures will result in satisfactory cosmesis. A satisfactory outcome requires that the surgeon communicate realistic expectations to the patient and family.

When planning surgery in patients with skeletal dysplasias, important factors to consider include patient age; psychosocial factors; angular and rotational deformities; joint abnormalities; activities of daily living, including improved personal hygiene resulting from lengthening the upper extremities; the order that limb segments will be lengthened; and the number and placement of osteotomies.

Dr. Mackenzie or an immediate family member is a member of a speakers' bureau or has made paid presentations on behalf of Smith & Nephew and Biomet; serves as an unpaid consultant to Biomet and Smith & Nephew; and has received research or institutional support from DePuy and Biomet. Dr. Cornes or an immediate family member serves as a board member, owner, officer, or committee member of Asociación Argentina de Ortopedia y Traumatología.

PATIENT AGE

Cattaneo et al[6] suggest that patients younger than 10 years not undergo limb lengthening because the bone is short, the percentage of lengthening can be limited, and the patient may require a second lengthening in the same limb. Once skeletal maturity is achieved, the discrepancy or length to be achieved can be measured and addressed precisely. Ganel et al[7] take the opposite approach. They recommend starting treatment as early as possible to achieve maximal height before starting school to avoid psychologic problems.

PSYCHOSOCIAL FACTORS

The physician, family, and patient need time to discuss all possible options, and all information must be provided before the lengthening. The physician should be assured that the patient and family can tolerate the surgery mentally, emotionally, and socially.[8] Postoperative care of the patient is time-consuming, and the caregivers need to understand the responsibilities required. Caregivers also must understand the lengthening process and the need for physical therapy and care of the frame. The patient needs to be realistic about the expectations and how to optimize the goals of the surgery.

Hrutkay and Eilert[9] described psychologic problems, from anxiety to suicidal intentions, that can occur during the limb-lengthening process. Most of the problems appeared in patients undergoing long hospitalizations and included depression, anxiety, anorexia nervosa, and feelings of guilt. Reactions such as noncompliance, dependence, and regression were seen in 18% of the patients. Participation in group psychotherapy during treatment helps prevent these problems. Psychologic problems are seen especially in bilateral lengthening, probably because patients are severely handicapped during this procedure.[10] Little evidence exists that psychologic problems persist after lengthening.

ANGULAR AND ROTATIONAL DEFORMITIES

The correction of angular or rotational deformities needs to be addressed along with the length adjustment to attain optimal function. Fixator choice and the method of lengthening are determined by structural considerations (eg, realignment of significant angulation and rotational deformity is best done with a gradual

technique and a circular fixator) and the goals of the surgery.

JOINT ABNORMALITIES

Articular surface abnormalities are present in many skeletal dysplasias. Typical joint abnormalities include those seen in spondyloepiphyseal dysplasia, caused by mutations in type II collagen, encoded by gene COL2A1, and in multiple epiphyseal dysplasia, caused by mutations in type IX collagen, encoded by COL9A2.[1] Other dysplasias, such as pseudoachondroplasia, have mutations in cartilage oligomeric matrix protein (COMP) that alter the architecture of the cartilage, resulting in premature degeneration and often requiring patients to undergo joint arthroplasty during the third decade of life.[2] Extensive limb lengthening and the resultant increased compressive forces across the joints in disorders with an abnormal articular surface may result in acceleration of cartilage degeneration.

Periarticular deformities are secondary to physeal and epiphyseal abnormalities, the deformed skeleton, weight bearing, and ligamentous laxity.[11] Surgical correction of these deformities is indicated when malalignment, subluxation, or dislocation is present. The goals of treatment are not only limb lengthening but also the reduction of pain caused by these joint abnormalities.

When planning surgery, it is necessary to align the mechanical axis and correct joint malalignment. The joint line can be easily discerned in older children, but arthrography is suggested in younger children because of the variable epiphyseal ossification.[12]

ACTIVITIES OF DAILY LIVING AND IMPROVED PERSONAL HYGIENE

One of the goals in lengthening is to improve the individual's activities of daily living because the short extremities present certain difficulties in accomplishing normal movement patterns and interaction with the environment. The person with short stature and short limbs has difficulty with hygiene, cooking, dressing, transportation, and movement. Limb lengthening can increase the overall stature to be closer to the median height of adults (50th percentile: ~176 cm for men, ~163 cm for women) and improve the function and satisfaction of activities of daily living. Humeral lengthening is an important consideration in achondroplasia, to improve reach and allow independent hygiene.

THE ORDER OF LIMB SEGMENT LENGTHENING
Several different methods have been described: ipsilateral limbs, bilateral segments (tibial, femoral, or both), and crossed or linear lengthening. Each has distinct advantages and disadvantages.

In ipsilateral limb lengthening, the femur and tibia are lengthened simultaneously. This results in a significant discrepancy between sides until the opposite limb is lengthened. One advantage is that this discrepancy encourages the patient to continue with the limb-lengthening process. A disadvantage is that concurrent femoral and tibial lengthenings cause increased stress on the neurovascular structures, musculotendinous units, and joints compared with other techniques.[13]

Bilateral Limb Lengthening
In bilateral lower limb lengthening, both tibias are lengthened first, followed by both femora (**Figure 1**). Because both limbs are lengthened at the same time, no significant length discrepancies result. Proportional appearance of the limb may be affected if the patient does not continue with subsequent procedures. Recently, Paley and others (personal communication, August 30, 2008, Baltimore, MD) have advocated bilateral concurrent femoral and tibial lengthening.

Crossed or Linear Lengthening
In crossed or linear lengthening, one femur and the contralateral tibia are lengthened concurrently. This technique avoids creating a large LLD and reduces the forces across the knee joint. Like ipsilateral lengthening, crossed lengthening encourages the surgeon and the patient to complete the program.[13]

BENEFITS OF LIMB LENGTHENING
Limb lengthening for skeletal dysplasias improves function but also is prophylactic and therapeutic. Lengthening reduces hyperlordosis of the lumbar spine[13] and may reduce the likelihood of spinal stenosis in achondroplasia. Realignment should reduce forces across the joints.

OSTEOTOMY
The number of osteotomies performed will depend on the required length. Two osteotomies may be used for longer lengthenings and may make the deformity correction easier. Bifocal osteotomies result in reduced healing indexes but increased complications.[14]

PREDICTING ADULT HEIGHT
Predicting the final height in patients with skeletal dysplasias allows the family and patient to decide among different treatment options such as limb lengthening or growth hormone treatment. The use of general developmental charts is not appropriate for patients with skeletal dysplasias. Two similar methods are used for prediction of adult height in patients with achondroplasia: the Horton[15] and Nehme[4] databases. Achondroplasia height multipliers were calculated from both databases, showing that final height in achondroplasia is percentile-independent and sex-dependent.[15] Height prediction methods are not available for the other types of skeletal dysplasias. Growth rates in patients with achondroplasia are slower than in unaffected individuals.

SURGICAL PROCEDURES
The Ilizarov Method of Distraction Osteogenesis
The Ilizarov method of distraction osteogenesis[13] involves the application of a circular ring fixator with tensioned wires and half pins. The assembly consists of two rings placed at metaphyseal sites at either end of the bone and connected by graduated telescopic rods. In a two-level osteotomy, the same frame is applied with the addition of a ring between the osteotomies. The purpose is to correct LLDs and angular, rotational, and multilevel deformities. Limb function is maintained with weight bearing and aggressive physical therapy.

The duration of the treatment depends on the amount of lengthening planned. Cattaneo et al[6] reported a mean treatment duration of 12.8 months in the tibia and 7.8 months in the femur from the initiation of the lengthening to the removal of the fixator (mean, 14 to 18 cm lengthened).

The Vilarrubias Method
The Vilarrubias method[13] of lengthening uses a monolateral fixator. Elongation starts with simultaneous bilat-

FIGURE 1

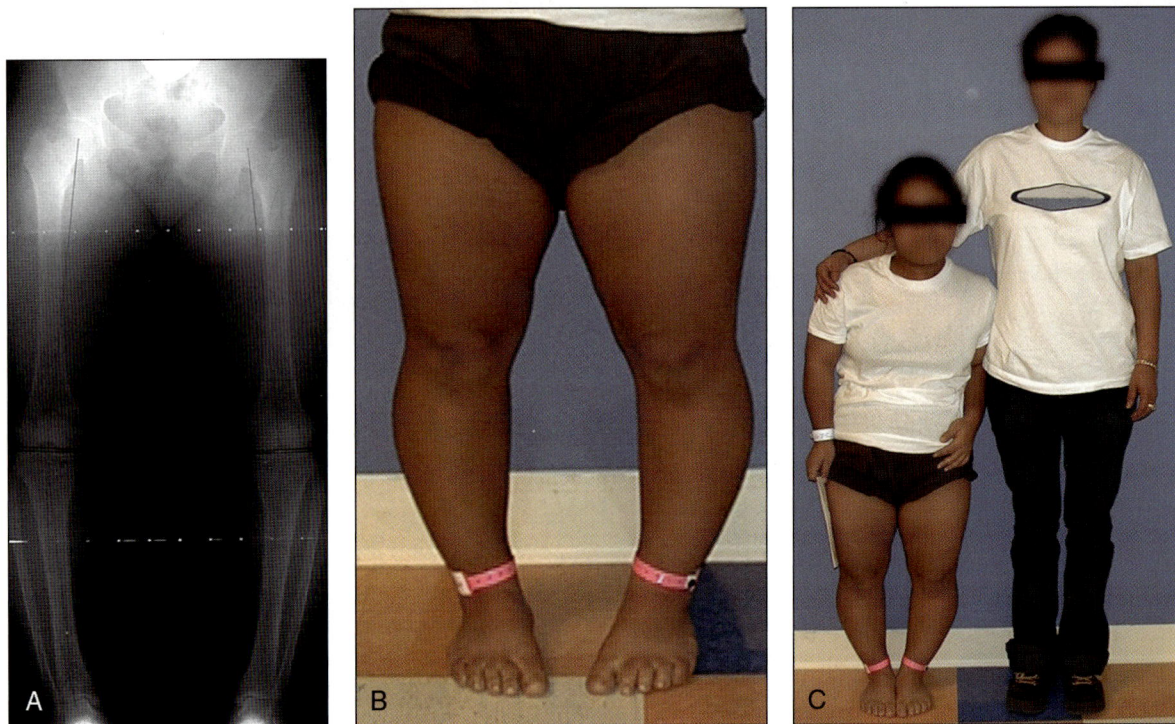

Images of a 15-year-old girl with hypoachondroplasia, short stature, and bilateral varus deformity. Preoperative AP hip-knee-ankle radiograph (**A**) and clinical photographs (**B, C**).

(continued)

eral tibial lengthening and Achilles tendon percutaneous lengthening while keeping the ankle joint at 90° in a cast boot. Humeral or femoral lengthening is the next stage. For the femoral lengthening, the proximal pins are inserted off-axis in the sagittal plane. Once the femoral osteotomy is performed, the proximal femur is extended to create a 20° apex anterior angular osteotomy to correct the hip flexion contracture and relieve lumbar hyperlordosis. The patient is not allowed to bear weight during the distraction. The duration of the treatment is similar to that using the Ilizarov technique.

DeBastiani Method

The DeBastiani method[16] is based on the physiologic principles of distraction osteogenesis described by Ilizarov[13] but differs in that lengthening is achieved by callotasis, in which the subperiosteal osteotomy is per-

formed with multiple drill holes and is completed with an osteotome. A lightweight, dynamic monolateral fixator is applied. Partial weight bearing and physical therapy are allowed immediately postoperatively. Distraction usually starts between 10 and 15 days after frame application. The dynamic axial compression is thought to promote corticalization of the new bone.

POSTOPERATIVE REHABILITATION

When indicated, weight bearing and physical therapy should start immediately after surgery to encourage mobilization. Physical therapy is necessary at least three times per week (ideally, every day) to maintain joint range of motion. Isometric exercises and active mobilization of the joints also are recommended.[13] Follow-up is every 2 weeks during the period of distraction and monthly during the consolidation phase. The external

FIGURE 1 (*continued*)

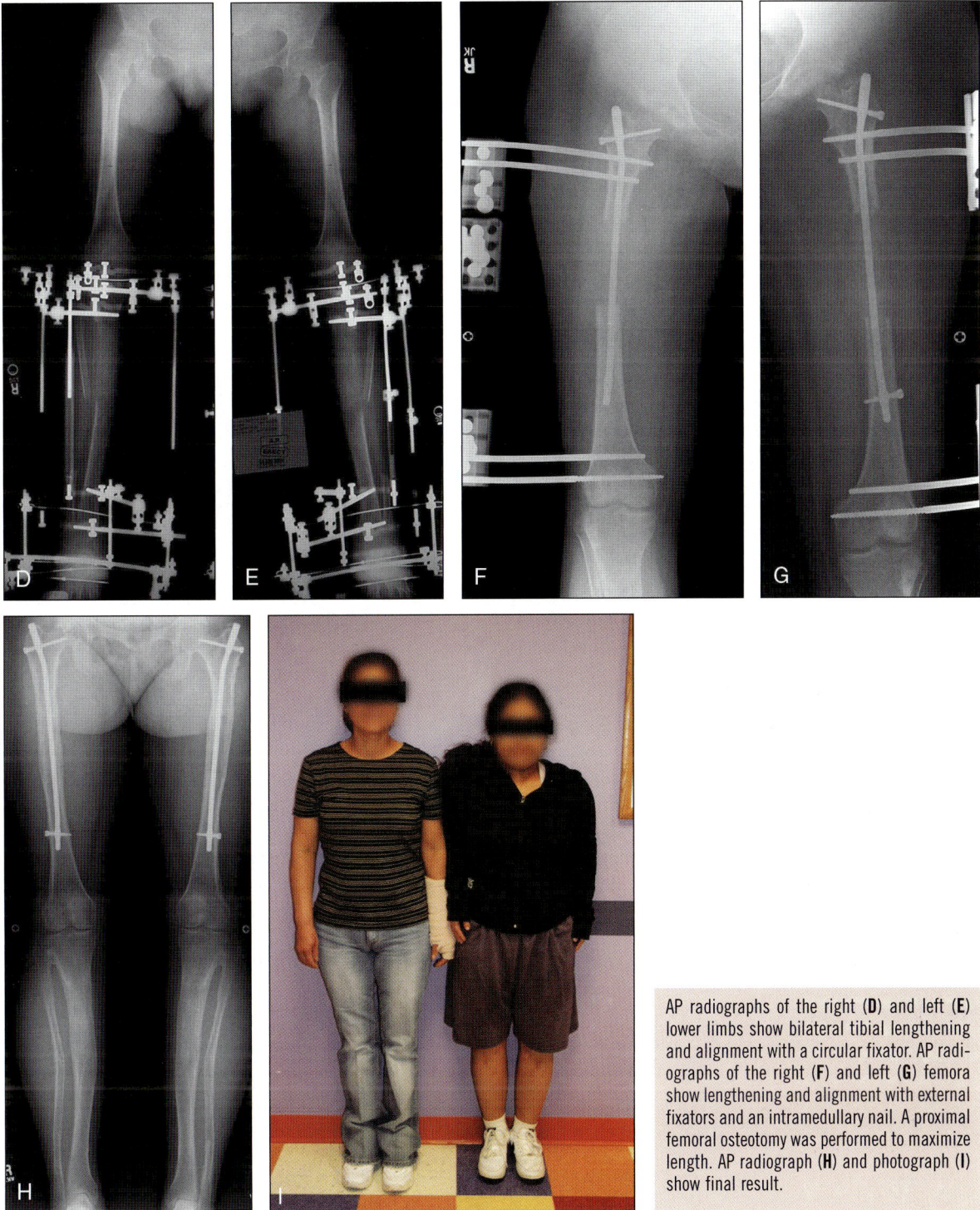

AP radiographs of the right (**D**) and left (**E**) lower limbs show bilateral tibial lengthening and alignment with a circular fixator. AP radiographs of the right (**F**) and left (**G**) femora show lengthening and alignment with external fixators and an intramedullary nail. A proximal femoral osteotomy was performed to maximize length. AP radiograph (**H**) and photograph (**I**) show final result.

fixator is dynamized and removed at the end of this process.[17]

COMPLICATIONS

Information on complications occurring with limb lengthening in skeletal dysplasias is limited. The most common complications are pin-tract infections, joint stiffness, excessive soft-tissue tension, and nerve injury. Others include premature consolidation, angular deformity, and failure to preserve gain in length.[18] Higher rates of complications and additional surgeries are seen with aggressive lengthening.[19]

LENGTHENING IN OSTEOGENESIS IMPERFECTA

In the most severe cases of osteogenesis imperfecta (OI), the more stable fixation provided by a circular frame is preferred. The half pins used with monolateral fixation can be a problem with the thinner diameter of bone associated with OI.[19] Fixator removal should be delayed until the regenerate bone clearly appears radiographically mature. After the frame has been removed, the limb should be protected by an intramedullary nail or by external support such as a cast brace.[18] The risk of complications with lengthening is higher in patients who are still incurring frequent fractures.

SUMMARY AND CONCLUSIONS

The decision to perform lengthening in skeletal dysplasias depends on many factors, including the extent of LLD, angular deformities, and physiologic factors. Emotional stability needs to be assessed to determine if the patient can tolerate this treatment. The different types of skeletal dysplasias respond differently to lengthening, but little information exists on optimal treatment strategies. Outcomes and complications vary because physicians often do not understand the differences among the many variations of skeletal dysplasias.

REFERENCES

1. Baitner AC, Maurer SG, Gruen MB, Di Cesare PE: The genetic basis of the osteochondrodysplasias. *J Pediatr Orthop* 2000;20(5):594-605.

2. Carter EM, Raggio CL: Genetic and orthopedic aspects of collagen disorders. *Curr Opin Pediatr* 2009;21(1): 46-54.

3. Fairbank T: *An Atlas of General Affections of the Skeleton.* Baltimore, MD, Williams & Wilkins, 1953.

4. Paley D, Matz AL, Kurland DB, Lamm BM, Herzenberg JE: Multiplier method for prediction of adult height in patients with achondroplasia. *J Pediatr Orthop* 2005;25 (4):539-542.

5. Rubin P: On organizing a dynamic classification of bone dysplasias. *Arthritis Rheum* 1964;7:693-708.

6. Cattaneo R, Villa A, Catagni M, Tentori L: Limb lengthening in achondroplasia by Ilizarov's method. *Int Orthop* 1988;12(3):173-179.

7. Ganel A, Horoszowski H, Kamhin M, Farine I: Leg lengthening in achondroplastic children. *Clin Orthop Relat Res* 1979(144):194-197.

8. Saleh M, Burton M: Leg lengthening: Patient selection and management in achondroplasia. *Orthop Clin North Am* 1991;22(4):589-599.

9. Hrutkay JM, Eilert RE: Operative lengthening of the lower extremity and associated psychological aspects: The Children's Hospital experience. *J Pediatr Orthop* 1990;10(3):373-377.

10. Correll J: Surgical correction of short stature in skeletal dysplasias. *Acta Paediatr Scand Suppl* 1991;377:143-148.

11. Kopits SE: Orthopedic complications of dwarfism. *Clin Orthop Relat Res* 1976(114):153-179.

12. Inan M, Jeong C, Chan G, Mackenzie WG, Glutting J: Analysis of lower extremity alignment in achondroplasia: Interobserver reliability and intraobserver reproducibility. *J Pediatr Orthop* 2006;26(1):75-78.

13. Vilarrubias JM, Ginebreda I, Jimeno E: Lengthening of the lower limbs and correction of lumbar hyperlordosis in achondroplasia. *Clin Orthop Relat Res* 1990(250): 143-149.

14. Bell DF, Boyer MI, Armstrong PF: The use of the Ilizarov technique in the correction of limb deformities associated with skeletal dysplasia. *J Pediatr Orthop* 1992;12(3):283-290.

15. Horton WA, Rotter JI, Rimoin DL, Scott CI, Hall JG: Standard growth curves for achondroplasia. *J Pediatr* 1978;93(3):435-438.

16. De Bastiani G, Aldegheri R, Renzi Brivio L: The treatment of fractures with a dynamic axial fixator. *J Bone Joint Surg Br* 1984;66(4):538-545.

17. Myers GJ, Bache CE, Bradish CF: Use of distraction osteogenesis techniques in skeletal dysplasias. *J Pediatr Orthop* 2003;23(1):41-45.

18. Ring D, Jupiter JB, Labropoulos PK, Guggenheim JJ, Stanitsky DF, Spencer DM: Treatment of deformity of the lower limb in adults who have osteogenesis imperfecta. *J Bone Joint Surg Am* 1996;78(2):220-225.

19. Saldanha KA, Saleh M, Bell MJ, Fernandes JA: Limb lengthening and correction of deformity in the lower limbs of children with osteogenesis imperfecta. *J Bone Joint Surg Br* 2004;86(2):259-265.

CHAPTER *16*

TREATMENT OF SOFT-TISSUE CONTRACTURES

HAROLD J.P. VAN BOSSE, MD

INTRODUCTION

Contractures of the knee joints have many etiologies. They can be congenital, as a result of pterygium syndromes, meningomyelocele or sacral agenesis, tibial hemimelia, or arthrogryposis; or acquired, as a result of neuromuscular disorders, trauma, burns, septic arthritis, juvenile idiopathic arthritis, hemophilia, poliomyelitis, or fibrosis resulting from intramuscular injections. Contractures can have combined congenital and acquired causes, as seen in skeletal dysplasias and dwarfism syndromes. Although not a true shortening of the limb, a severe flexion contracture of the knee functions as one and is one of the most difficult problems causing gait disturbances.[1] The flexed-knee gait has a shortened stride length, and the center of gravity permanently falls posterior to the knee, fatiguing the extensor mechanism and profoundly disrupting gait mechanics.[2-5] Isolated ankle or hip contractures can be compensated for by other lower extremity joints or the lumbar spine, but knee contractions cannot easily be compensated for. The knee's central position in the limb reduces the energy efficiency of gait. For severe contractures in both children and adults, gradual extension of knee contracture using an external fixator is an important treatment option.[6,7]

CLINICAL EVALUATION

Knee

The quality of a contracture can be described as having a soft end point, much like hyperextending a metacarpophalangeal joint, or a hard end point, similar to the elbow at terminal extension. A soft end point will show significant improvement immediately as a result of a soft-tissue procedure, whereas a hard end point will show less improvement acutely.

Subluxation of the tibia on the femur, either posterior or rotatory, can be identified either clinically or radiographically. Lateral radiographs of the knee in flexion and extension define the knee's range of motion and can demonstrate any tendency to tibial hinging or subluxation. If an external fixator is used to correct the contracture, the subluxation can be addressed by acutely reducing the subluxation at the time of frame application, followed by gradual extension of the knee. Repair of posttraumatic ligamentous injury should be performed after contracture correction, rather than before.

Hip

Hip deformities and contractures can pose challenging obstacles to the correction and maintenance of knee flexion contractures, as well as to the patient's ability to

---

sit and ambulate after correction; therefore, they should be addressed first. Proximal femoral osteotomies and occasionally soft-tissue releases are used to treat hip deformities such as extension contractures, flexion contractures greater than 30°, and rotation contractures that prohibit positioning the knee directly anteriorly. Treating the knee first makes it difficult to maintain knee correction while treating the hip.

Foot and Ankle

The primary consideration in regard to the foot and ankle during gradual extension of knee contracture by external fixator is whether the foot needs to be stabilized during joint distraction. In particular, the ankle may be at risk for developing an equinus contracture, necessitating extension of the frame to include the foot. Occasionally, a foot deformity needs to be addressed as well, requiring frame extension for simultaneous deformity correction, either gradually or acutely.

Soft Tissue

Acute correction of a knee flexion contracture in the presence of scarring of the popliteal space, skin grafts, or a compromised neurovascular status may lead to skin necrosis, neurapraxias, or vascular embarrassment, even in a mild knee flexion contracture.[8-10] In these cases, gradual extension of knee contracture by external fixator is the safer option, and these findings should be considered when planning surgical incisions or pin sites. The rate of contracture distraction may need to be decreased to protect soft-tissue viability.

CONTRACTURE AND DEFORMITY EVALUATION

When both a knee contracture and a coronal plane deformity exist, the contribution of each to the total limb malalignment is difficult to differentiate. The extremity is difficult to position anatomically for standard AP radiographs of the femur, tibia, or knee, and the flexed knee creates projectional distortions, leading to imprecise angular measurements.[11] Instead, positioning the patient prone for individual tibia and femur PA radiographs allows each segment to be placed much closer to the film cassette. The best strategy for surgical correction is to address the knee flexion contracture first, after which corrective osteotomies can be accurately planned.

On lateral radiographs, the distal femoral and proximal tibial joint orientation, as measured by the posterior distal femoral and posterior proximal tibia angles,[12] helps determine if a deformity is entirely the result of a contracture or if it has a bony procurvatum/recurvatum component.

TREATMENT OPTIONS

Patients with normal hip strength and ankle function often can tolerate a knee flexion contracture less than 20°.[1] They compensate by leaning forward with the hip locked in extension and using the plantar flexors to stabilize the ankle, bringing the body's center of gravity anterior to the knee and augmenting the quadriceps function.[1,4] Bracing with knee-ankle-foot orthoses or floor reaction ankle-foot orthoses may improve gait efficiency when quadriceps and ankle weakness is present.

In contractures that are less than 20° with a soft end point, hamstring lengthening may be the only procedure necessary, but only when the popliteal angle is greater than the flexion contracture preoperatively. If hip extension strength is weak preoperatively, a gracilis or semitendinosus tendon transfer to the distal femur can help prevent a crouched gait.[13] In walking children with cerebral palsy, contractures of up to 30° may resolve with hamstring lengthening alone. Adult knees can rapidly develop intracapsular fibrosis; therefore, hamstring lengthening alone is recommended only for recent contractures less than 20°. I prefer a percutaneous release of the gracilis and semitendinosus just above the knee flexion crease and open muscle-sparing tenotomies of the semimembranosus and biceps femoris through 3- to 4-cm incisions at the junction of the middle and distal thirds of the thigh.

Posterior knee capsular releases are effective in adults and children to treat contractures less than 20° with a hard end point and no hamstring tightness. They also can be used in conjunction with hamstring lengthenings and/or gastrocnemius tenotomies for contractures between 20° and 30° that exhibit a soft end point and hamstring tightness. The technique for posterior knee capsular releases is discussed below.

Supracondylar femoral extension osteotomies are useful in both adults and children. In children, they are suitable for contractures as small as 20° to 30° and as large as 45° with a hard end point. Distal femoral osteotomies have been reported to correct contractures up to 90°,[14,15] but potential complications include neurovascular stretch injury, nonphysiologic weight bearing on the posterior femoral condyles, and unacceptable recurrence rates of 0.9° per month.[14,16,17] Shortening the femur at the osteotomy site can avoid neurovascular injury but will create or exacerbate a limb-length discrepancy. In adults, the risk of complications limits the indications for supracondylar femoral extension osteotomies to contractures of 30° or less. Attention to alignment is important to avoid recurvatum or coronal plane deformities.[18] I prefer to use a 95° condylar blade plate through a lateral approach to the distal femur. The blade is inserted parallel to the distal femoral condyles as seen on the AP view, and the plate portion is aligned with the tibial shaft as seen on the lateral view, with the knee in its fullest extension. Either a transverse or an anterior-based isosceles triangular closing-wedge osteotomy is performed, shortening the femur as little as possible.

INDICATIONS FOR EXTERNAL FIXATION

Although gradual extension of knee contracture using an external fixator is an excellent tool for correction of knee flexion contractures of essentially any size,[6,7,19-21] it is best suited for contractures too large to treat safely by other means. The advantages of the technique are that gradual rather than acute correction reduces the risk of neurovascular injury, tibial subluxation can be addressed during contracture correction, and no femoral shortening is required, even with large deformities. The webbed and contracted skin and fascia of pterygia can be gradually stretched, essentially resolving the soft-tissue web once the knee is fully extended. The main drawbacks of the technique are its technical difficulty, patient and family acceptance, and inconvenience. Soft tissues in children are often more pliant than in adults, even in congenital contractures. Adults can develop intra-articular fibrosis rapidly, even when contractures are initially extracapsular, making the contractures more resistant to correction with simple soft-tissue procedures. Indications, therefore, are contractures greater than 40° in children and greater than 30° in adults. In an effort to prevent recurrence or proximal tibial procurvatum bending, I always perform a posterior capsule and/or tendon release concurrently. Other authors have not always found this nec-

FIGURE 1

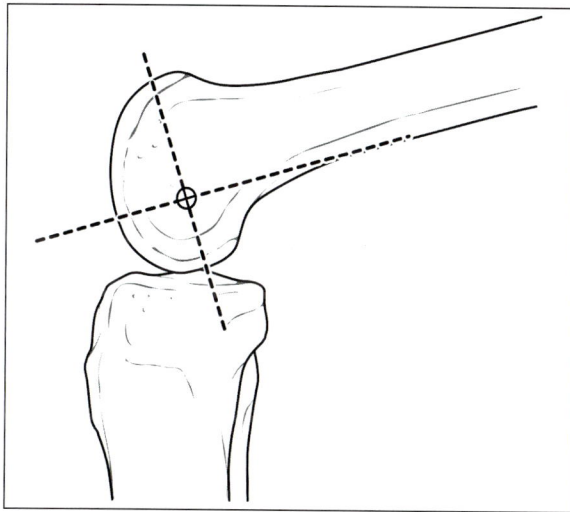

Drawing of the knee shows the flexion-extension axis at the junction of a line drawn along the posterior femoral cortex and a line drawn through the widest anterior-posterior dimension of the femoral condyles.

essary.[7,21] After gradual extension of the knee contracture using an external fixator, the total arc of motion is usually less than it was preoperatively. Intensive physical therapy can restore most or all of the motion.[6]

SURGICAL TECHNIQUES
Approximation of Knee Center of Rotation

A temporary guidewire is placed through the knee's center of rotation to facilitate accurate hinge placement. The true center of rotation cannot be defined, but it can be approximated by an axis that runs through the origins of the medial and lateral collateral ligaments.[22] Intraoperatively, the knee is positioned such that its lateral projection on the image intensifier has the posterior and distal femoral condyles exactly overlapping (approximately 3° of external rotation); an arthrogram may help visualize the condyles in young children. The intersection of the posterior femoral diaphyseal cortical line and the greatest anterior-posterior dimension of the femoral condyles is identified both medially and laterally (**Figure 1**).[21] A 1.8-mm Ilizarov transfixion wire is

FIGURE 2

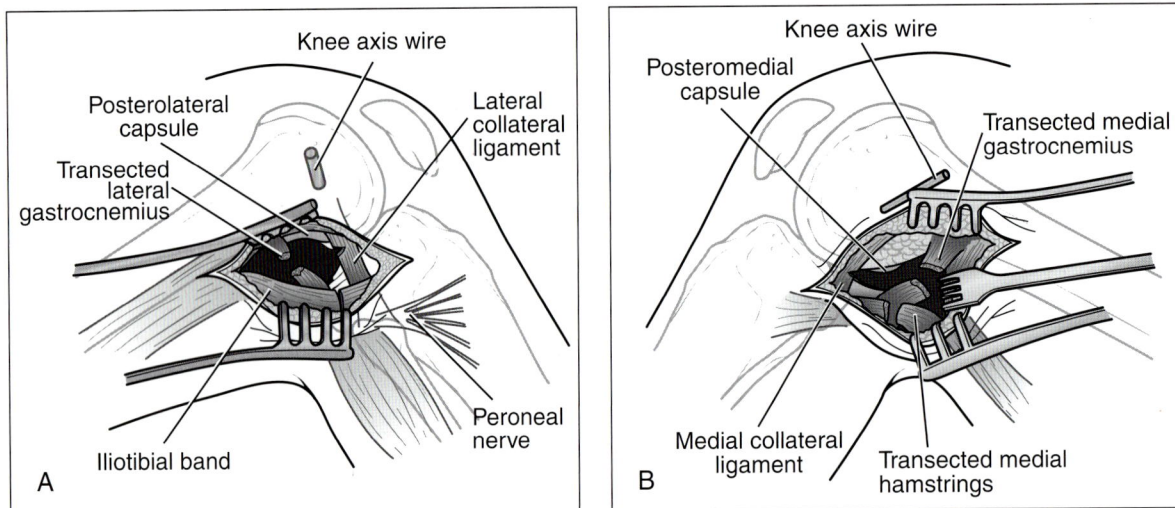

Posterior knee release. **A**, Exposure through the lateral incision. Note that the posterior halves of the iliotibial band and the lateral collateral ligament are transected. **B**, Exposure through the medial incision. Note that the posterior half of the medial collateral ligament is transected.

drilled through the axis, in a medial-to-lateral direction, protruding 3 to 6 cm on either side of the knee. It is better to place the wire slightly anteriorly and inferiorly; posterior placement will exacerbate the tendency to tibial subluxation, and proximal placement will lead to anterior femorotibial impingement in full extension. If subluxation is identified during correction, the lateral knee radiograph is evaluated for a shift in hinge axis of the frame in relation to the axis of the knee. The knee is then flexed until the tibia aligns well with the femur, followed by a realignment of the axes.

Posterior Knee Release

The leg is formally prepared and draped to the level of the anterior superior iliac spine. No tourniquet is used. With the knee flexed to 90°, lateral and medial 4- to 8-cm incisions are made parallel to the operating table, centered over the palpable posterior femoral condyle.[23] Exposure is begun laterally, splitting the fascia lata in line with its fibers, with the anterior portion kept anterior to the knee axis (**Figure 2, A**). The posterior portion of the fascia lata is transected distally. The lateral hamstrings are identified, as is the common peroneal nerve. The biceps femoris tendon can be transected or length-ened by tenotomy at the tendomuscular junction. Soft tissues are bluntly elevated off the posterior capsule until a finger can be passed to at least the middle of the knee. The lateral gastrocnemius muscle and tendon appear as a tight structure posterior to the capsule. The tendon is transected; the muscle is divided only if needed for exposure. The posterolateral corner of the capsule is incised, staying superior to the lateral meniscus. The capsulotomy is extended anteriorly, sectioning the posterior half of the lateral collateral ligament. Posteriorly, the capsule is incised as far medially as possible. If the posterior geniculate is transected, the wound is packed for 5 minutes to attain hemostasis.

The medial hamstrings are identified through the medial incision, and the gracilis and semitendinosus are tenotomized (**Figure 2, B**). The tendon of the semimembranosus is incised, leaving the underlying muscle intact. The posterior capsule is exposed, and the medial head of the gastrocnemius is treated similarly to the lateral head. The posteromedial joint capsule is incised, as is the posterior half of the medial collateral ligament, staying superior to the meniscal attachments. The capsulotomy is then completed posteriorly. If the posterior cruciate ligament is found to be tethering during knee extension, it can easily be transected. It is unusual to find significant instability of the collateral or cruciate ligaments after correction.[24] Only the skin is closed, in two layers, and without a drain.

Ilizarov Application

A femoral cage (two rings separated by four threaded rods) is affixed to the femur. Caudal to the distal ring, a medial and lateral Ilizarov universal joints are positioned in line with the knee axis wire. A tibial cage is hung from the universal joints with short, threaded rods. Distally, the tibial cage is affixed to the tibia by a transverse wire in the coronal plane. Proximally, another wire is passed, but this one is attached anteriorly to the proximal ring so that as the wire is tensioned, it pulls the tibia forward on the femur, thereby preventing posterior subluxation during contracture correction (**Figure** 3). Additional points of fixation are then added. By lengthening the threaded rods that connect the knee axis universal joints to the tibial cage, the knee joint is distracted 5 to 10 mm. A telescopic rod is used to motor the frame, either in distraction posteriorly or in compression anteriorly; an anterior rod is more convenient for sitting.

Occasionally, full rings cannot be used on the distal femur and proximal tibia, because of either ring impingement posteriorly with large flexion contractures or the soft-tissue webbing of pterygia. Instead, an anterior partial ring is used as a drop ring either in addition to or as a substitution for the periarticular full rings, providing better support for the hinges (**Figure** 4).

Postoperative Care

Correction is begun 1 week after surgery. A modified method of similar triangles is used to calculate a rate of correction between 1° and 2° per day, adjusted to the patient's tolerance.[25] Stiff knees with a hard end point and low total arc of motion require a slower rate of distraction for patient comfort and to reduce chances of periarticular fracture. The frame is maintained an additional 4 weeks at full extension. At frame removal, the leg is measured for a knee-ankle-foot orthosis with locking knee hinges. The leg is then placed in a cast in full extension, molded to prevent posterior tibial subluxation. The knee is often ligamentously unstable at frame removal; this resolves by the time of cast removal. The cast is removed after 2 to 4 weeks, and knee-ankle-foot

FIGURE 3

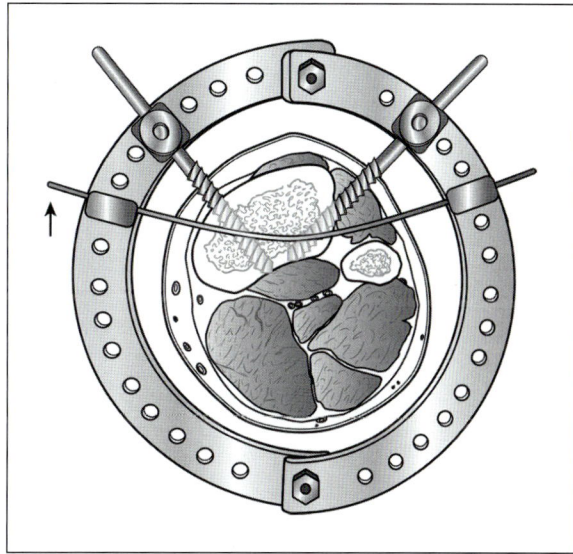

Drawing shows tensioning of the proximal tibia anteriorly. An Ilizarov wire (arrow) is attached anteriorly to the ring before tensioning the wire.

orthosis use is begun immediately. Use of the knee-ankle-foot orthosis is initially continuous, as physical therapy helps regain knee motion. Then the orthosis is used only at night, as the patient gains knee extension strength.

COMPLICATIONS

The most common significant problems encountered with gradual extension of knee contractures using external fixation are posterior tibial subluxation, recurrence of contracture, fractures, and stiff knees. Recurrences often are preceded by tibial subluxation and need to be treated with reapplication of the Ilizarov frame. Fractures can be avoided by using half-pin widths between 25% and 33% of the diameter of the bone isthmus, avoiding unicortical pins, and being aware of any limitations of hip range of motion, which could lead to excessive stress on the femur with intraoperative positioning. Periarticular bending fractures, which occur during contracture correction, are minimized by ensuring an adequate posterior release.

FIGURE 4

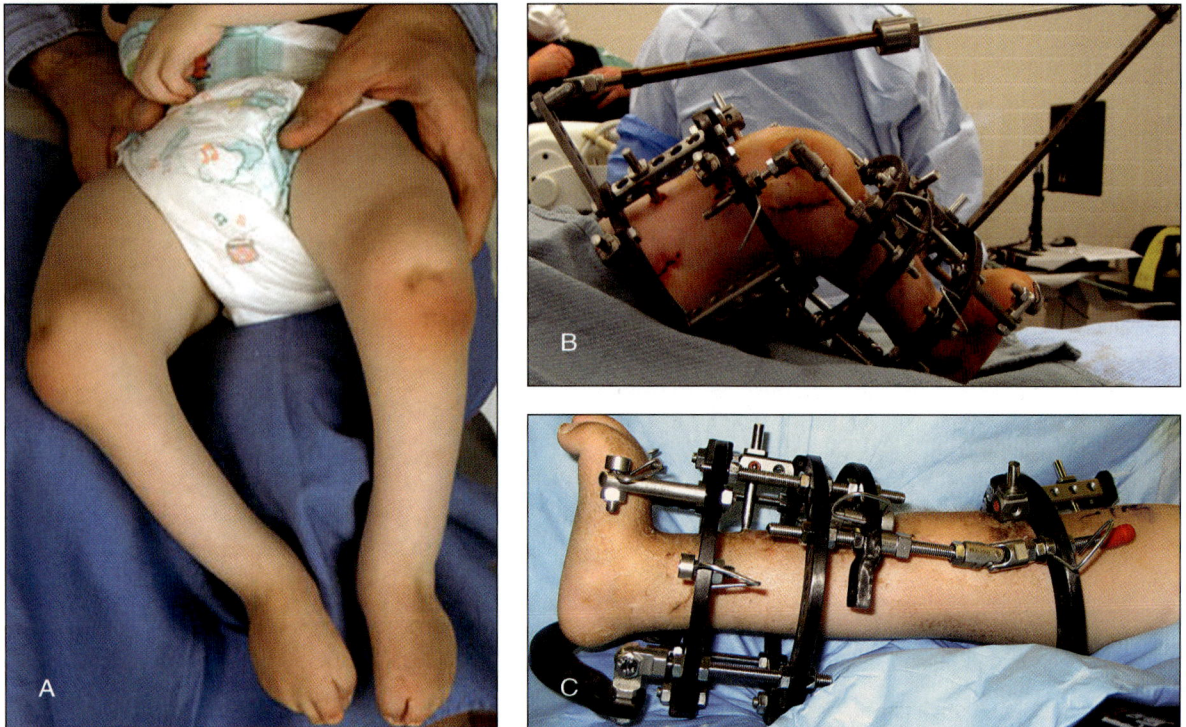

Clinical photographs of a 28-month-old boy with arthrogrypotic knee flexion contractures of 60°. An Ilizarov external fixator with a proximal tibial drop ring was used because of the patient's size. Photographs obtained preoperatively (**A**), immediately postoperatively (**B**), and at frame removal 3.5 months postoperatively (**C**). Note the proximal tibial drop ring, to prevent impingement behind the knee.

In cases of knee stiffness, the intracapsular and extracapsular components both need to be addressed. Intracapsular release can be performed through lateral and anteromedial incisions, releasing the lateral and medial patellar retinacula, suprapatellar pouch, and any intraarticular adhesions.[26,27] Extracapsular contractures are addressed by using Judet-type elevating quadricepsplasties,[26] quadriceps lengthenings,[9] or a combination of the two.[9,28,29] An elevating quadricepsplasty involves extraperiosteal release of the quadriceps off the femur and the lateral intermuscular septum. In extensive cases, the vastus lateralis is released from the greater trochanter and the rectus femoris is released from the pelvis. Quadriceps lengthening procedures can be achieved by V-Y lengthenings[9] or a more extensive release of the medial and lateral vasti from the quadriceps tendon, reattaching them more proximally, possibly combined with a rectus femoris tendon lengthening.[9,28] Occasionally, an immobile patella may require release after correction of the contracture, to improve active extension.

REFERENCES

1. Perry J: Contractures: A historical perspective. *Clin Orthop Relat Res* 1987(219):8-14.

2. Hoffer MM, Swank S, Eastman F, Clark D, Teitge R: Ambulation in severe arthrogryposis. *J Pediatr Orthop* 1983;3(3):293-296.

3. Kettelkamp DB, Johnson RJ, Smidt GL, Chao EY, Walker M: An electrogoniometric study of knee motion in normal gait. *J Bone Joint Surg Am* 1970;52(4): 775-790.

4. Levangie PK, Norkin CC: *Gait, in Joint Structure and Function: A Comprehensive Analysis.* Philadelpha, PA, FA Davis, 2001, pp 454-463, 477-478.

5. Perry J, Antonelli D, Ford W: Analysis of knee-joint forces during flexed-knee stance. *J Bone Joint Surg Am* 1975;57(7):961-967.

6. van Bosse HJ, Feldman DS, Anavian J, Sala DA: Treatment of knee flexion contractures in patients with arthrogryposis. *J Pediatr Orthop* 2007;27(8):930-937.

7. Hosny GA, Fadel M: Managing flexion knee deformity using a circular frame. *Clin Orthop Relat Res* 2008;466 (12):2995-3002.

8. Bhan S, Rath S: Modified posterior soft tissue release for management of severe knee flexion contracture. *Orthopedics* 1989;12(5):703-708.

9. Dias LS: Surgical management of knee contractures in myelomeningocele. *J Pediatr Orthop* 1982;2(2):127-131.

10. Heydarian K, Akbarnia BA, Jabalameli M, Tabador K: Posterior capsulotomy for the treatment of severe flexion contractures of the knee. *J Pediatr Orthop* 1984; 4(6):700-704.

11. Koshino T, Takeyama M, Jiang LS, Yoshida T, Saito T: Underestimation of varus angulation in knees with flexion deformity. *Knee* 2002;9(4):275-279.

12. Paley D: Sagittal plane deformities, in *Principles of Deformity Correction.* Berlin, NY, Springer, 2002, pp 155-163.

13. Eggers GW: Transplantation of hamstring tendons to femoral condyles in order to improve hip extension and to decrease knee flexion in cerebral spastic paralysis. *J Bone Joint Surg Am* 1952;34-A(4):827-830.

14. DelBello DA, Watts HG: Distal femoral extension osteotomy for knee flexion contracture in patients with arthrogryposis. *J Pediatr Orthop* 1996;16(1):122-126.

15. Saleh M, Gibson MF, Sharrard WJ: Femoral shortening in correction of congenital knee flexion deformity with popliteal webbing. *J Pediatr Orthop* 1989;9(5):609-611.

16. Parikh SN, Crawford AH, Do TT, Roy DR: Popliteal pterygium syndrome: Implications for orthopaedic management. *J Pediatr Orthop B* 2004;13(3):197-201.

17. Thomas B, Schopler S, Wood W, Oppenheim WL: The knee in arthrogryposis. *Clin Orthop Relat Res* 1985(194):87-92.

18. Asirvatham R, Mukherjee A, Agarwal S, Rooney RJ, Ellis RD, Watts HG: Supracondylar femoral extension osteotomy: Its complications. *J Pediatr Orthop* 1993;13(5):642-645.

19. Brunner R, Hefti F, Tgetgel JD: Arthrogrypotic joint contracture at the knee and the foot: Correction with a circular frame. *J Pediatr Orthop B* 1997;6(3):192-197.

20. Damsin JP, Ghanem I: Treatment of severe flexion deformity of the knee in children and adolescents using the Ilizarov technique. *J Bone Joint Surg Br* 1996;78 (1):140-144.

21. Herzenberg JE, Davis JR, Paley D, Bhave A: Mechanical distraction for treatment of severe knee flexion contractures. *Clin Orthop Relat Res* 1994(301):80-88.

22. Hollister AM, Jatana S, Singh AK, Sullivan WW, Lupichuk AG: The axes of rotation of the knee. *Clin Orthop Relat Res* 1993(290):259-268.

23. Murray C, Fixsen JA: Management of knee deformity in classical arthrogryposis multiplex congenita (amyoplasia congenita). *J Pediatr Orthop B* 1997;6(3): 186-191.

24. Södergård J, Ryöppy S: The knee in arthrogryposis multiplex congenita. *J Pediatr Orthop* 1990;10(2): 177-182.

25. Herzenberg JE, Waanders NA: Calculating rate and duration of distraction for deformity correction with the Ilizarov technique. *Orthop Clin North Am* 1991; 22(4):601-611.

26. Ali AM, Villafuerte J, Hashmi M, Saleh M: Judet's quadricepsplasty, surgical technique, and results in limb reconstruction. *Clin Orthop Relat Res* 2003(415): 214-220.

27. Ebraheim NA, DeTroye RJ, Saddemi SR: Results of Judet quadricepsplasty. *J Orthop Trauma* 1993;7(4): 327-330.

28. Burnei G, Neagoe P, Margineanu BA, Dan DD, Bucur PO: Treatment of severe iatrogenic quadriceps retraction in children. *J Pediatr Orthop B* 2004;13(4):254-258.

29. Hosalkar HS, Jones S, Chowdhury M, Hartley J, Hill RA: Quadricepsplasty for knee stiffness after femoral lengthening in congenital short femur. *J Bone Joint Surg Br* 2003;85(2):261-264.

CHAPTER 17

MANAGEMENT OF PREMATURE PHYSEAL ARREST

TIMOTHY P. CAREY, MD

INTRODUCTION

The treatment of musculoskeletal problems in children requires a thorough knowledge and understanding of the structural and functional characteristics of the immature skeleton. The primary distinguishing characteristic of the pediatric skeleton is the growth plate, or physis, which is present at the end of all long bones. Although our knowledge of physeal physiology continues to evolve, the anatomy has been well described.[1-3]

Injury to the physis is a well-recognized complication of childhood injury.[4-9] Most growth plate disturbances seen clinically are a result of traumatic injuries, although physeal injury can be seen secondary to infection, thermal injury, irradiation, and other causes.[10-14]

Complete cessation of growth secondary to physeal injury can lead to significant limb-length discrepancy (LLD) in a growing child, and techniques to deal with this are well described elsewhere in this monograph. Premature partial physeal arrest presents unique challenges because the functioning growth plate that remains can be tethered by the area of physeal bar formation, leading to progressive angular deformities, possible articular surface distortions, and relative limb shortening.[15,16]

Physeal bar (or bridge) formation can occur shortly after physeal injury, but clinically significant findings may not be apparent for some time, depending on the location of the bar and rate of growth of the involved physis.[17-19] Not all physeal bars lead to growth disturbance or deformity, so physicians must not only have a high index of suspicion for physeal bars, they must also ensure adequate follow-up of at-risk cases until resumption of normal growth is confirmed.[20] In addition, identified partial physeal arrest must be managed, taking into consideration the anatomy of the injury, the physiology of the patient, and the technical resources of the surgeon.

ETIOLOGY

The anatomy of the growth plate is well described. A columnar arrangement of chondrocytes traverses the space between the epiphyseal subchondral bone and the bone of the metaphysis. Four zones are identified from the epiphysis to the metaphysis: germinal, proliferative, hypertrophic, and provisional calcification. The germinal and proliferative zones are characterized by proliferation of small chondrocytes with abundant surrounding matrix composed of collagen, proteoglycans, and glycoproteins. With longitudinal growth, the

Dr. Carey or an immediate family member is a member of a speakers' bureau or has made paid presentations on behalf of Allergan, and has received research or institutional support from Arthrex, the Canadian Institutes of Health Research (CIHR), the Canadian Orthopaedic Foundation, DePuy, Johnson & Johnson, London Health Sciences Center, Merck, Medtronic Sofamor Danek, Smith & Nephew, Surgical Monitoring Associates, Stryker, and Synthes.

FIGURE 1

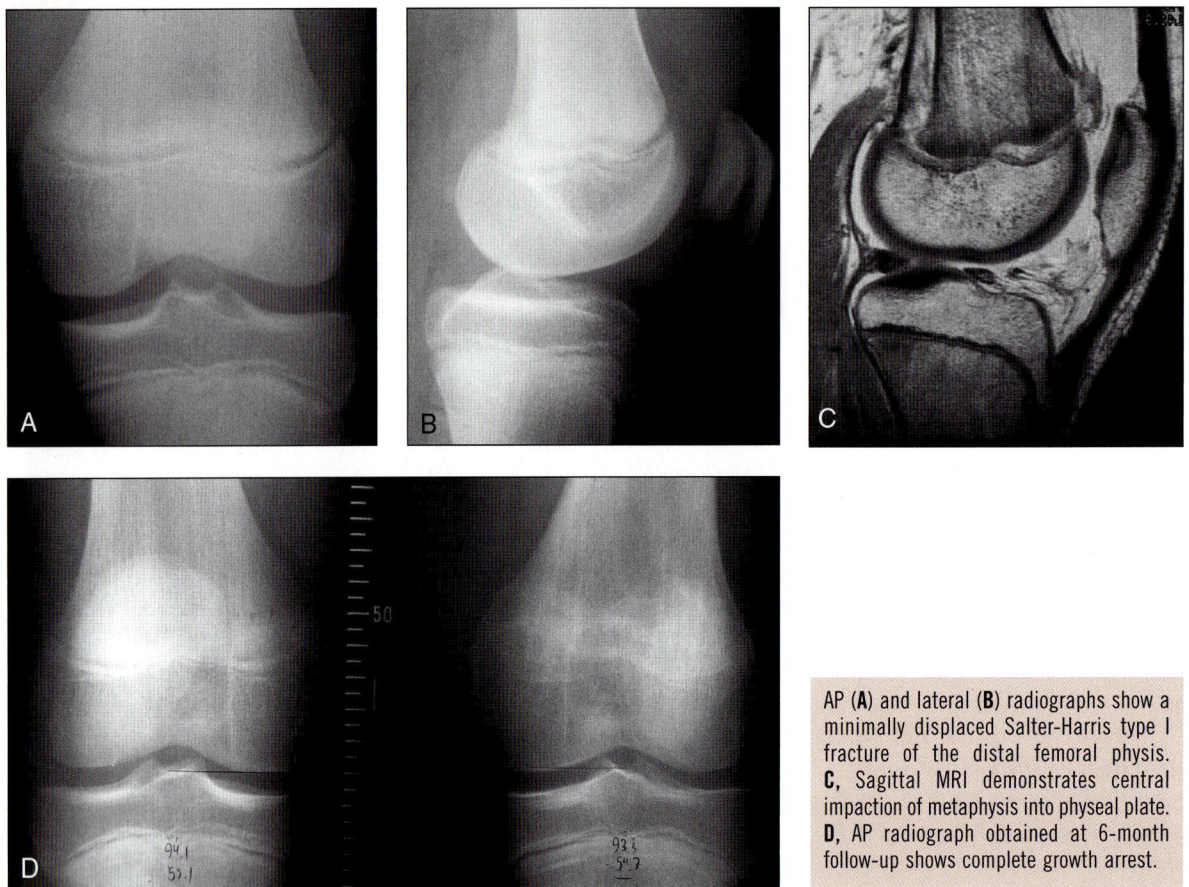

AP (**A**) and lateral (**B**) radiographs show a minimally displaced Salter-Harris type I fracture of the distal femoral physis. **C,** Sagittal MRI demonstrates central impaction of metaphysis into physeal plate. **D,** AP radiograph obtained at 6-month follow-up shows complete growth arrest.

cells mature and become hypertrophic, and there is correspondingly less matrix in the hypertrophic zone. Cell death and matrix calcification occur, followed by vascular invasion and the formation of primary bone trabeculae. Latitudinal growth is governed by the zone of Ranvier, an area of fibroblasts, chondroblasts, and osteoblasts at the edge of the physis. Mechanical support of the physis is provided by the ring of Lacroix, a tough fibrous structure at the periphery of the physis that is in continuity with the periosteum and perichondrium.[21]

Epiphyseal vessels often gain access to the cartilage-covered epiphysis via the perichondrium and are therefore at risk for disruption with physeal separation. Epiphyseal vessel disruption can lead to growth distur-

bance by affecting the germinal zone chondrocytes, whereas vascular injury to the metaphyseal circulation affects normal bone formation but does not directly affect chondrocyte proliferation.[22-24]

A physeal bar is an osseous connection between the metaphyseal and epiphyseal bone. Direct damage to the growth plate cartilage as a result of trauma is the most common mechanism. Displacement of a fracture through the growth plate in such a manner that epiphyseal and metaphyseal bone can heal in contact is another possible mechanism of bar formation.[16] The growth plate is involved in 15% to 30% of all pediatric fractures. Premature physeal arrests, however, occur in only about 10% of these physeal injuries.[6,7,9]

FIGURE 2

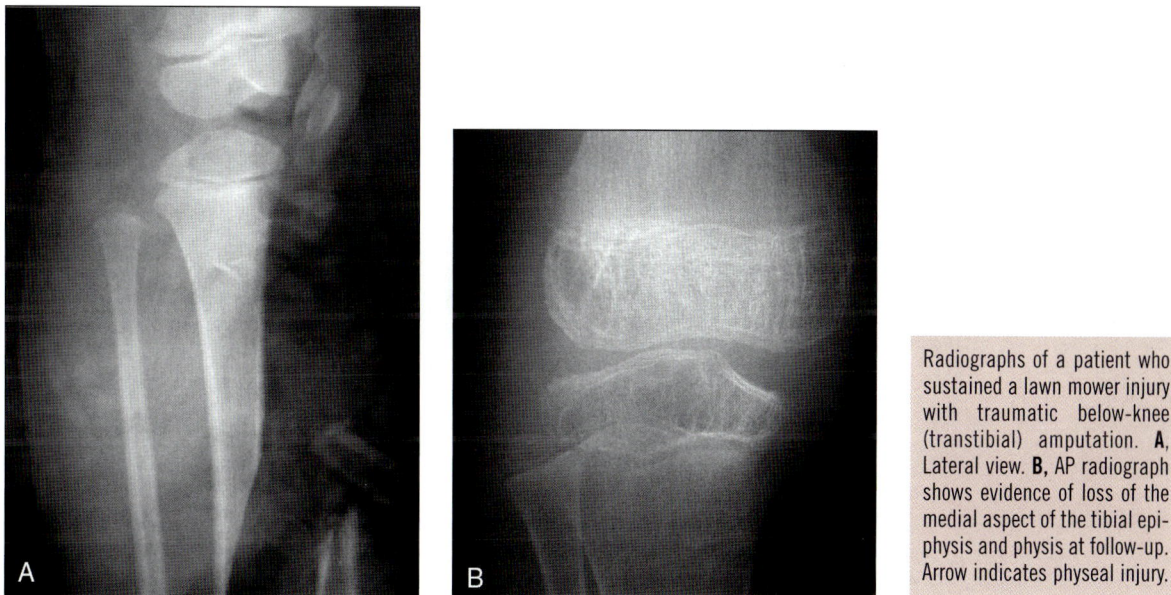

Radiographs of a patient who sustained a lawn mower injury with traumatic below-knee (transtibial) amputation. **A,** Lateral view. **B,** AP radiograph shows evidence of loss of the medial aspect of the tibial epiphysis and physis at follow-up. Arrow indicates physeal injury.

The mostly widely used classification system for physeal fractures is the Salter-Harris system, which both describes physeal injury and is prognostic of the risk of subsequent growth arrest, with an increasing incidence seen in fracture types III, IV, and V. Fracture type V and the Rang modification type VI are, by definition, growth arrests.[25] The Salter-Harris system, however, is not the sole predictor of the risk of subsequent growth arrest because clinically that risk also depends on the site of injury, mechanism of injury, and method of treatment. The influence of these factors is best demonstrated by distal femoral physeal fractures, which demonstrate high rates of growth disturbance even in relatively low-risk fracture patterns (eg, Salter-Harris types I and II).[26,27] The relatively high incidence of growth disturbance at this location suggests that physeal anatomy also may be an independent risk factor. The large surface area and significant undulations of this physis are evolutionary adaptations to the shear forces that the location is subjected to, and they are thought to increase stability and resistance to displacement.[18,28] Consequently, more energy is required to cause displacement, so when displacement does occur, this greater force can result in significant damage to the physis. The significant undulations of the physis can create areas of contact or crush injury that traverse the entire width of the growth plate, a concept that Ogden included in his modification of the Salter-Harris fracture classification system. The recognition that certain fracture patterns cause impaction of the metaphysis into the physis are reflected in Ogden's[29] subcategories (eg, type IC and IID fractures) (**Figure 1**). Experimentally, it also has been demonstrated that the fracture line in physeal fractures often propagates across the entire width of the physis, as opposed to failing solely through the weaker hypertrophic zone, as some supposed.[19,29-31]

Peterson[32] also modified physeal fracture classification systems to recognize growth arrest patterns not readily described by the Salter-Harris system. Additions include fractures of the metaphysis extending to the physis (type I) and slice fractures, where parts of the epiphysis and physis are lost (type VI) (**Figure 2**).

The Salter-Harris classification system is well established in the literature and assists greatly in the description of physeal injuries. The modifications described by Ogden and Peterson are useful because they recognize that injury patterns are occasionally more complicated than they initially appear. Optimum clinical practice

FIGURE 3

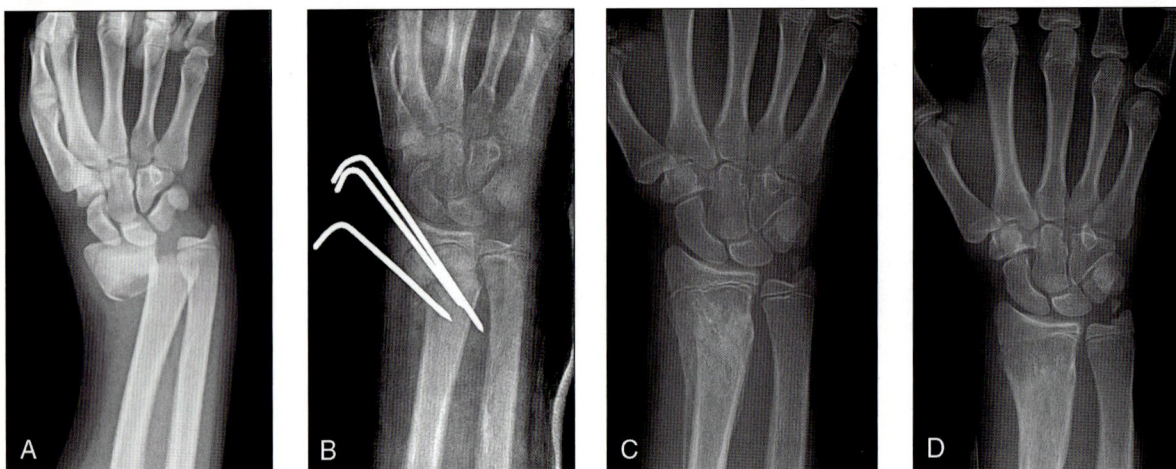

PA radiographs of a patient who sustained a displaced metaphyseal fracture of the distal radius and ulna. **A,** Preoperative view. **B,** Appearance after treatment with a closed reduction and percutaneous pinning. **C,** Appearance after pin removal. **D,** Central growth arrest, possibly a result of internal fixation, is demonstrated at 1-year follow-up.

requires evaluation of all available information related to both the fracture and the patient, including recognition of fracture patterns and locations that are at a higher risk of growth disturbance.

In addition to the effects of location, treatment of the injury can adversely affect the outcome of physeal injuries. To avoid further injury to the physis during fracture reduction, optimal treatment is required, including adequate patient analgesia and relaxation, a judicious use of force, and the avoidance of multiple repeated attempts at reduction.[33] Residual fracture displacement has been correlated with subsequent risk of growth disturbance in injuries of the distal tibial physis. An increased gap at the level of the physis, presumably created by entrapped periosteum, seemed to be a modifiable risk for fracture in one series.[34,35]

Internal fixation is not required in the management of most physeal fractures but it must be used with caution when it is indicated. Traversing the physis with fixation should be avoided whenever possible; if required, smooth pins should be used, to minimize the risk of growth plate injury. Although difficult to quantitate in clinical situations, it has been suggested experimentally that avoiding injuring more than 7% of the surface area of the physis is a useful guideline[36,37] (**Figure 3**).

Occasionally, a growth disturbance develops in physes not directly involved at the time of injury. This could be the result of an unrecognized type V injury or a direct vascular injury to the epiphyseal circulation. Similarly, repetitive microtrauma seen in some overuse syndromes has been associated with premature physeal closure.[15,38,39]

Other mechanisms of injury include infection and tumor. Disseminated infective processes seem to have the highest risk for growth complications. Multifocal neonatal osteomyelitis and meningococcemia are well recognized as having the potential for serious long-term sequelae with respect to longitudinal bone growth; microvascular emboli that cause vascular injury to the physis have been implicated as the etiology.[40,41] Direct invasion of the growth plate by a tumor or tumor-like process also has been described.[11]

Rarely, growth disturbances are due to unusual mechanisms such as isolated vascular injury in a limb or thermal or electrical injuries. Irradiation used for treatment of malignant lesions also has the risk of physeal injury[10] (**Table 1**).

FIGURE 4

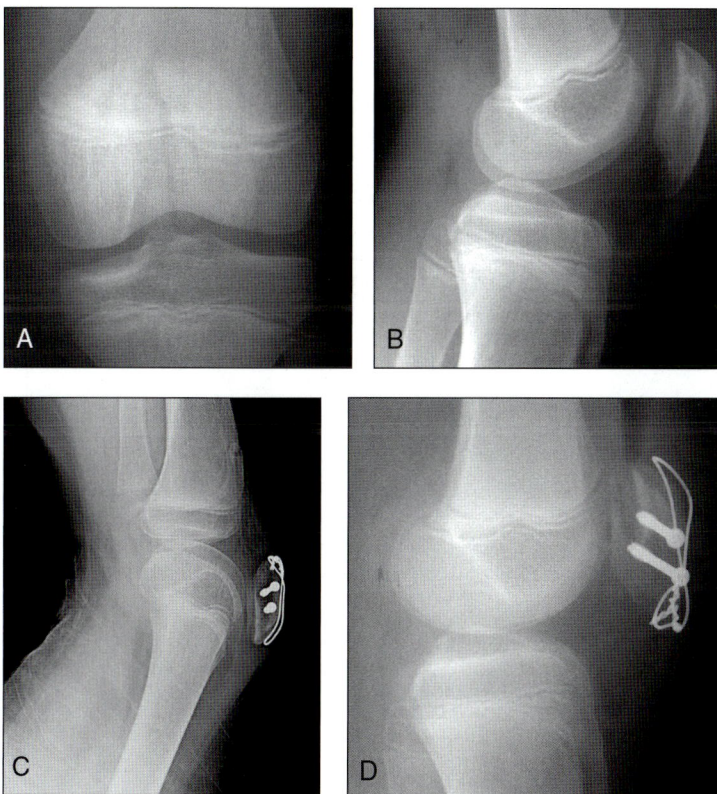

Radiographs of a patient who sustained a comminuted patellar fracture in motocross bike accident. Preoperative AP (**A**) and lateral (**B**) views. **C**, Lateral radiograph obtained after treatment with internal fixation. **D**, Lateral weight-bearing radiograph obtained at 1-year follow-up shows anterior growth arrest at the proximal tibial physis.

EVALUATION AND CLASSIFICATION

One of the most significant complications of physeal fractures is premature physeal growth arrest. As discussed above, multiple factors are implicated; unfortunately, even with appropriate treatment, growth arrest and physeal bar formation can occur. A high index of suspicion for physeal arrest is required in certain injury patterns and close follow-up is mandatory in these situations[42,43] (**Figure 4**).

The hallmark of premature growth arrest is a demonstrated failure of normal longitudinal growth, best documented on radiographs. The undulating, three-dimensional nature of the physis can make complete visualization on any one radiographic view a challenge. Occasionally, a physeal arrest will be obvious as an area of sclerotic bone traversing the physis, but many times

TABLE 1   **Etiologies of Premature Physeal Arrest***

Trauma
Associated with nonphyseal fractures
Physeal fractures
Repetitive microtrauma
Infection
Disseminated (eg, meningococcemia)
Local (eg, osteomyelitis)
Iatrogenic intraoperative injury/internal fixation
Tumor
Thermal injury
Vascular insufficiency
Irradiation

*Causes listed in order of prevalence.

FIGURE 5

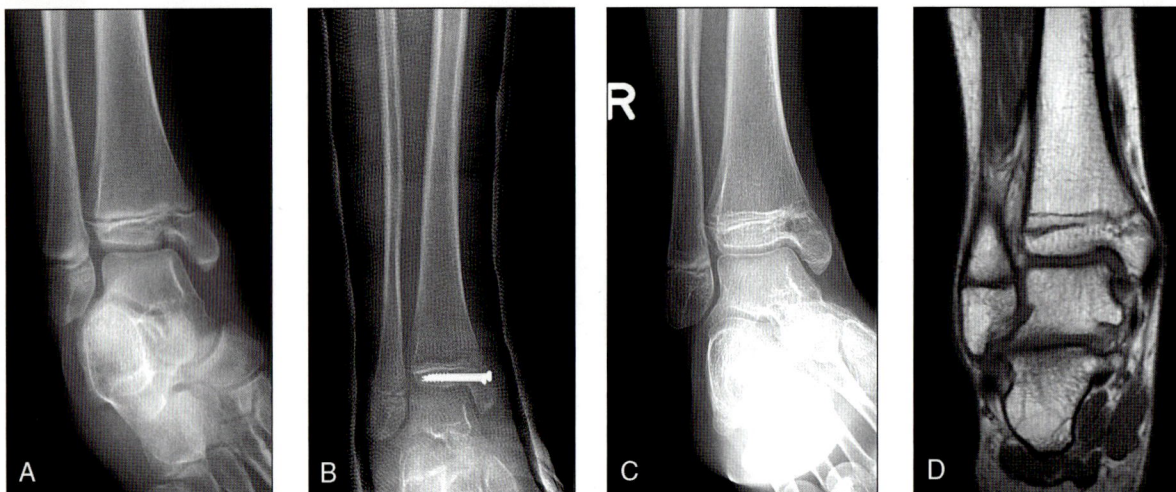

Images of a patient who sustained a Salter-Harris type IV fracture of the medial malleolus. **A,** Preoperative AP radiograph. **B,** AP view obtained after transepiphyseal internal fixation. **C,** AP view obtained at follow-up demonstrates linear arrest. Note converging growth arrest line. **D,** Coronal T1-weighted MRI shows physeal bar and growth arrest line.

it is not seen distinctly. Asymmetry in the appearance of growth arrest lines is a useful sign. These subtle horizontal markings in the trabecular bone of the metaphysis denote a period of relatively slow growth occurring around the time of injury. As normal growth rates are reestablished, these radiographic features should maintain a parallel relationship to the physis and move away as growth proceeds. Alterations in normal physeal growth can present as asymmetry, and convergence of the line with the physis indicates a complete growth arrest.[44,45] Other signs of growth arrest include angular deformity, epiphyseal distortion, and shortening (**Figure 5**).[46,47]

When a premature growth arrest is suspected based on clinical and radiographic results, further imaging to better characterize the arrest is usually indicated. Plain tomographic imaging has been supplanted by CT, and fine-cut CT scans with coronal and sagittal reconstruction are useful to help identify areas of bony bridges between metaphyseal and epiphyseal bone.[20,48,49]

MRI has proved extremely sensitive in helping evaluate the physis and demonstrating the extent of physeal bars, which can give some indication of the relative health of the adjacent physis. This is especially useful in nontraumatic growth disturbances, where one may see more widespread physeal disorganization.[50] MRI techniques continue to evolve with experience, and sequences that demonstrate cartilage optimally (eg, three-dimensional spoiled gradient-echo recalled images with fat saturation) are indicated in the evaluation of physeal bars.[45,51-53] Complete imaging is required for treatment decisions and should include weight-bearing long-leg radiographs to assess alignment, scanograms to accurately determine LLDs, and bone age determination.

Growth arrest can be classified by etiology and location. Etiologic classification is useful as a prognostic factor because surgical treatment of physeal arrests is more likely to be successful with posttraumatic bars and in infantile Blount disease. Restoration of normal growth is less predictable with other etiologies, presumably because of greater involvement of the physis with these processes (**Table 1**).

Classification by location of the area of arrest relative to the remaining intact physis is helpful for surgical planning. Physeal bars can be divided into three main subgroups: peripheral bars, linear bars, and central bars [36] (**Figure 6**).

Peripheral (type I) bars occur along the margin of the physis and are due to injury to the zone of Ranvier; because of their location, they can cause significant angular deformity over a relatively short period. Linear (type II) bars are created by a bony bridge extending through the physis from one side to another, with normal physis on either side of the bridge. Linear bars are commonly seen above the medial corner of the ankle mortise after Salter-Harris IV injuries of the medial malleolus. Central (type III) bars cause tethering of the physis with resultant alterations in normal physeal and joint anatomy, LLD, and variable angular deformity, depending on the eccentricity of the lesion.

TREATMENT

The management of premature physeal growth arrest requires a consideration of all the variables discussed above. Every attempt should be made to provide optimal treatment of physeal injuries at the outset. Management of children's fractures involving the growth plate requires appropriate protection of the physis during reduction maneuvers, strict criteria for acceptable reduction, appropriate fixation techniques when indicated, and potentially prophylactic techniques for inserting interposition material when operating on high-risk fracture patterns (eg, type IV and VI injuries).[54]

The treatment approach for established growth disturbances depends on whether restoration of normal growth at the injured physis is achievable. Treatment options include the following: no treatment, completion of growth arrest with epiphysiodesis, physeal bar excision, and angular correction/lengthening. No treatment is appropriate when little growth remains and the projected length discrepancy/angular deformity is deemed acceptable.

If treatment is considered necessary, the ideal treatment is to restore normal growth at the site of injury. Physeal bar excision is an attractive option and can restore growth, but it is a technically demanding procedure with variable results.[55-57] Other techniques for managing length discrepancies and angular deformities exist and often are more appropriate. The first treatment question to answer, therefore, is whether the patient is a candidate for physeal bar excision. Location of the

FIGURE 6

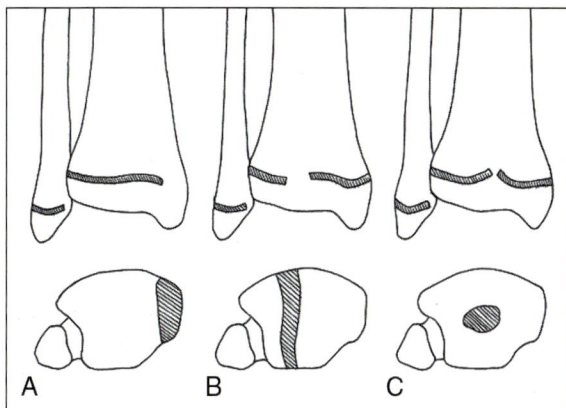

Anterior (top) and cross-section (bottom) drawings of the Peterson classification of physeal bridges. Shaded areas: peripheral (**A**), elongated (**B**), and central (**C**). Note the tenting of the physis (top drawings) caused by peripheral growth. (Reproduced with permission from Khoshal KI, Keifer GN: Physeal bridge resection. *J Am Acad Orthop Surg* 2005;13[1]:51.)

physis involved is an important factor because anatomic constraints make certain physes extremely difficult to access safely (eg, proximal femur). In addition, the amount of potential growth to be restored needs to be calculated. Traditionally, more than 2 years of remaining growth has been regarded as necessary to make bar resection worthwhile, but given the significant variation in growth rates of different physes, an accurate calculation of growth remaining at the involved physis is a more appropriate determination. A completely normal growth rate is rarely restored by means of bar excision, and premature closure after a seemingly successful procedure occurs quite frequently.[56]

An additional requirement for bar excision is sufficient remaining normal physeal area to produce continued longitudinal growth. Physeal bar excision merely removes the bony bridge between the epiphysis and metaphysis and leaves a void in this area of the physis. At least 50% of the normal surface area of the physis is considered a minimum requirement for longitudinal growth, although clinical experience would suggest that this may be an overly optimistic estimation; some authors consider bars occupying more than 25% of the physeal surface area nonresectable.[57] An additional risk

FIGURE 7

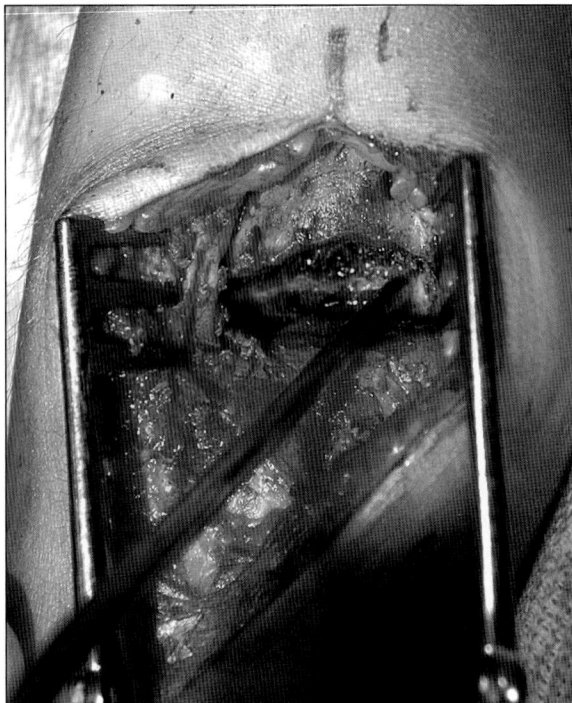

Intraoperative photograph of physeal bar resection of distal tibia demonstrates complete visualization of the physis at the base of the resection cavity.

with larger areas of resection is potential failure of the overlying epiphyseal bone with loading, particularly if a nonstructural interposition material is used.

If the area of physeal arrest is considered unresectable, two treatment options are available: completion of the growth arrest, if necessary to prevent further asymmetric growth and resultant deformity; and corrective osteotomy, if the angular deformity is significant. Often these options are performed as a combined procedure. In situations where there is a matched bone, epiphysiodesis of that bone also must be performed to prevent development of deformity secondary to continued growth (eg, performing a distal fibular epiphysiodesis for a complete growth arrest of the distal tibia to prevent a progressive varus angulation developing at the ankle).[58-60] Treatment also includes calculation and management of the final LLD. Lengthening techniques

and angular correction combined with lengthening are frequently necessary and are described elsewhere in this monograph. Contralateral epiphysiodesis can be performed to manage less significant discrepancies, or in combination with lengthening for severe degrees of discrepancy.

Surgical resection of physeal bars is considered in cases that meet the above inclusion criteria. Careful preoperative planning is necessary to determine the exact location and size of the bony bar so the surgical excision can be performed efficiently and with the least amount of damage to surrounding tissues. Access to the bar depends on the location. The use of a metaphyseal window is required for most central bars, although in cases where a significant angular deformity is present, a corrective osteotomy can be used to gain access. Peripheral bars are accessed by means of direct exposure with resection of the overlying periosteum.[42]

The bone comprising the physeal bar is often very sclerotic, and it can be extremely difficult at times to identify the plane of the physis. Intraoperative fluoroscopy is mandatory, and the ability to visualize the exposed physis as the excision proceeds is crucial to prevent excess removal of normal juxtaphyseal bone. For central and linear bars in particular, the surgical field is a deep cavity, and adequate lighting and a dry field are of paramount importance. Use of a headlight and, occasionally, a "dry" arthroscope or dental mirror will help ensure adequate visualization of the intact physeal cartilage circumferentially at the end of the procedure. A combination of rongeurs, angled and straight curets, and a high-speed burr may all be required to facilitate removal of the sclerotic bone[61] (**Figure 7**).

Once an adequate resection has been achieved, some form of interposition material must be placed in the cavity to prevent reformation of the bony bridge between metaphysis and epiphysis. Although several materials have been used historically, at present, the two choices are an autologous fat graft or polymethylmethacrylate (PMMA). Fat, harvested locally or distantly, is readily available and theoretically may remain viable long term. Fat can sometimes be difficult to secure in the bed of resection, however, and it is difficult to ensure that it stays with the epiphysis during growth. In addition, fat provides no structural support. PMMA does provide support, and it can be inserted in a "collar button" fash-

FIGURE 8

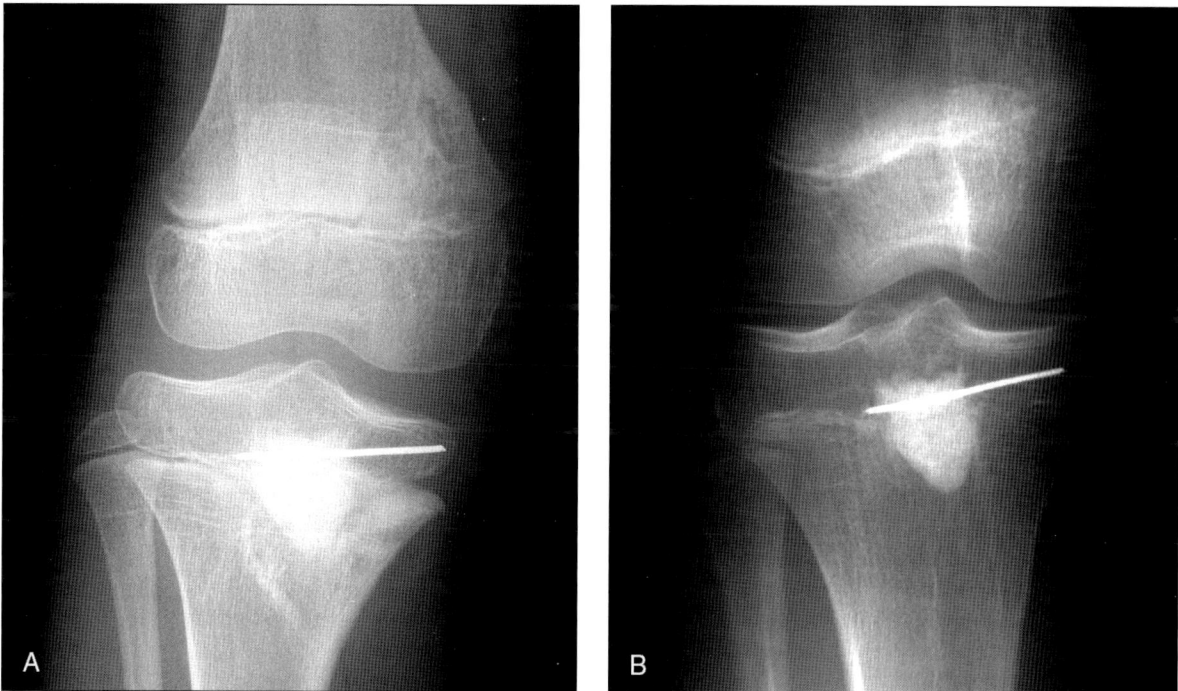

AP radiographs obtained after resection of a central physeal bar in the proximal tibia and insertion of polymethylmethacrylate (PMMA) interposition material demonstrate the position of the PMMA plug immediately postoperatively (**A**) and at 2-year follow-up (**B**). Note that the position of the PMMA plug in the epiphysis was maintained.

ion by means of slight undercutting of the epiphyseal bone to ensure the cement plug stays adherent to the epiphysis with growth and continues to block transphyseal bone formation. A low-temperature cement minimizes the risk of local thermal injury, and the radiopaque quality facilitates long-term radiographic follow-up. Metallic markers placed in the epiphysis and metaphysis also make assessing subsequent growth easier, and the epiphyseal pin can often help anchor the cement plug (**Figure 8**).[36]

With a significant angular deformity, an additional decision is whether to perform a corrective osteotomy at the time of bar resection. Spontaneous improvement of angular deformity after bar excision has been reported but is inconsistent. A corrective osteotomy can usually be performed at the time of physeal surgery without too much difficulty, particularly in areas with little tolerance for residual deformity (eg, coronal plane deformity at the ankle), and is indicated for angular deformities greater than 10° to 20°.[36,55,62]

Close follow-up is required to monitor the success of the procedure because even when growth is restored, early physeal closure or bar reformation can occur. Reported success rates vary considerably, probably because of the varying etiologies, locations, and extent of bar formation included in these reviews.[57,62-64]

REFERENCES

1. Bright RW: Operative correction of partial epiphyseal plate closure by osseous-bridge resection and silicone-rubber implant: An experimental study in dogs. *J Bone Joint Surg Am* 1974;56(4):655-664.

2. Craig JG, Cody DD, Van Holsbeeck M: The distal femoral and proximal tibial growth plates: MR imaging, three-dimensional modeling and estimation of area and volume. *Skeletal Radiol* 2004;33(6):337-344.

3. Birch JG, Herring JA, Wenger DR: Surgical anatomy of selected physes. *J Pediatr Orthop* 1984;4(2):224-231.

4. Aitken AP: Fractures of the epiphyses. *Clin Orthop Relat Res* 1965(41):19-23.

5. Mann DC, Rajmaira S: Distribution of physeal and nonphyseal fractures in 2,650 long-bone fractures in children aged 0-16 years. *J Pediatr Orthop* 1990;10(6): 713-716.

6. Mizuta T, Benson WM, Foster BK, Paterson DC, Morris LL: Statistical analysis of the incidence of physeal injuries. *J Pediatr Orthop* 1987;7(5):518-523.

7. Peterson HA, Madhok R, Benson JT, Ilstrup DM, Melton LJ III: Physeal fractures: Part I. Epidemiology in Olmsted County, Minnesota, 1979-1988. *J Pediatr Orthop* 1994;14(4):423-430.

8. Rang MC: Injuries of the epiphyses, the growth plate, and the perichondrial ring, in *Children's Fractures*, ed 2. Philadelphia, PA, JB Lippincott, 1983, pp 10-25.

9. Worlock P, Stower M: Fracture patterns in Nottingham children. *J Pediatr Orthop* 1986;6(6):656-660.

10. Peterson HA, Wood MB: Physeal arrest due to laser beam damage in a growing child. *J Pediatr Orthop* 2001;21(3):335-337.

11. Stanton RP, Abdel-Mota'al MM: Growth arrest resulting from unicameral bone cyst. *J Pediatr Orthop* 1998;18(2):198-201.

12. Hernandez J Jr, Peterson HA: Fracture of the distal radial physis complicated by compartment syndrome and premature physeal closure. *J Pediatr Orthop* 1986;6(5):627-630.

13. Kruse RW, Tassanawipas A, Bowen JR: Orthopedic sequelae of meningococcemia. *Orthopedics* 1991; 14(2):174-178.

14. Langenskiöld A: Growth disturbance after osteomyelitis of femoral condyles in infants. *Acta Orthop Scand* 1984;55(1):1-13.

15. Bowler JR, Mubarak SJ, Wenger DR: Tibial physeal closure and genu recurvatum after femoral fracture: Occurrence without a tibial traction pin. *J Pediatr Orthop* 1990;10(5):653-657.

16. Cass JR, Peterson HA: Salter-Harris Type-IV injuries of the distal tibial epiphyseal growth plate, with emphasis on those involving the medial malleolus. *J Bone Joint Surg Am* 1983;65(8):1059-1070.

17. Berson L, Davidson RS, Dormans JP, Drummond DS, Gregg JR: Growth disturbances after distal tibial physeal fractures. *Foot Ankle Int* 2000;21(1):54-58.

18. Lombardo SJ, Harvey JP Jr: Fractures of the distal femoral epiphyses: Factors influencing prognosis. A review of thirty-four cases. *J Bone Joint Surg Am* 1977;59(6):742-751.

19. Ogden JA, Ganey T, Light TR, Southwick WO: The pathology of acute chondro-osseous injury in the child. *Yale J Biol Med* 1993;66(3):219-233.

20. Young JW, Bright RW, Whitley NO: Computed tomography in the evaluation of partial growth plate arrest in children. *Skeletal Radiol* 1986;15(7):530-535.

21. Ogden JA: Anatomy and physiology of skeletal development, in *Skeletal Injury in the Child*. Philadelphia, PA, WB Saunders, 1990, p 930.

22. Trueta J, Amato VP: The vascular contribution to osteogenesis: Part III. Changes in the growth cartilage caused by experimentally induced ischaemia. *J Bone Joint Surg Br* 1960;42-B:571-587.

23. Trueta J, Morgan JD: The vascular contribution to osteogenesis: Part I. Studies by the injection method. *J Bone Joint Surg Br* 1960;42-B:97-109.

24. Ecklund K, Jaramillo D: Patterns of premature physeal arrest: MR imaging of 111 children. *AJR Am J Roentgenol* 2002;178(4):967-972.

25. Salter RB: Injuries of the epiphyseal plate. *Instr Course Lect* 1992;41:351-359.

26. Beals RK: Premature closure of the physis following diaphyseal fractures. *J Pediatr Orthop* 1990;10(6): 717-720.

27. Hresko MT, Kasser JR: Physeal arrest about the knee associated with non-physeal fractures in the lower extremity. *J Bone Joint Surg Am* 1989;71(5):698-703.

28. Riseborough EJ, Barrett IR, Shapiro F: Growth disturbances following distal femoral physeal fracture-separations. *J Bone Joint Surg Am* 1983;65(7):885-893.

29. Ogden JA: Skeletal growth mechanism injury patterns. *J Pediatr Orthop* 1982;2(4):371-377.

30. Smith DG, Geist RW, Cooperman DR: Microscopic examination of a naturally occurring epiphyseal plate fracture. *J Pediatr Orthop* 1985;5(3):306-308.

31. Wattenbarger JM, Gruber HE, Phieffer LS: Physeal fractures: Part I. Histologic features of bone, cartilage, and bar formation in a small animal model. J *Pediatr Orthop* 2002;22(6):703-709.

32. Peterson HA: Physeal fractures: Part II. Two previously unclassified types. *J Pediatr Orthop* 1994;14(4):431-438.

33. Egol KA, Karunakar M, Phieffer L, Meyer R, Wattenbarger JM: Early versus late reduction of a physeal fracture in an animal model. *J Pediatr Orthop* 2002;22(2):208-211.

34. Gruber HE, Phieffer LS, Wattenbarger JM: Physeal fractures: Part II. Fate of interposed periosteum in a physeal fracture. *J Pediatr Orthop* 2002;22(6):710-716.

35. Phieffer LS, Meyer RA Jr, Gruber HE, Easley M, Wattenbarger JM: Effect of interposed periosteum in an animal physeal fracture model. *Clin Orthop Relat Res* 2000(376):15-25.

36. Peterson HA: Partial growth plate arrest and its treatment. *J Pediatr Orthop* 1984;4(2):246-258.

37. Guille JT, Yamazaki A, Bowen JR: Physeal surgery: Indications and operative treatment. *Am J Orthop (Belle Mead NJ)* 1997;26(5):323-332.

38. Albanese SA, Palmer AK, Kerr DR, Carpenter CW, Lisi D, Levinsohn EM: Wrist pain and distal growth plate closure of the radius in gymnasts. *J Pediatr Orthop* 1989;9(1):23-28.

39. Carter SR, Aldridge MJ: Stress injury of the distal radial growth plate. *J Bone Joint Surg Br* 1988;70(5):834-836.

40. Grogan DP, Love SM, Ogden JA, Millar EA, Johnson LO: Chondro-osseous growth abnormalities after meningococcemia: A clinical and histopathological study. *J Bone Joint Surg Am* 1989;71(6):920-928.

41. Jacobsen ST, Crawford AH: Amputation following meningococcemia: A sequela to purpura fulminans. *Clin Orthop Relat Res* 1984(185):214-219.

42. Ogden JA: Management of growth mechanism injuries and arrest, in *Skeletal Injury in the Child.* New York, NY, Springer-Verlag, 2000.

43. Craig JG, Cramer KE, Cody DD, et al: Premature partial closure and other deformities of the growth plate: MR imaging and three-dimensional modeling. *Radiology* 1999;210(3):835-843.

44. Ogden JA: Growth slowdown and arrest lines. *J Pediatr Orthop* 1984;4(4):409-415.

45. Futami T, Foster BK, Morris LL, LeQuesne GW: Magnetic resonance imaging of growth plate injuries: The efficacy and indications for surgical procedures. *Arch Orthop Trauma Surg* 2000;120(7-8):390-396.

46. Kasser JR: Physeal bar resections after growth arrest about the knee. *Clin Orthop Relat Res* 1990(255):68-74.

47. Lalonde KA, Letts M: Traumatic growth arrest of the distal tibia: A clinical and radiographic review. *Can J Surg* 2005;48(2):143-147.

48. Loder RT, Swinford AE, Kuhns LR: The use of helical computed tomographic scan to assess bony physeal bridges. *J Pediatr Orthop* 1997;17(3):356-359.

49. Carlson WO, Wenger DR: A mapping method to prepare for surgical excision of a partial physeal arrest. *J Pediatr Orthop* 1984;4(2):232-238.

50. Carey J, Spence L, Blickman H, Eustace S: MRI of pediatric growth plate injury: Correlation with plain film radiographs and clinical outcome. *Skeletal Radiol* 1998;27(5):250-255.

51. Lohman M, Kivisaari A, Vehmas T, Kallio P, Puntila J, Kivisaari L: MRI in the assessment of growth arrest. *Pediatr Radiol* 2002;32(1):41-45.

52. Sailhan F, Chotel F, Guibal AL, et al: Three-dimensional MR imaging in the assessment of physeal growth arrest. *Eur Radiol* 2004;14(9):1600-1608.

53. Jaramillo D, Connolly SA, Vajapeyam S, et al: Normal and ischemic epiphysis of the femur: Diffusion MR imaging study in piglets. *Radiology* 2003;227(3):825-832.

54. Foster BK, Hansen AL, Gibson GJ, Hopwood JJ, Binns GF, Wiebkin OW: Reimplantation of growth plate chondrocytes into growth plate defects in sheep. *J Orthop Res* 1990;8(4):555-564.

55. Williamson RV, Staheli LT: Partial physeal growth arrest: Treatment by bridge resection and fat interposition. *J Pediatr Orthop* 1990;10(6):769-776.

56. Hasler CC, Foster BK: Secondary tethers after physeal bar resection: A common source of failure? *Clin Orthop Relat Res* 2002(405):242-249.

57. Rathjen KE, BJ: Physeal injuries and growth disturbances, in Kasser JR, Beaty JH, eds: *Rockwood and Wilkins' Fractures in Children.* Philadelphia, PA, Lippincott Williams & Wilkins, 2005, p 1200.

58. Green WT, Anderson M: Skeletal age and the control of bone growth. *Instr Course Lect* 1960;17:199-217.

59. Anderson M, Green WT, Messner MB: Growth and predictions of growth in the lower extremities. *J Bone Joint Surg Am* 1963;45-A:1-14.

60. Anderson M, Messner MB, Green WT: Distribution of lengths of the normal femur and tibia in children from one to eighteen years of age. *J Bone Joint Surg Am* 1964;46:1197-1202.

61. Khoshhal KI, Kiefer GN: Physeal bridge resection. *J Am Acad Orthop Surg* 2005;13(1):47-58.

62. Ogden JA: The evaluation and treatment of partial physeal arrest. J Bone Joint Surg Am 1987;69(8):1297-1302.

63. Birch JG: Surgical technique of physeal bar resection. *Instr Course Lect* 1992;41:445-450.

64. Peterson H: Physeal injuries and growth arrest, in Beaty JH, Kasser JR, eds: *Rockwood and Wilkins' Fractures in Children.* Philadelphia, PA, Lippincott Williams & Wilkins, 2001, pp 91-138.

CHAPTER 18

TREATMENT OF SEGMENTAL BONE LOSS DUE TO TRAUMA

DAVID W. LOWENBERG, MD

INTRODUCTION

The increased incidence of high-energy trauma has resulted in the need for improved methods of treatment of segmental defects in long bones. Many methods have been used over time, with varying success rates, but autologous grafting remains the gold standard. Autologous grafting for segmental defects uses massive cancellous grafting, avascular fibular transfers, vascularized free osseous transfers (with or without an accompanying soft-tissue envelope), and tibiofibular synostoses.[1-9] These methods have their limitations, however, depending on the health of the soft-tissue envelope and the total amount of bone defect. Graft hypertrophy and refracture have remained huge issues in patients treated with these methods. In the larger series[5,6,9] using free vascularized fibular transfers, graft hypertrophy is reported to take 18 months, thus necessitating protected weight bearing. A deep infection rate in the range of 10% is reported, and major complications occur in 8% to 30% of patients in series using large nonvascularized bone grafts.

Treatment of segmental defects with allograft bone, including demineralized allogenic bone matrix, has had mixed results and currently does not represent the standard of care.[10]

Newer ceramics appear promising for filling segmental defects. Studies on their efficacy, however, remain limited to rabbit and sheep models.[11-14] Their value in clinical practice is limited to case reports, and no controlled studies have been reported.

Few studies have compared the efficacy of bone transport with that of grafting procedures. Cierny and Zorn[15] looked at two subsets of patients with segmental defects of the tibia after débridement. In one group, the defect was treated with bone transport; in the other group, conventional methods of treatment with massive cancellous grafts and tissue transfers were used. The overall success rate (95%) was the same in the two groups. The bone transport group, however, had a lower incidence of complications (33% versus 60%) and 23 fewer days of hospitalization, representing a cost savings of $30,000 per patient. Platz et al[16] more recently reported the value of bone transport as compared with free vascularized fibular transfer for treatment of lower extremity defects and found that defects smaller than 12 cm were better treated with bone transport, whereas defects greater than 12 cm were better treated with a free vascularized fibular transfer. Some recent unpublished work presented at meetings on the use of titanium cages filled with bone graft is promising, but it is too early to

Dr. Lowenberg or an immediate family member serves as a board member, owner, officer, or committee member of the Limb Length and Reconstruction Society and the California Pacific Medical Center; is a member of a speakers' bureau or has made paid presentations on behalf of Stryker; and serves as a paid consultant to or is an employee of Stryker.

FIGURE 1

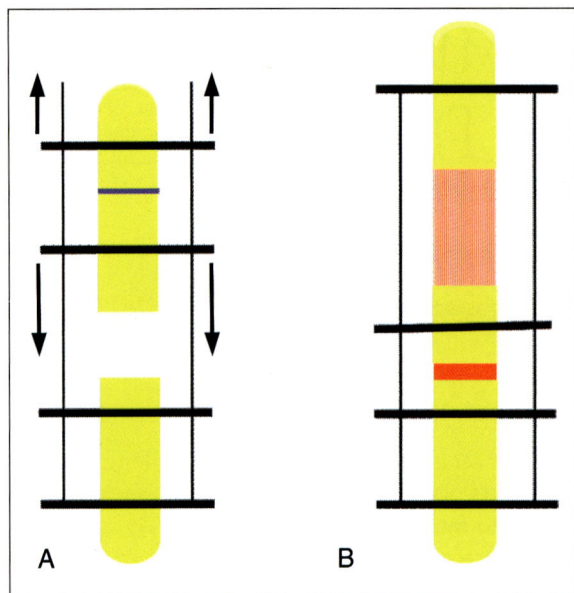

Schematic shows a ring fixator used for transport (**A**), then converted to a lengthener (**B**). (Adapted with permission from Kevin Louie, MD, California Pacific Medical Center, San Francisco, CA.)

say whether this will replace the other accepted methods of treatment.

The best treatment for severe, traumatic injuries to the lower extremity clearly involves attaining early restoration of a healthy soft-tissue envelope followed by restitution of the bone segment. The best results occur when alignment and limb length both are achieved with a healed bone; Lowenberg et al,[17] Gopal et al,[18] and McKee et al[19] have reported good long-term clinical outcomes when these goals are met.[20] These studies show the need for aggressive free-tissue transfer or rotational muscle coverage, which provides a means to effectively restore the bone segment, regardless of the method used. Among these series, bone transport seems to result in the most predictable restoration of limb length and alignment.

SELECTION OF PATIENTS

Ideal candidates for bone transport are those with a diaphyseal defect of the long bones of the lower extremities. Although bone transport is more easily performed in the tibia, it also can be successful in the femur. If a joint is involved, the patient must be made aware of potential posttraumatic arthritis despite limb salvage. The patient also may require bridging of the joint during the process to prevent contracture. If significant destruction of the ankle joint exists, the patient might have a better outcome with primary arthrodesis of the joint.

Because the process of bone transport is rather thorough and demanding of patients, it is recommended that the patient be evaluated by a psychiatrist or psychologist for any underlying mental health issues. If the patient is deemed a viable candidate, these practitioners can aid the patient with issues that may arise during the treatment process, such as depression.

PREOPERATIVE PLANNING

Proper preoperative planning includes careful evaluation of the soft-tissue envelope. I readily consider a limb viable for a soft-tissue augmentation procedure (free muscle transfer) if the existing soft-tissue envelope is extremely atrophic in an isolated location. I have found this helps with bone healing as well. Therefore, if any concern exists regarding the patency of vessels to the limb, digital subtraction angiography or CT angiography is often performed.

Radiographs also are necessary, to determine the amount of bone deficiency. This is not as straightforward as it might seem, because atrophic bone ends often exist, which must be trimmed back to viable bone ends. In many traumatized limbs, a limb-length discrepancy (LLD) may exist. Performing a bone transport also allows for the rare opportunity to correct LLD and deformity (including rotational deformity) during the process. Therefore, during the preoperative templating process, radiographic studies, including a 51-inch–cassette AP weight-bearing (when possible) view from hip to ankle or a CT scanogram of both lower extremities, are quite useful in determining comparative absolute limb-length segments.

The actual bone deficiency in an affected limb is the sum of the measured defect plus the amount of resected, nonviable bone ends plus the measured LLD. The beauty of bone transport methodology is that with proper treatment of a corticotomy site, the frame can be converted to a lengthener upon completion of bone transport. Once the defect is filled, the LLD often can be corrected as well (**Figure 1**).

FIGURE 2

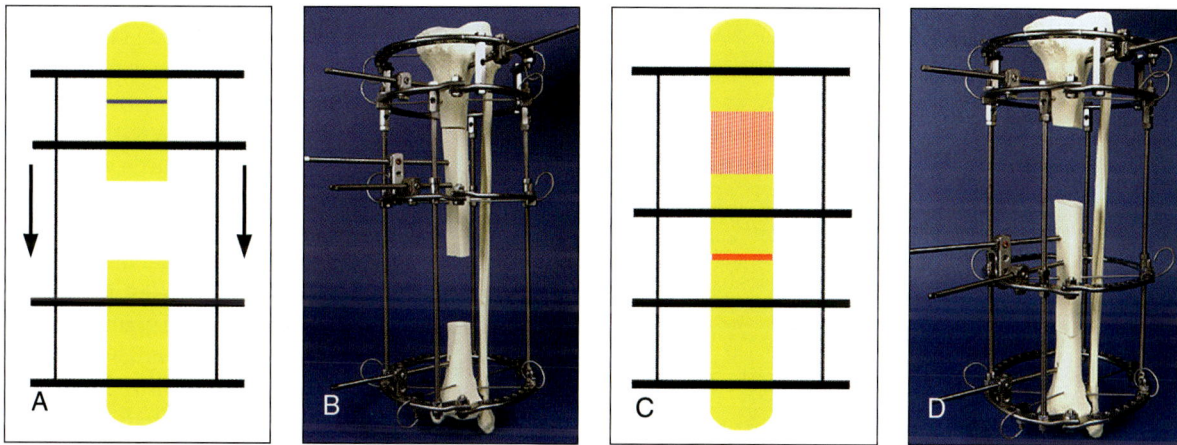

Schematic (**A**) and model (**B**) show a basic circular ring fixation system for standard bone transport prior to the transport of the intercalary middle segment. Schematic (**C**) and model (**D**) show bone transport at the time of docking following completion of transport. (Adapted with permission from Kevin Louie, MD, California Pacific Medical Center, San Francisco, CA.)

SURGICAL TECHNIQUE

It is best to preconstruct the ring fixator before its application to the affected limb when possible. When mounting a frame for bone transport, I frequently follow classic Ilizarov concepts when possible, using two rings per fixation block segment. In its classic form, this would mean two proximal rings and two distal rings, with a single ring between the two sets to act as the transport segment. In essence, the proximal and distal fixation blocks represent stationary segments, and the transport ring is the mobile segment (**Figure 2**). Transport of a long bone can be successfully performed in an antegrade or retrograde fashion, depending on the location of the healthiest bone. The key to creating good regenerate bone is the existence of a healthy soft-tissue envelope at the site of the corticotomy, with resultant healthy and well-perfused bone at this site.

The preconstructed frame is then mounted to the limb in an orthogonal fashion. I have found this easiest to do by balancing the frame off two reference wires. The first wire is placed at a proximal site (in the tibia, at the proximal tibial physeal scar), the frame is slipped onto the limb, and the second reference wire is placed at a distal site (in the tibia, at the distal tibial physeal scar).

Using an image intensifier, the frame is then balanced to the limb, lining up the segments to allow accurate bone transport. Alternately, this can be performed with reference half pins.

The frame is mounted and fixed to the limb once the frame is balanced to the limb. The transport ring is then fixed to the limb. On the tibia, normally this is done with two wires and a half pin, but this also can be performed with half pins only, depending on the surgeon's preference.

Last, a corticotomy is performed. Ideally the corticotomy is made near the metaphyseal-diaphyseal junction of a long bone, but from a technical point of view, it can be performed anywhere on a limb segment. As with limb lengthening, various corticotomy techniques can be used, and appropriate latency times must be respected before transport is initiated.

Although I prefer performing bone transport with a moving ring segment, it can also be performed via pull-through wires (**Figure 3**). The technical benefit of this technique is that it involves a single site where each wire is pulled through the skin. Greater soft-tissue dissection often is required to place the wires, however, and the pull-through technique has inherent instability, unlike the ring transport method.

FIGURE 3

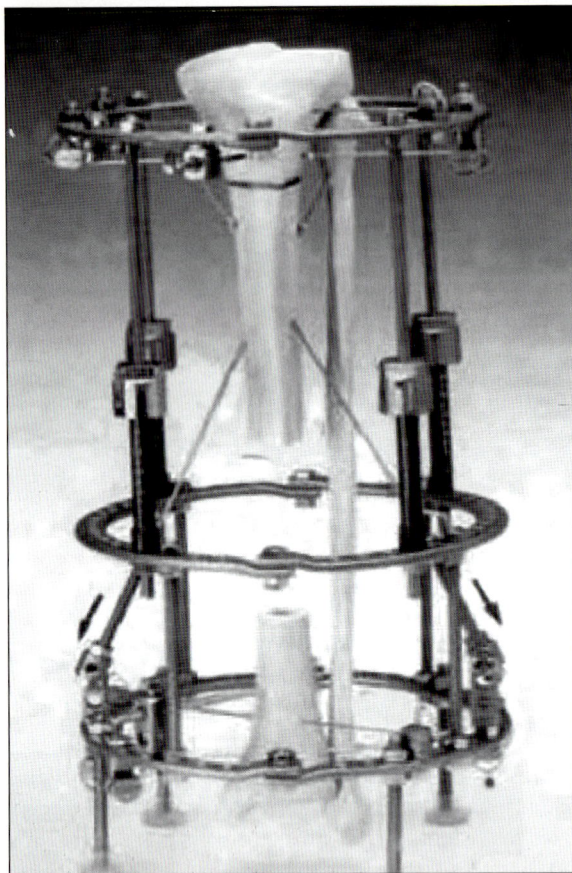

Model demonstrates wire transport technique. At the completion of transport, definitive fixation of the transport segment at the docking site should be performed via wire or pin fixation at a ring added to this level. (Reproduced with permission from Kevin Louie, MD, California Pacific Medical Center, San Francisco, CA.)

Transport also can be performed over an intramedullary rod. I have found this most useful at the femoral level. One must be exceedingly careful that a pin or wire does not contact or come too close to the intramedullary rod, as intramedullary osteomyelitis can occur. As a result, I do not use this technique in the tibia.

Docking

The act of the bone ends coming into apposition at the conclusion of transport is referred to as docking. Once transport is completed and docking occurs, the surgeon must then manage the docking site. The preferred method of docking site management used in the United States involves formally opening up the docking site, removing the invaginated fibrous tissue interzone, freshening the bone ends, and, often, bone grafting of the docking site. This process, although distinctly in contrast to the original Russian techniques, has reduced the incidence of nonunion at the docking site.[21,22] With this method of docking site management, the incidence of nonunion at the docking site should be less than 10%. I still prefer to use autologous iliac crest grafting at this site because of failure experienced with other methods. At my institution, a union rate of 95% is reproducibly achieved at the docking site using this method. In fact, when these guidelines are followed, the docking site almost always heals before the regenerate bone is healed to the extent that allows for frame removal.

Using the transport ring, a certain amount of compression (until wire deflection is noted) can then be applied across the docking site to increase stability at the apposed bone ends. Care should be taken not to overcompress this site, however, as this can lead to necrosis of the grafted bone ends.

At the time of the docking, any residual limb shortening can be addressed. By cutting the transport rods between the segment crossing the regenerate section of the frame and replacing them with lengthening devices between the transport ring and accompanying fixation block, the fixator is converted to a lengthener. When performing this on the tibia, one must be sure that proximal and distal tibiofibular fixation is present and that discontinuity of the fibular shaft exists. If the fibular shaft is healed, a fibular osteotomy must be performed during this surgical setting.

Frame Management After Docking

Following the docking procedure, if no lengthening is required, the limb is managed in the static phase while the regenerate bone heals. At this point, management is the same as it would be for handling any regenerate gap, including the need for appropriate limb dynamization before fixator removal.

If limb lengthening is performed, then the frame and limb are managed in the same manner as a lengthening of that limb segment. The surgeon must follow the healing of both the regenerate bone and the docking site to determine when sufficient healing has occurred to allow for frame removal. Occasionally, one site will be delayed far longer than the other (ie, failure of regenerate healing as compared with docking site healing). Rarely, the surgeon may elect to selectively dynamize or even remove the frame at one or the other of these limb segments in these instances.

ACUTE SHORTENING VERSUS BONE TRANSPORT

In the 1980s, when surgeons in Western Europe and North America learned of the Ilizarov method, many thought that this would be their Holy Grail for the treatment of all segmental defects associated with limb trauma. These surgeons thought that these traumatized limbs could be acutely shortened to simultaneously eliminate any bone deficit as well as achieve soft-tissue closure without the need for tissue transfer. As the principles of distraction osteogenesis and traumatized soft-tissue management were better understood, however, it became apparent that this procedure was not the panacea for these devastating limb injuries. Acute shortening of the limb did not allow for the safe closure of many of the soft-tissue defects that were present because many of them occurred in a vertical direction along the course of the limb. When limbs are acutely shortened, a "fish mouth" deformity of the soft-tissue envelope is often created. Often, these deformities are very hard to close and can be rather disfiguring.

Another problem was that when a traumatized limb was acutely shortened, microvascular and arteriolar kinking occurred about the shortened soft-tissue envelope.[23] This led to acute devascularization of the surrounding soft-tissue envelope and death of the previously viable soft tissue, worsening the problems of the limb to a much greater degree than normal. Many surgeons soon realized that in an acutely traumatized limb, the greatest shortening that could safely be tolerated was about 2.5 cm. In fact, at my institution we tested this during many operations by placing oxygen tension probes on patients' toes while the limb was acutely shortened. In nearly every case, the oxygen tension to the skin distal to the site of injury dropped rather precipitously once the shortening reached 2.5 to 3.0 cm. Hence, in the acutely traumatized limb, acute shorten-

ing greater than 3 cm has a very limited role at best and should be performed with extreme caution.

The last problem to become apparent was that when a limb segment is shortened in one region and lengthened in another, the limb segment mechanics are altered because the muscle length for the affected limb segment is not preserved. In fact, the limb is often shortened at the tendinous portion and lengthened at the muscular portion, or vice versa. Because of the significant scar tissue created with this procedure, limb biomechanics and muscle function are inferior to that achieved when the initial limb and muscle length is preserved.

For all the reasons listed above, most surgeons experienced in the use of distraction osteogenesis and limb salvage prefer maintaining limb length when possible. The bone defect is then corrected via bone transport rather than acute shortening followed by lengthening.

PITFALLS AND COMMON ERRORS

In my experience performing bone transport for the past 20 years, I overcame many hurdles during the early learning curve. One lesson that bears repeating is the need for bone grafting at the docking site, which became quite apparent to many surgeons performing this surgery in the early 1990s. Green et al[21,22] were the first to describe this technique, as the need for bone grafting at the docking site was not reported by surgeons in Italy or the countries formerly part of the Eastern Bloc. Bone grafting is now uniformly accepted in North America as a necessary step in performing bone transport.

Another common pitfall is not building enough structural support and stability into the frame. For a tibial transport, the transport ring usually requires two diverging half pins or two wires and an off-ring half pin. Using fewer pins may result in a "windshield wiper" effect on the regenerate bone. This problem is one of many associated with a pure pull-through wire technique and might represent one of the reasons for the poor regenerate bone formation that can result from this technique.

Another error is using too rapid a transport rate. The surgeon must diligently follow these patients with regular radiographic exams. If the regenerate bone shows any signs of "hourglassing" (assuming an hourglass-like shape), the transport rate must be reduced immediately.

FIGURE 4

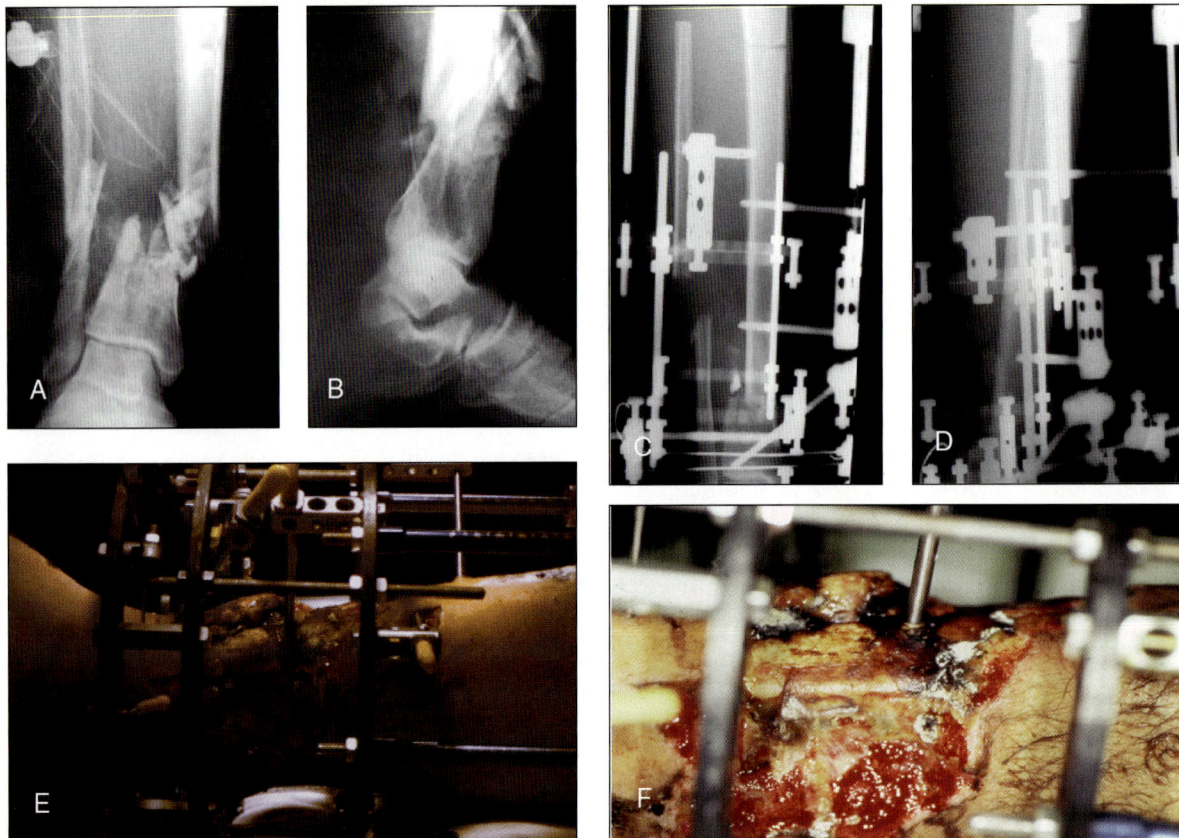

A 24-year-old man sustained isolated Gustilo and Anderson grade IIIB open right distal tibial and fibular fractures during a motorcycle collision with a motor vehicle. Initial AP (**A**) and lateral (**B**) radiographs. AP (**C**) and lateral (**D**) radiographs show treatment with primary application of a circular fixator with fibular osteotomy and 8 cm of acute limb shortening. **E** and **F**, Clinical photographs of the soft-tissue envelope at the fracture level and shortening. Arteriolar compromise with resultant necrosis of the envelope developed over the next 10 days.

(continued)

If hourglassing occurs, many surgeons prefer to stop transport for several days to allow the regenerate bone to recover and heal. For optimal results, the regenerate bone should appear a bit wider than the host bone above and/or below it ("reverse hourglassing") because this is a sign of healthy regenerate bone forming. One must remember that in these severely traumatized limbs, significant arterial and venous compromise often exists, so these limbs do not always respond the same as limbs undergoing simple lengthenings.

Another similar issue involves proper preoperative evaluation of the soft-tissue envelope before the initiation of bone transport. The key to successful bone transport is a healthy soft-tissue envelope. I have had cases of failure of the docking site to heal despite multiple bone grafting attempts. These failures directly resulted from an atrophic soft-tissue envelope. Union was achieved by free-tissue transfer that brought a vascular supply to the bone at the docking site.

Careful examination of the limb for atrophic skin over the bone and for skin tightly adherent to the bone should be performed, as both can adversely affect bone

FIGURE 4 (*continued*)

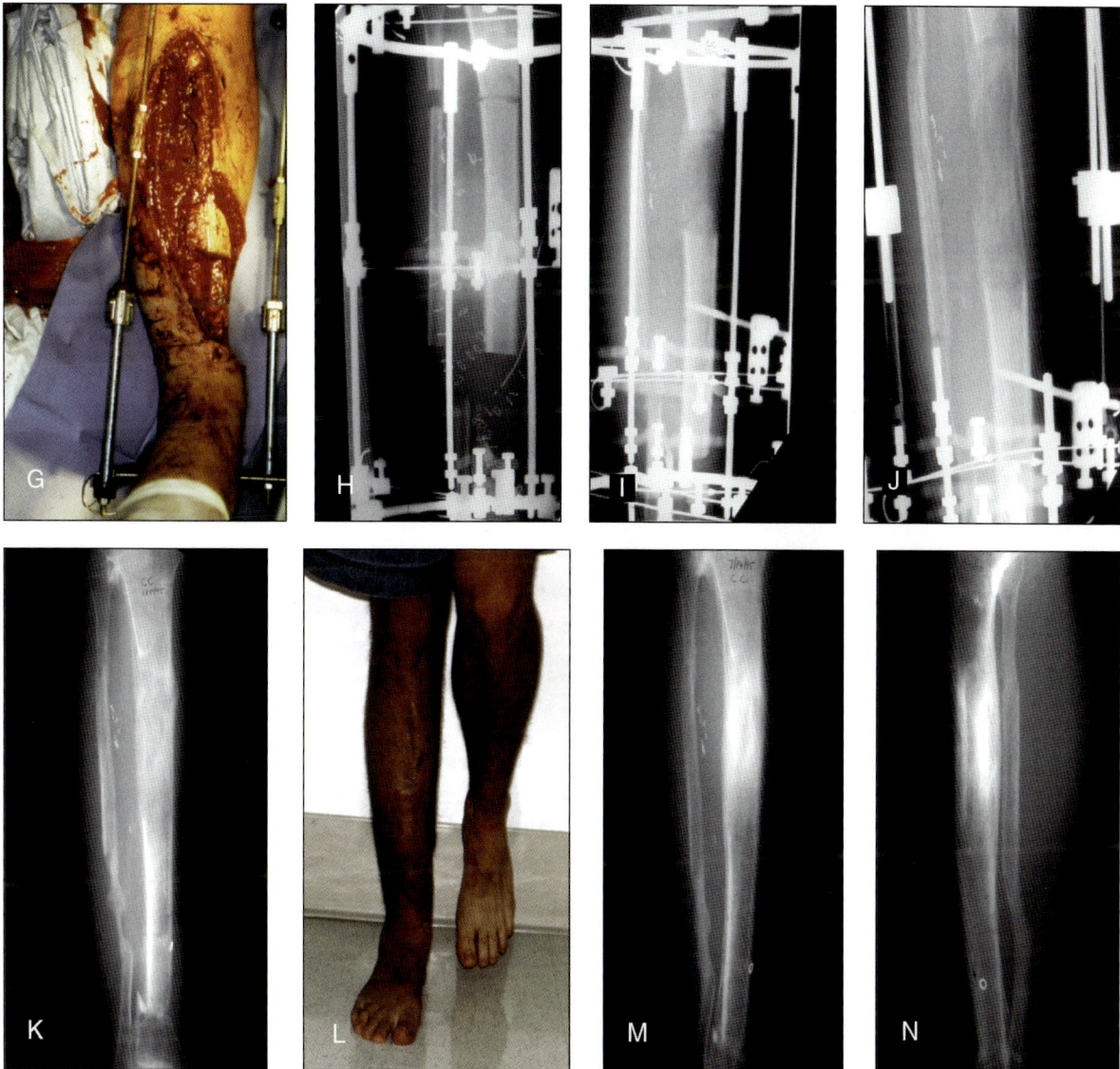

G, Intraoperative photograph of resection of necrotic bone and soft tissue. The patient was left with a 15.5-cm bone defect, including the shortening that was previously present. **H,** AP radiograph obtained after free-flap placement and bone transport to treat the bone defect. **I,** AP radiograph obtained near the end of bone transport shows the defect was eliminated with bone transport. **J,** AP radiograph obtained at the time of docking. Iliac crest bone grafting was performed, and the frame was converted to a lengthener. AP radiograph (**K**) and clinical photograph (**L**) obtained after 13 months of treatment, when the fixator was removed. Restoration of limb length and a healed functional leg were achieved. AP (**M**) and lateral (**N**) radiographs obtained 1 year following fixator removal show a healed limb. The patient returned to work and resumed normal function. At 13-year follow-up, the patient works full-time, functions normally, and skis for recreation. (Reproduced with permission from Lowenberg DW, Feibel RJ, Louie KW, Eshima I: Combined muscle flap and Ilizarov reconstruction for bone and soft tissue defects. *Clin Orthop Relat Res* 1996;332:37-51.)

transport. If this atrophic or adherent skin must be elongated with the transport segment, the soft-tissue envelope tends to further thin. This can lead to chronic breakdown of this envelope over time, creating long-term problems for the patient. **Figure 4** best illustrates the capability of bone transport, the ability to incorporate limb lengthening into the process, and the danger of acute shortening of the traumatized limb. One must follow the basic principles outlined above when performing bone transport for traumatic reconstruction. In general, the success rate remains very high with proper technique. In my experience, limbs that would otherwise have been amputated are saved and have good long-term clinical results.[19]

REFERENCES

1. Goldstrohm GL, Mears DC, Swartz WM: The results of 39 fractures complicated by major segmental bone loss and/or leg length discrepancy. *J Trauma* 1984;24(1): 50-58.

2. Banic A, Hertel R: Double vascularized fibulas for reconstruction of large tibial defects. *J Reconstr Microsurg* 1993;9(6):421-428.

3. Christian EP, Bosse MJ, Robb G: Reconstruction of large diaphyseal defects, without free fibular transfer, in Grade-IIIB tibial fractures. *J Bone Joint Surg Am* 1989;71(7):994-1004.

4. Salibian AH, Anzel SH, Salyer WA: Transfer of vascularized grafts of iliac bone to the extremities. *J Bone Joint Surg Am* 1987;69(9):1319-1327.

5. Shapiro MS, Endrizzi DP, Cannon RM, Dick HM: Treatment of tibial defects and nonunions using ipsilateral vascularized fibular transposition. *Clin Orthop Relat Res* 1993(296):207-212.

6. Weiland AJ, Moore JR, Daniel RK: Vascularized bone autografts: Experience with 41 cases. *Clin Orthop Relat Res* 1983(174):87-95.

7. Yaremchuk MJ, Brumback RJ, Manson PN, Burgess AR, Poka A, Weiland AJ: Acute and definitive management of traumatic osteocutaneous defects of the lower extremity. *Plast Reconstr Surg* 1987;80(1):1-14.

8. Doi K, Kawakami F, Hiura Y, Oda T, Sakai K, Kawai S: One-stage treatment of infected bone defects of the tibia with skin loss by free vascularized osteocutaneous grafts. *Microsurgery* 1995;16(10):704-712.

9. Hierner R, Wood MB: Comparison of vascularised iliac crest and vascularised fibula transfer for reconstruction of segmental and partial bone defects in long bones of the lower extremity. *Microsurgery* 1995;16(12):818-826.

10. Ehrnberg A, De Pablos J, Martinez-Lotti G, Kreicbergs A, Nilsson O: Comparison of demineralized allogeneic bone matrix grafting (the Urist procedure) and the Ilizarov procedure in large diaphyseal defects in sheep. *J Orthop Res* 1993;11(3):438-447.

11. Mastrogiacomo M, Corsi A, Francioso E, et al: Reconstruction of extensive long bone defects in sheep using resorbable bioceramics based on silicon stabilized tricalcium phosphate. *Tissue Eng* 2006;12(5):1261-1273.

12. Bloemers FW, Blokhuis TJ, Patka P, Bakker FC, Wippermann BW, Haarman HJ: Autologous bone versus calcium-phosphate ceramics in treatment of experimental bone defects. *J Biomed Mater Res B Appl Biomater* 2003;66(2):526-531.

13. Blokhuis TJ, Wippermann BW, den Boer FC, et al: Resorbable calcium phosphate particles as a carrier material for bone marrow in an ovine segmental defect. *J Biomed Mater Res* 2000;51(3):369-375.

14. Wippermann B, Donow C, Schratt HE, den Boer FC, Blokhuis T, Patka P: The influence of hydroxyapatite granules on the healing of a segmental defect filled with autologous bone marrow. *Ann Chir Gynaecol* 1999;88(3):194-197.

15. Cierny G III, Zorn KE: Segmental tibial defects: Comparing conventional and Ilizarov methodologies. *Clin Orthop Relat Res* 1994(301):118-123.

16. Platz A, Werner CM, Künzi W, Trentz O, Meyer VE: Reconstruction of posttraumatic bony defects of the lower extremity: callotaxis or free vascularized fibula graft? *Handchir Mikrochir Plast Chir* 2004;36(6): 397-404.

17. Lowenberg DW, Feibel RJ, Louie KW, Eshima I: Combined muscle flap and Ilizarov reconstruction for bone and soft tissue defects. *Clin Orthop Relat Res* 1996(332): 37-51.

18. Gopal S, Giannoudis PV, Murray A, Matthews SJ, Smith RM: The functional outcome of severe, open tibial fractures managed with early fixation and flap coverage. *J Bone Joint Surg Br* 2004;86(6):861-867.

19.   McKee MD, Yoo DJ, Zdero R, et al: Combined single-stage osseous and soft tissue reconstruction of the tibia with the Ilizarov method and tissue transfer. *J Orthop Trauma* 2008;22(3):183-189.

20.   Horton KM, Brooks D, Buntic RF, Louie KM, Buncke GM, Lowenberg DW: Outcome analysis of combined Ilizarov bone transport and immediate free tissue transfer for lower extremity salvage. *Annual Meeting of American Society of Plastic Surgeons,* San Francisco, CA, October 8, 2006.

21.   Green SA, Jackson JM, Wall DM, Marinow H, Ishkanian J: Management of segmental defects by the Ilizarov intercalary bone transport method. *Clin Orthop Relat Res* 1992(280):136-142.

22.   Green SA: Skeletal defects: A comparison of bone grafting and bone transport for segmental skeletal defects. *Clin Orthop Relat Res* 1994(301):111-117.

23.   Lowenberg DW, Van der Reis W: Acute shortening for tibia defects: When and where. *Tech Orthop* 1996;11:210-215.

CHAPTER 19

TREATMENT OF SEGMENTAL BONE LOSS DUE TO INFECTION

GEORGE CIERNY III, MD
DOREEN DiPASQUALE, MD

INTRODUCTION

Over the past 2 decades, new insights into the pathophysiology of musculoskeletal infection have transformed its management.[1-9] Therapeutic milestones include versatile methods of skeletal fixation and tissue transference, limb lengthening through distraction, local depot therapies, patient-at-risk treatment strategies, and new antimicrobials to address an ever-changing microbiosphere. The prospective matching of treatment options to factors common to the natural history of infection, however, provided the foundation for successful limb salvage protocols.[2,10,11]

The time-related process by which an acute infection becomes chronic parallels the biologic mechanisms inherent to microbial colonization. Once free-floating (planktonic) microorganisms attach to nonviable surfaces (necrotic tissue, foreign materials) in the wound, they create colony-forming units and secrete a protective matrix (biofilm) to enhance growth and provide an immunity to antimicrobials and host defenses.[4,12,13] To cure such a biofilm infection, all substrates for microbial attachment must be excised.[14,15] The location of the infection, the patient's medical condition, the physician's skills, and the potential impact of treatment will determine if it is to be palliative or curative, limb-sparing or ablative.

The protocol used to treat adult osteomyelitis first establishes a live, clean, manageable wound (**Table 1**). Débridement is the unchallenged cornerstone of successful treatment. Soft tissues are resected to supple, well-perfused margins. Bone is tangentially excised until the surface bleeds with a uniform, haversian pattern (the "paprika sign"),[16] after which the live wound is protected from further injury with dressings, coverage, and stabilization, and homeostasis is maintained with optimization of the host response to both treatment and infection.

Following débridement and resuscitation, reconstruction must address the following issues in every case: the integrity of the bony segments, mechanical stability, and soft-tissue coverage.[17] Although a live, clean wound will heal both primarily and by secondary intention, an open-wound environment nevertheless creates obstacles to treatment: components of the reconstruction also must be live to be able to withstand the presence of pathogens; access to well-vascularized surfaces (for bone grafting) is limited because of the compromised soft-tissue envelope. Methods meeting these criteria include external fixation strategies, open cancellous bone grafting,[18] acute shortening osteosynthesis,[19] vascularized bone flaps,[20] and open methods of internal bone lengthening (eg, bone transport).[21]

TABLE 1 Treatment Protocol for Adult Osteomyelitis[a]

Stage	Protocol
Patient history and examination	
Immediate medical history	Mechanism and time of injury; treatment history (surgical procedures, previous culture/sensitivities, antibiotic regimes)
Past medical history	Comorbidities,[11] cognitive and functional assessment, allergies, medications
Physical examination	Body habitus, gait, ambulatory aids; anatomic site; wounds, scars, tissue defects; extremity examination; neurovascular status
Preoperative testing	Laboratory values (full metabolic panel, CBC with differential, coagulation panel, UA, ESR, CRP), diagnostic tests (vascular indices; angiography, ultrasonography; tissue oxygen tension measurements [$TcPO_2$]), imaging (radiography, MRI, CT, nuclear, PET), tissue biopsies
Clinical staging	Anatomic type (I, medullary; II, superficial; III, localized; IV, diffuse); physiologic host class (A, B, C)
Treatment format	Limb salvage, amputation, palliation (no treatment), suppression (early infections only)
Host optimization (reversal of all amenable comorbidities)	
First surgery	
Single-stage treatment	Débridement, culture, biopsy, stabilization, systemic antibiotics
	Dead-space management: wound management (secondary intention healing, primary closure, delayed closure), antibiotic depots (beads, gels)
First stage of two- or three-stage treatment	Débridement, cultures, biopsy, systemic antibiotics
	Double set-up (change instruments, re-prep, re-drape, new gowns/gloves)
	Temporary fixation
	Dead-space management: wound management (secondary intention healing, primary closure, delayed closure), antibiotic depots (beads, spacers, gels, or impregnated implants)
Outpatient follow-up	Monitor wound healing, laboratory values (ESR, CRP, albumin, prealbumin), physical rehabilitation
Second surgery	
Definitive reconstruction	Prophylactic antibiotics
	Débridement, cultures, biopsy (negative = no infection)
	Double set-up (change instruments, re-prep, re-drape, new gowns/gloves)
	Reconstruction: bone grafts, internal or external fixation, prosthetic implants, antibiotic depots (beads, spacers, or gels)
Second stage of two- or three-stage treatment	Prophylactic antibiotics
	Débridement, cultures, biopsy (positive = infection)
	Double set-up (change instruments, re-prep, re-drape, new gowns/gloves)
	Temporary fixation
	Dead-space management: wound management (secondary intention healing, primary closure, delayed closure), antibiotic depots (beads, spacers, gels, or impregnated implants)
Third surgery	
Definitive reconstruction	Prophylactic antibiotics
	Débridement, cultures, biopsy (negative = no infection)
	Double set-up (change instruments, re-prep, re-drape, new gowns/gloves)
	Reconstruction (bone grafts, internal or external fixation, prosthetic implants)
	Antibiotic depots (beads, spacers, or gels)

TABLE 1 (*continued*)

Stage	Protocol
Third stage of four-stage treatment	Prophylactic antibiotics Débridement, cultures, biopsy (positive = infection) Double set-up (change instruments, re-prep, re-drape, new gowns/gloves) Temporary fixation Dead-space management: wound management (secondary intention healing, primary closure, delayed closure), antibiotic depots (beads, spacers, gels, or impregnated implants)
Fourth surgery (limited to biologic solutions: fusion, amputation, resection arthroplasty, etc)	
Outpatient follow-up	Monitor wound healing Laboratory values (ESR, CRP obtained at 3 mo) Biyearly checkups (× 2)

CBC = complete blood count, UA = urinalysis, ESR = erythrocyte sedimentation rate, CRP = C-reactive protein.

[a] The 1983[14] treatment algorithm for adult osteomyelitis augmented in 1987[10] with the addition of depot antibiotic therapies to safeguard the staged reconstruction of complex débridement defects using methods of both internal and external fixation.

(Adapted from Cierny GC, DiPasquale D: Adult osteomyelitis, in Cierny G III, McClaren AC, Wongworawat MD, eds: *Orthopaedic Knowledge Update: Musculoskeletal Infection.* Rosemont, IL, American Academy of Orthopaedic Surgeons, 2009, p 144.)

On the other hand, it is crucial to provide adequate and supple wound coverage when vital structures (vessels, nerves, tendons) are exposed, the wound bed is too feeble to heal on its own, or reconstruction requires a sterile field (surgical implants, massive bone grafts)[22] (**Figure 1**). In the latter scenario, reconstruction usually is staged to follow a course of local antibiotic therapy.[23-25] The high concentrations of antibiotics created by an antibiotic depot (beads, spacers) implanted into a closed, dead space will eliminate or kill pathogens that persist following débridement, safeguard a primary closure, and maintain a workable dead space for later use in the reconstruction (the "spacer effect"). Once the wound heals and the patient recovers, the depot is removed, the dead space is reclaimed, and the reconstruction is performed as with a clean surgical procedure.[26]

Although transposition flaps and free-tissue transfers are the methods of choice to restore significant soft-tissue deficits in the extremities, flaps sometimes fail and/or circumstances preclude their use. In those cases, bone transport and combined methods of shortening

and lengthening (by means of compression and distraction, respectively) are valuable tools in the armamentarium of salvage surgeons.

RECONSTRUCTION USING DISTRACTION OSTEOGENESIS

By 1990, Ilizarov's principles of skeletal fixation, deformity correction, and distraction osteogenesis had revolutionized the science, art, and practice of limb salvage[27-29] (**Table 2**). When used following a thorough débridement, these methods literally transformed residual limb segments into a self-healing mechanism, restoring alignment, length, and substance (bone and soft tissue). The method of bone transport is the internal lengthening of bone for the purpose of eliminating intercalary bony defects.[22] Compared with conventional techniques, bone transport has several advantages: (1) The process is nontraumatic and well-suited for use in both healthy and compromised hosts; (2) the regenerate bone and transport segments are live and match the anatomic site in structure and volume; (3) there are no statistical differences in outcomes using open versus

FIGURE 1

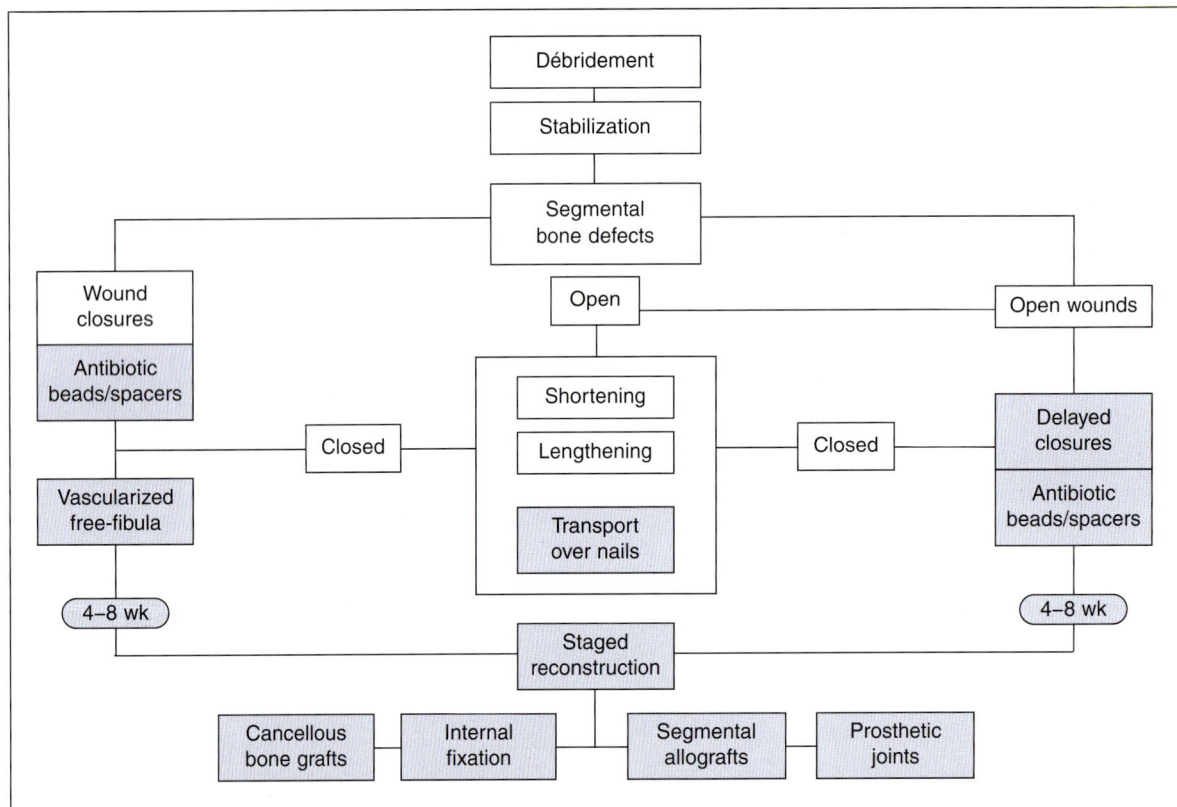

Treatment algorithm for segmental bone loss due to osteomyelitis. Restoration of the soft-tissue envelope and/or use of a two- or three-stage reconstruction (shaded boxes) will increase treatment options when managing composite bony and soft-tissue defects following débridement. Wound healing through secondary intention is discouraged except when performing an acute shortening or an open method of internal lengthening (bone transport). (Adapted from Cierny G III, DiPasquale D: Treatment of chronic infection. *J Am Acad Orthop Surg* 2006;14[10]:S105-S110.)

TABLE 2 Segmental Bone Defects: Methods of Reconstruction[a]

Method	Incidence of Use (%)
Internal fixation allografts, prosthetic joints	32
Distraction osteogenesis[b]	25
External fixation, bone grafts[b]	16
Vascularized bone grafts	11
Permanent acrylic spacers	8

[a] The various methods used to reconstruct 314 consecutively managed bony defects in patients with chronic osteomyelitis treated 2000 to 2008 (Atlanta and San Diego). The permanent spacers used in this series were composites of antibiotic-impregnated bone cements (polymethylmethacrylate) reinforced with medullary nails (REOrthopaedics, San Diego, CA).
[b] Includes all cases (41%) in which the Ilizarov principles[27-29] were exclusively used.

FIGURE 2

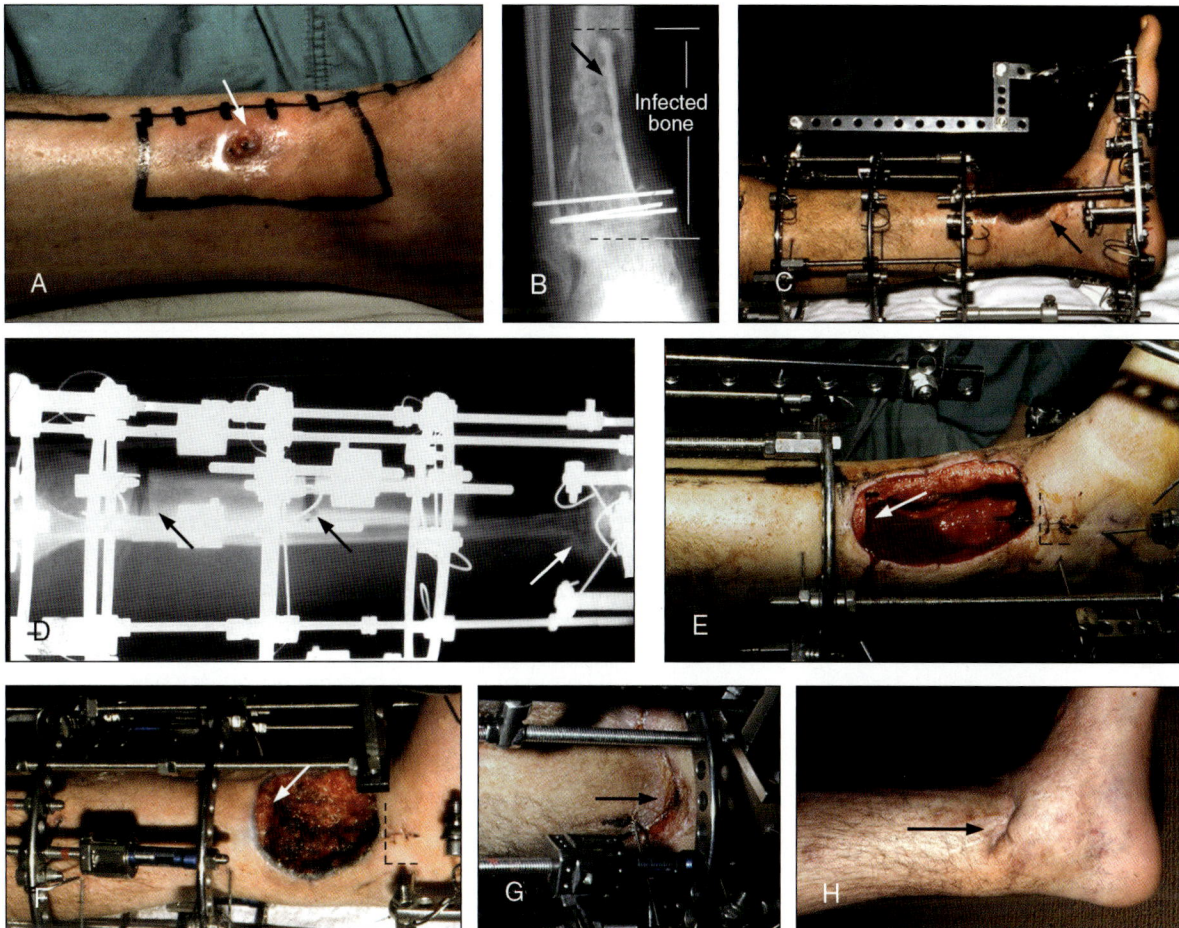

Chronic osteomyelitis (stage IVB) of the distal tibia and talus. **A,** Clinical photograph shows atrophic scars and a draining fistula (arrow) associated with an infected nonunion of the distal tibia and septic arthritis of the ankle. The inked box represents the anticipated soft-tissue defect. **B,** AP radiograph shows a sequestered cortex (arrow) and the anticipated débridement defect (area between the dashed lines). **C,** Photograph obtained following resection and fixation shows loose packing of the open wound (arrow). **D,** Lateral radiograph shows two corticotomies (black arrows) and docking surface at the talus, distally (white arrow). **E,** Photograph obtained at the first dressing change shows the resection defect, the docking end of the tibia (arrow), and the docking site (dashed lines) located distal to its corresponding soft-tissue margin. **F,** As the bifocal transport progressed, the dimensions of the open wound lessened. The distal end of the tibia (arrow) is well aligned with the talar docking site (dashed lines). **G,** Right before contact, the bone surfaces were contoured and the transposed soft-tissue margin was de-epithelialized (arrow) before it passed beneath the overhanging soft tissues at the docking site. **H,** Photograph of the healed docking site (arrow) at the end of treatment.

(continued)

closed wound protocols; (4) soft-tissue defects are simultaneously eliminated; and (5) length can be restored once docking is complete[21] (**Figure 2**). The disadvantages to bone transport are as follows: (1) the process is difficult to master, is time consuming, and requires constant surveillance; (2) the rate of distraction is deduced subjectively using radiographs and biofeedback mechanisms; and (3) patient compliance is paramount to success. Complications of treatment include healing disturbances at the docking sites and in regen-

FIGURE 2 (*continued*)

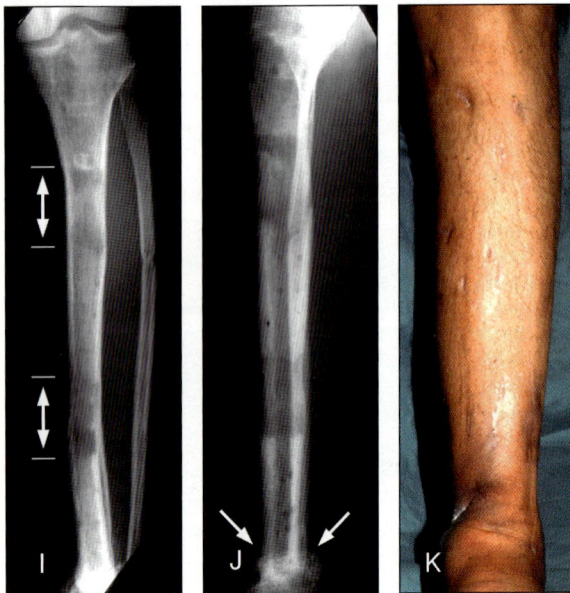

AP (**I**) and lateral (**J**) radiographs show the fully restored limb length, with complete consolidation of the two areas of regenerate bone (double-headed arrows), and solid union at the docking site (arrows). **K**, Clinical appearance of the limb and docking site at 2-year follow-up.

TABLE 3 **Contraindications to Bone Transport**

General Conditions[a]	Host Factors[b]
Defect too large	Neural compromise
Injury too extensive	RSD paraplegia spacticity psychosis
Deficient reserves	Noncompliance
Preexisting hardware	Chronic edema
No therapeutic advantage	Radiation injury, regional ischemia, ≥3 comorbidities

[a] General conditions refer to management options, same-limb deficiencies (ie, purchase for fixation) and preexisting conditions (same-limb total joint arthroplasty).
[b] Host factors are conditions affecting the ability to use clinical feedback mechanisms to monitor the rate of distraction, patient compliance, and insurmountable obstacles to wound healing.
RSD = reflex sympathetic dystrophy.

erate bone, septic sequelae from pin-site infections, premature consolidation of the regenerate bone, insufficiency fractures following frame removal, and joint stiffness and axial deformities at the end of treatment. Contraindications to this method are listed in **Table 3**.

OPEN WOUND BONE TRANSPORT
Indications
Open methods of bone transport eliminate the need for specialty skills (flap surgery) and the surgical morbidity of complex, conventional reconstructions, thereby broadening the indications for limb salvage. Open methods have several disadvantages, however: care for large, open wounds is required; creative surgical approaches are needed when bone grafting the docking site; and there is an increased incidence of secondary infections (**Figure 2**). For these reasons, closed rather than open methods of transport are recommended following

removal of an infected intramedullary nail, protecting the reamed transport segment and corticotomy from contamination.

Technique
Once a live wound has been established, the limb is reprepared, a frame is applied, the limb is held to length, and the segments are aligned for transport.[22] The wound is dressed with a layer of petrolatum gauze and moist gauze sponges. In 2 or 3 days, the patient is returned to the operating room for reinspection and a corticotomy. Thereafter, the dressings are changed (wet to dry) on the ward. Systemic antibiotics are stopped by day 6 or 7.

After a delay of 5 days, bone transport (in adults) is initiated at a distraction rate of 0.5 to 0.75 mm/d until the transport segment is within 10 mm of docking. The bone ends and soft tissues are then contoured to optimize contact and distraction is continued until the docking site is compressed.[22] If a limb-length discrepancy still exists, the fixator can be converted to a lengthening construct.

Once the soft tissues have healed, the docking site is bone grafted opposite the previous wound. During this exposure, care must be taken to avoid injury to vessels and nerves that are displaced during bone transport or a shortening. Thereafter, consolidation of the regenerate bone and docking site is monitored accordingly.

CLOSED WOUND BONE TRANSPORT
Advantages and Disadvantages

When faced with a composite bony or soft-tissue defect, restoration of the soft-tissue envelope will protect vital structures from desiccation, decrease the risk for secondary infection, facilitate early bone grafting of the docking site(s), and increase therapeutic options with the use of antibiotic depots and two-stage protocols (**Figure 1**). Disadvantages of the closed method include the following: (1) complex wound closures and repeat exposures must be done within the confines of an external fixator; (2) a familiarity with the use of antibiotic depots is required; (3) an unobstructed transport alley (dead-space defect) must be maintained; (4) the wound must be monitored for closed-space infections; (5) pin-tract compromise to vascular pedicles and tenuous flaps is a risk (**Figure 3**).

Technique

Following débridement, the frame is applied, taking into consideration the size and type of coverage (local versus distant transfer) and antibiotic depot (rod, spacer, and/or beads) used. Because the soft tissues overlying the defect will bulge and become less pliable as the transport distance decreases, poorly positioned frame components and/or undersized rings will make reexposure difficult at the time of depot removal (2 to 4 weeks). If the gap is 2 cm or less, the bone ends are contoured and the site is bone grafted at the same time. Otherwise, the docking preparation is postponed until the segment is within 10 to 15 mm of contact. If necessary, transport can be reversed (in direction) to give more exposure. To prevent involution into the alley or dead-space defect during long transports, stent wires can be used to protect soft tissues until docking is complete (**Figure 3**, *B*).

Closed Wound Transport Over an Intramedullary Nail

Transport over a nail is a two-stage process.[30] The added stability of a locked nail simplifies the frame construct, improves patient tolerance, and shortens the time to frame removal (**Figure 4**). Disadvantages of transport over a nail include a relative increase in surgical-site infections, late cross-contamination of the nail with pin-tract pathogens, and the sequelae of infection (regenerate bone failures and docking site nonunions). As mentioned above, open transport over an intramedullary nail is discouraged.[30,31]

Technique

At the time of débridement/destabilization, a simple frame is applied. Pins at either end of the bone are placed peripheral to the central axis (**Figure 5**). Access "through" the frame is carefully maintained for inserting the nail and locking screws and to allow repeated exposures of the docking site. Unicortical drop wires are used to establish and maintain alignment (**Figure 5, *C* and *D***). Thereafter, an antibiotic depot is implanted and the wound is closed. If coverage is to be delayed, a dead space can be temporarily dressed with a bead pouch.[25]

Two to six weeks later, the limb is surgically prepared, the depot is removed, and the frame is converted to a transport construct. Transport pins are kept unicortical (out of the canal). If only half pins are used for transport, at least two are placed, ensuring that they are cantilevered to facilitate fore-and-aft movement on the nail. A solid nail 1.5 to 2.0 mm smaller than the isthmus is trialed to ensure an unobstructed passage. The corticotomy is then completed and the nail is inserted and locked into position. Locking screws and their insertion sites also must avoid contact with fixation pins.

After a delay of 4 to 5 days, distraction is initiated (0.75 mm/d) and adjusted as needed; 10 to 15 mm before contact, the wound is opened for contouring and bone grafting the docking surfaces. The frame can be removed once there is adequate consolidation of the regenerate bone to hold the segment in place. Alternatively, the transport segment can be locked using an interlocking screw or buried wire passed through a custom hole in the nail drilled prior to insertion.

Infection Sequelae

If an infection occurs during transport over a nail, cultures are obtained and any suspicious pins are removed. IV antibiotics are initiated and maintained. If signs of infection abate and the regenerate bone develops normally, the docking site is contoured and the bone is

FIGURE 3

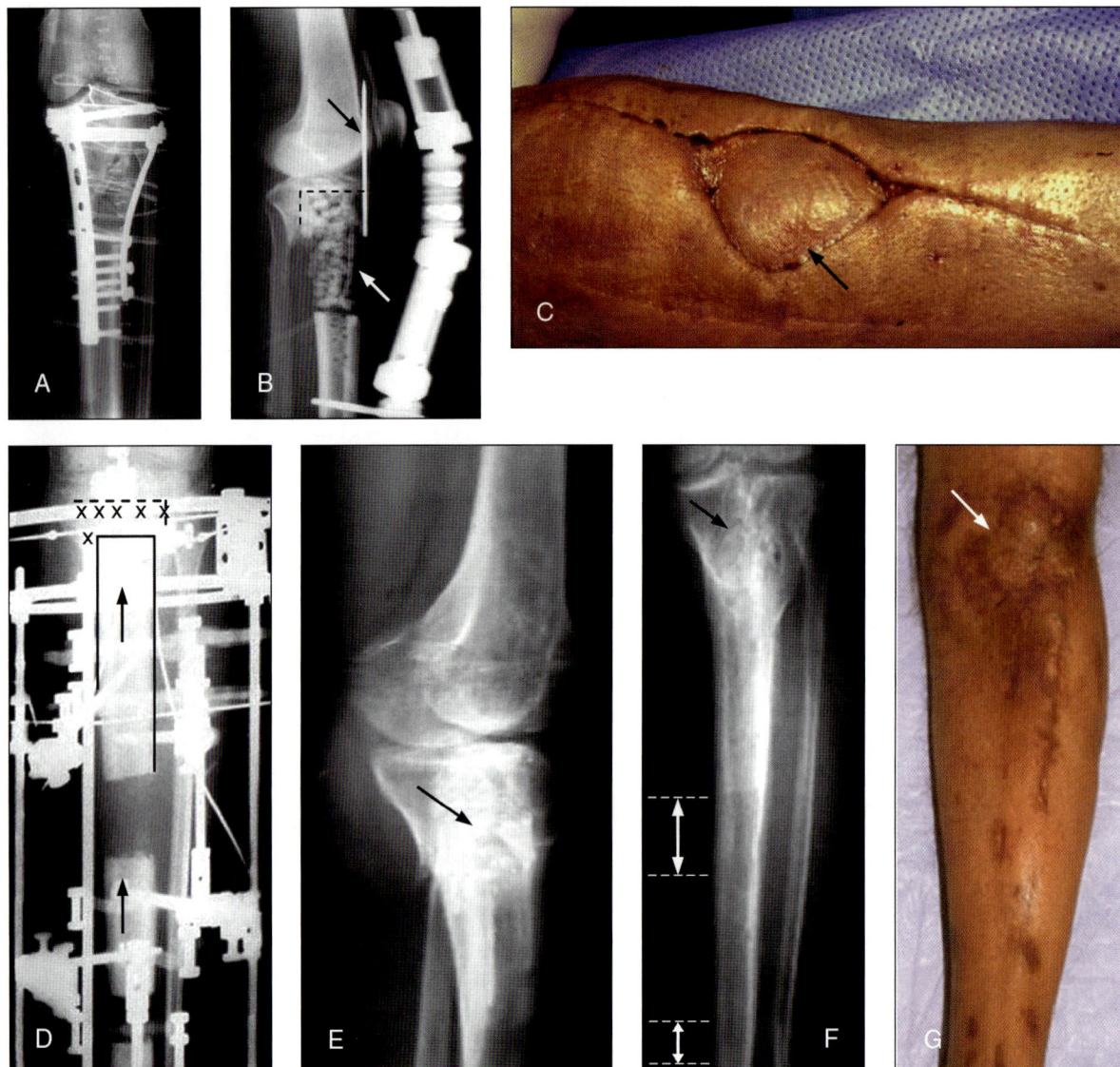

Patient with an infected nonunion of the tibia following dual-plate fixation. **A,** AP radiograph obtained at presentation shows the fixation and the metaphyseal fracture. **B,** Lateral radiograph obtained after débridement and initial stabilization with a spanning frame shows an 8.5-cm débridement defect extending to subchondral bone (dashed lines). A Steinmann pin (black arrow) holds soft tissues (extensor mechanism) out from the transport alley. Antibiotic beads (white arrow) dress the dead space. **C,** Photograph shows coverage attained with a gastrocnemius myoplasty and skin graft (arrow). **D,** Following wound healing, the docking site (dashed lines) was bone grafted (x) and a ring fixator was positioned for bifocal transport. The black arrows indicate the direction of transport, with the proximal segment outlined (black lines) to illustrate its relationship to the bone grafts (x) and the future docking site. Lateral (**E**) and AP (**F**) radiographs obtained at 2-year follow-up show union at the docking site (black arrow) and consolidation at both regenerates (white arrows). **G,** Final clinical photograph of the limb shows the healed myoplasty (arrow) and cosmetic profile of the reconstructed limb.

FIGURE 4

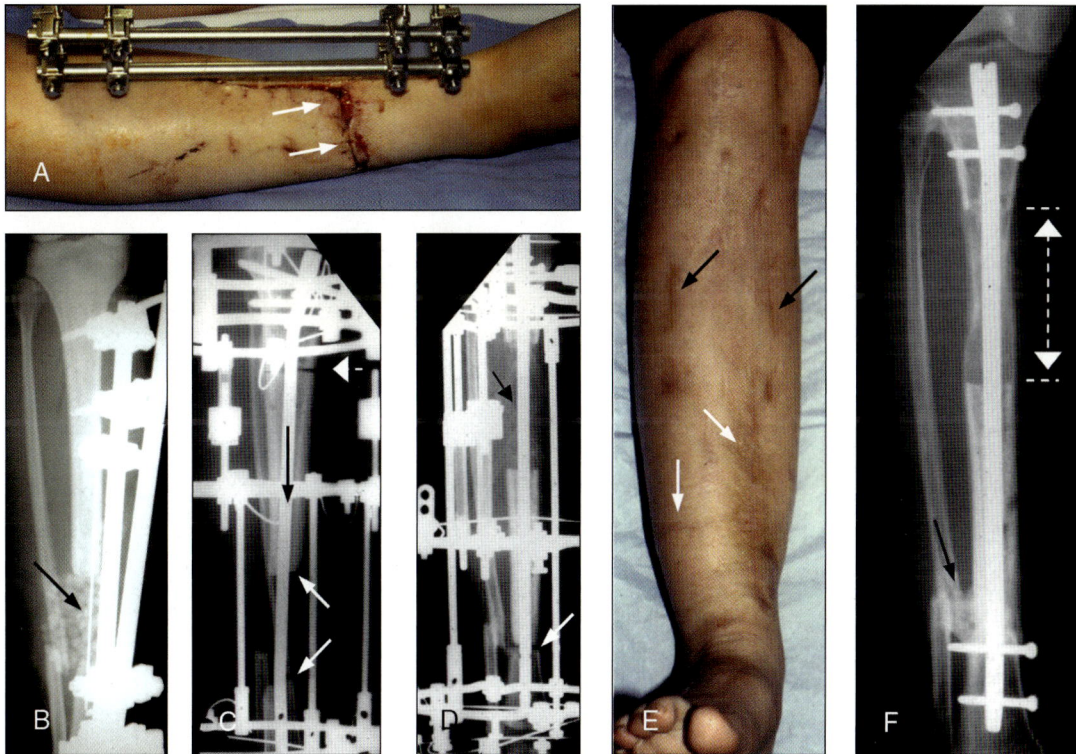

Patient with an infected tibial fracture. Photograph (**A**) and AP radiograph (**B**) show an infected tibial fracture in its original fixator following débridement, a 2.5-cm shortening, placement of antibiotic beads (black arrow), and loose approximation of the original wounds (white arrows). **C,** AP radiograph obtained 2 weeks later shows a transport over nail frame construct, the limb out to length, the direction of transport (black arrow), the true bony defect (white arrows), and the corticotomy (arrowhead). **D,** AP radiograph of the early consolidation (black arrow) at the time of docking (white arrow). **E,** Photograph of the limb shows surgical scars (white arrows) and transport tracks (black arrows) following frame removal. **F,** AP radiograph obtained at last follow-up shows regenerate consolidation (dashed arrow) and fibular cross-union (black arrow).

grafted as above. When an infection has been documented, the frame is not removed until healing is complete.

If, however, the regenerate bone fails to develop or the inflammation cannot be controlled with antibiotics and host optimization, transport is reversed until the corticotomy is compressed and closed. Then, drop wires are placed to control the segments, the nail is removed, the canal and alley are débrided, and the entire dead space is dressed with an antibiotic depot (beads, spacers, and/or an antibiotic rod).[32] The antibiotic coverage is adjusted according to culture sensitivities. Two to four weeks later, a new transport or conventional protocol is initiated.[17,21]

Docking Site Protocols

In our initial series of 21 bone transports (**Table 4**), bone ends were contoured at the time of débridement and docking took place without further preparation or exposure.[21] In that series, 29% of the protocols failed, (10% nonunions at the docking site, 19% failure of regenerate bone to heal). Regenerate bone failures occurred only in distractions 6 cm or longer. All healing disturbances resolved with retreatment (frame revi-

FIGURE 5

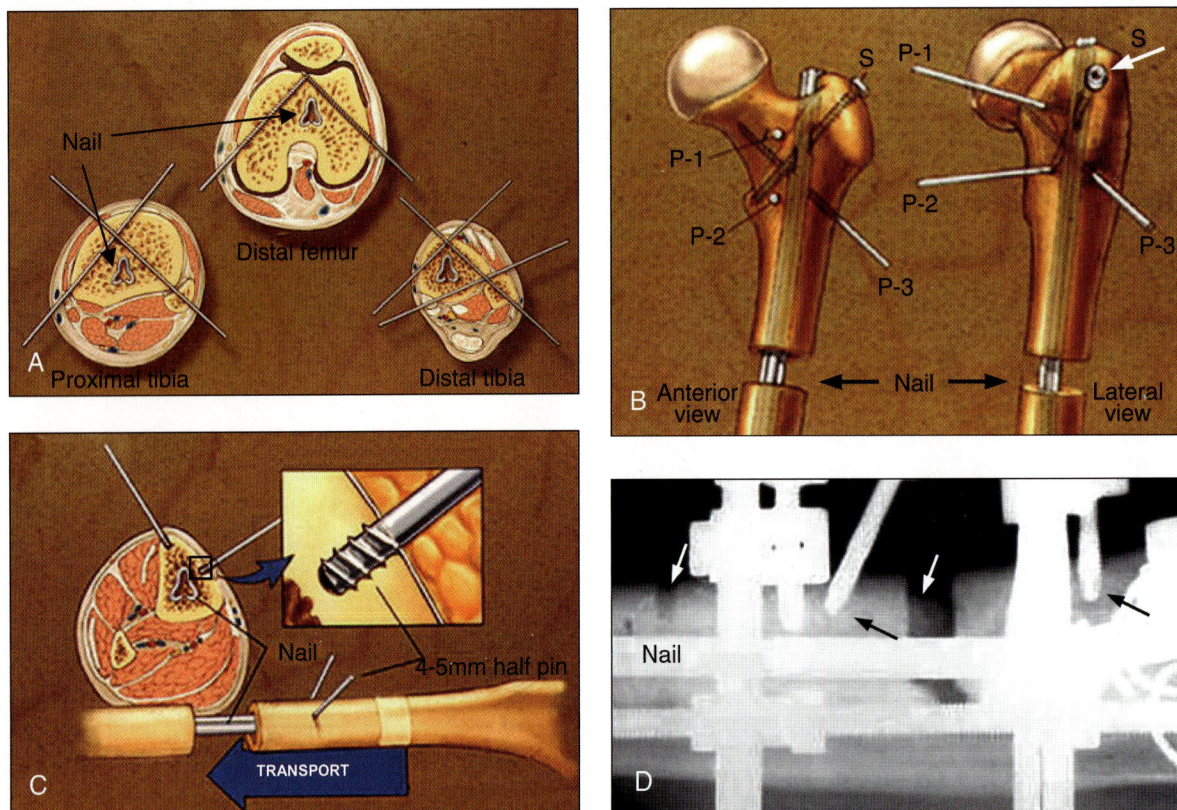

Transport over nail pin strategies. **A,** Cross-section illustrations of the tibia and distal femur show pins placed peripheral to the central axis, out of contact with the nail. **B,** Options for pin placement in the proximal femur (S = proximal interlocking screw) and the positions for half pins (P). **C,** Illustration shows unicortical/intracortical cantilevered half pins (inset) for the transport segment. **D,** Lateral radiograph of a tibia shows bifocal, unicortical half pin fixation (black arrows) and two separate regenerate bone sites (white arrows).

sions, realignment, and/or cancellous bone grafting) using the original fixator.

From 1992 to 1997, all docking sites were recontoured and/or bone grafted before contact and regenerate bone was not allowed to exceed 5 cm in length. As a result, there were significantly more bifocal transports in the second series (27%) than in the first (5%). These changes decreased the rate of regenerate failure from 19% to 7% but did not decrease the rate of docking site nonunion or the treatment time (**Table 4**). Again, all disturbances healed following retreatment using the original frame.

Our third (current) protocol follows guidelines from the second protocol with one exception: instead of waiting for nonunion or failure of the regenerate to fully manifest (6 to 9 months), intervention is initiated at the first sign of a healing disturbance (ie, no evidence of progressive healing on three consecutive radiographs obtained at 4-to 6-week intervals). The intervention, tailored to the anatomic site, physiologic condition of the host, and wound parameters, includes frame removals, new frames, and exchange fixation (external-to-internal, staged or immediate). The data on the first 54 patients treated on this third protocol are listed in

T A B L E 4 **Bone Transports**[a]

Parameter	1988 to 1991	1992 to 1997	1998 to 2003	Average (%)
Number of patients	21	64	52	137
Average defect size (cm)	6.5	7	6.3	6.5
Nonunions	2	7	0[b]	9(7)
Regenerate bone failures	4	6	0[b]	10(9)
Bifocal transports	1	17	10	28(20)
First treatment success (%)	71	80	77	76
Second treatment success (%)	96	94	98	96
Treatment time (months)	17.6	16.4	13.9	15.6

[a] Demographics and treatment outcomes for 137 patients who underwent bone transport from 1988 to 2004 to reconstruct a segmental defect that followed débridement for chronic infection.

[b] 11 early interventions.

Table 4. There were 10 (19%) docking site and three (5%) regenerate disturbances calling for 11 early interventions: seven locking nails (two with bone grafts); two locking plates with bone grafts; and two new frames augmented with marrow grafts. This stepped-up protocol has had a 100% success rate and has decreased the average time of treatment by 18%.

EXCHANGE FIXATION: EXTERNAL TO INTERNAL

When internal stabilization is performed to replace long-term external fixation, steps should be taken to prevent infectious sequelae.[31] At least 5 days before the exchange, all pins that have inflamed tracts or that are positioned within the surgical field are removed and cultures are obtained. Cavitary pin tracts are débrided (overreamed and/or overcuretted) and dressed with matchstick-shaped pieces of antibiotic-impregnated polymethylmethacrylate (PMMA) for 4 to 5 days. Pathogens are treated with bactericidal agents until inflammation resolves.

The new method of fixation (locked or limited-contact plates; solid locked nails) must take into account physician skills, the condition of the host, and the wound parameters. A primary exchange can be performed with an all-PMMA antibiotic rod[32] or with a standard nail coated with antibiotic-impregnated PMMA. Otherwise, definitive internal fixation is staged

to follow a 1- to 3-month course of local antibiotic therapy (**Table 1**). If signs of infection recur and/or healing does not progress, the host and lesion are restaged and a new protocol is initiated.[17]

ACUTE AND GRADUAL SHORTENING

When managing a resection defect up to 1.5 cm, primary apposition of the bone ends at the time of débridement is a well-accepted definitive reconstruction. Defects up to 4 cm may be restored by coupling an acute shortening with lengthening through a corticotomy placed outside the zone of injury (**Figure 6**). This method (bifocal compression/distraction) has several advantages over bone transport alone, including earlier stability and healing at the site of injury, immediate elimination of a coexisting soft-tissue deficit, and rapid mobilization of juxta-articular lesions otherwise prone to stiffness and/or joint contractures.[32,33] Disadvantages of this method include the sequelae of soft-tissue compression (vascular occlusion, nerve entrapment, tissue bulge, difficult wound closures, distal edema) and muscle weakness resulting from shortened musculotendinous units. In patients with deficits 4 cm or greater, an acute shortening also may be coupled with methods of transport and limb lengthening. The method of shortening to "contact" and then lengthening through the same site (monofocal compression/distraction) is prob-

FIGURE 6

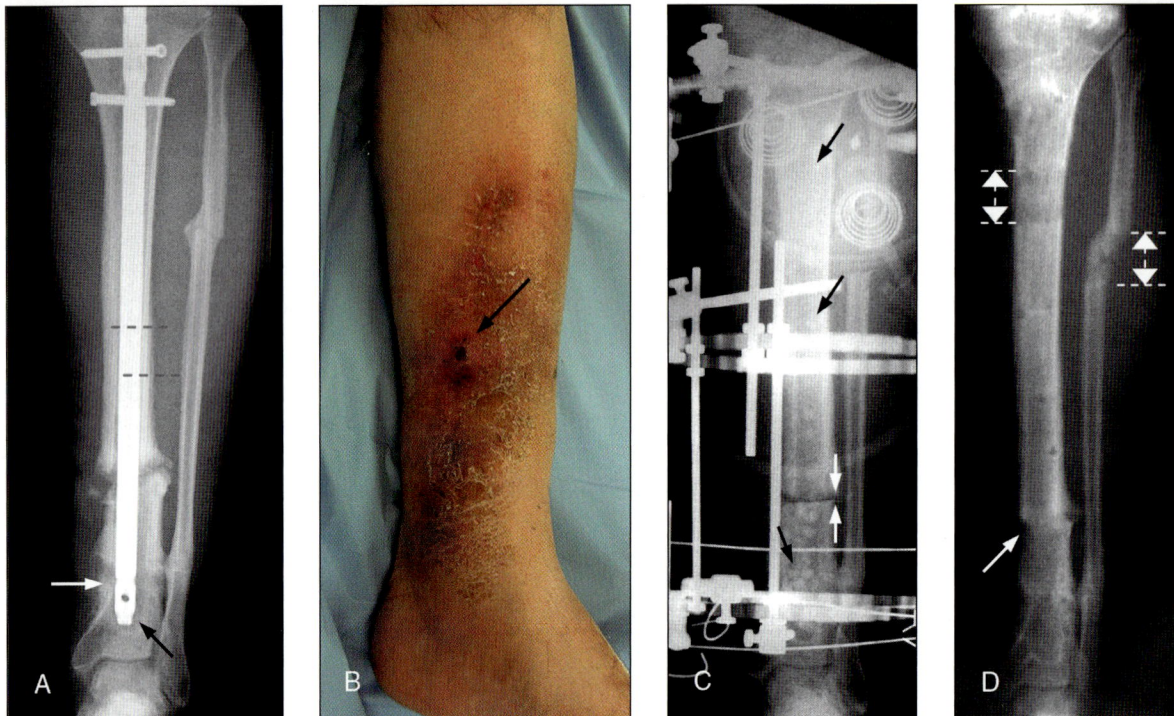

Bifocal compression/distraction. **A,** AP radiograph of an infected tibial nonunion with intramedullary fixation shows cavitation at a previous screw site (white arrow) and an intramedullary abscess (black arrow) at the tip of the nail. **B,** Clinical photograph of a draining fistula (arrow) and dystrophic skin changes on the medial leg. **C,** AP radiograph obtained following débridement/fixation shows that the limb was acutely shortened to docking (white arrows), allowing for an immediate closure over antibiotic beads (black arrows) placed throughout the canal. **D,** AP radiograph obtained following frame removal. Length was restored using a remote corticotomy (double-headed arrows); docking was augmented with intramedullary bone grafts (arrow) placed at the time of bead removal.

lematic and less reliable than when using multifocal techniques.[33-35]

CONCLUSIONS

The principles of sepsis surgery and transosseous bone lengthening (bone transport) are perfect partners in treatment protocols addressing bone loss as a sequela to infection: thorough débridement, coupled with host optimization, creates a live, clean wound that is both resilient and responsive; using distraction as a stimulus, bone transport generates the replacement parts needed to restore both form and function. Using these methods together, significant bone loss is no longer an obstacle to successful limb salvage.

REFERENCES

1. Chang CC, Merritt K: Infection at the site of implanted materials with and without preadhered bacteria. *J Orthop Res* 1994;12(4):526-531.

2. Cierny G III, Mader JT, Penninck JJ: A clinical staging system for adult osteomyelitis. *Clin Orthop Relat Res* 2003(414):7-24.

3. Gristina AG, Costerton JW: Bacterial adherence and the glycocalyx and their role in musculoskeletal infection. *Orthop Clin North Am* 1984;15(3):517-535.

4. Heppenstall RB, Goodwin CW, Brighton CT: Fracture healing in the presence of chronic hypoxia. *J Bone Joint Surg Am* 1997;58(8):1153-1156.

5. Mathes SJ, Alpert BS, Chang N: Use of the muscle flap in chronic osteomyelitis: Experimental and clinical correlation. *Plast Reconstr Surg* 1982;69(5):815-829.

6. Mathes SJ, Feng LJ, Hunt TK: Coverage of the infected wound. *Ann Surg* 1983;198(4):420-429.

7. Patzakis MJ, Wilkins J, Kumar J, Holtom P, Greenbaum B, Ressler R: Comparison of the results of bacterial cultures from multiple sites in chronic osteomyelitis of long bones: A prospective study *J Bone Joint Surg Am* 1994;76(5):664-666.

8. Perry CR, Pearson RL, Miller GA: Accuracy of cultures of material from swabbing of the superficial aspect of the wound and needle biopsy in preoperative assessment of osteomyelitis. *J Bone Joint Surg Am* 1991;73(5):745-749.

9. Whiteside LA, Lesker PA: The effects of extraperiosteal and subperiosteal dissection: Part I. On blood flow in muscle. *J Bone Joint Surg Am* 1978;60(1):23-26.

10. Cierny G III: Infected tibial nonunions (1981-1995): The evolution of change. *Clin Orthop Relat Res* 1999(360):97-105.

11. Cierny G III, DiPasquale D: Treatment of chronic infection. *J Am Acad Orthop Surg* 2006;14(Suppl 10):S105-S110.

12. Gristina AG: Biomaterial-centered infection: Microbial adhesion versus tissue integration. *Science* 1987;237(4822):1588-1595.

13. Costerton JW, Stewart PS, Greenberg EP: Bacterial biofilms: A common cause of persistent infections. *Science* 1999;284(5418):1318-1322.

14. Cierny G III, Mader JT: The surgical treatment of adult osteomyelitis, in Evarts C, McCollister MD, eds: *Surgery of the Musculoskeletal System.* New York, NY, Churchill Livingstone, 1983, pp 4814-4834.

15. Simpson AH, Deakin M, Latham JM: Chronic osteomyelitis: The effect of the extent of surgical resection on infection-free survival. *J Bone Joint Surg Br* 2001;83(3):403-407.

16. Sachs BL, Shaffer JW: Osteomyelitis of the tibia and femur: A critical evaluation of the effectiveness of the Papineau technique in a prospective study. *50th Annual Meeting Proceedings.* Rosemont, IL, American Academy of Orthopaedic Surgeons, 1983.

17. Cierny GC III, DiPasquale D: Adult osteomyelitis, in Cierny G, McClaren AC, Wongworawat MD, eds: *Orthopaedic Knowledge Update: Musculoskeletal Infection.* Rosemont, IL, American Academy of Orthopaedic Surgeons, 2009, p 138.

18. Papineau LJ: Osteocutaneous resection-reconstruction in diaphyseal osteomyelitis. *Clin Orthop Relat Res* 1974(101):306.

19. Sales de Gauzy J, Vidal H, Cahuzac JP: Primary shortening followed by callus distraction for the treatment of a posttraumatic bone defect: Case report. *J Trauma* 1993;34(3):461-463.

20. Yajima H, Tamai S, Mizumoto S, Inada Y: Vascularized fibular grafts in the treatment of osteomyelitis and infected nonunion. *Clin Orthop Relat Res* 1993(293):256-264.

21. Cierny G III, Zorn KE: Segmental tibial defects: Comparing conventional and Ilizarov methodologies. *Clin Orthop Relat Res* 1994(301):118-123.

22. Lowenberg DW, Feibel RJ, Louie KW, Eshima I: Combined muscle flap and Ilizarov reconstruction for bone and soft tissue defects. *Clin Orthop Relat Res* 1996(332):37-51.

23. Cierny G III, Nahai F: Soft tissue reconstruction of the lower leg: Part I. *Perspect Plast Surg* 1988;1(1):1-32.

24. Cierny G III, Nahai F: Dialogue: Lower extremity reconstruction: Part II. *Perspect Plast Surg* 1988;1(2):76-78.

25. Henry SL, Seligson D: Management of open fractures and osteomyelitis with the antibiotic beads pouch technique. *South Med J* 1990;83:98-104.

26. Cierny G III: Managing the débridement defect, in Coombs R, Fitzgerald R, eds: *Infection in the Orthopaedic Patient.* London Press, Butterworth Publishers, 1988.

27. Ilizarov GA: The tension-stress effect on the genesis and growth of tissues: Part I. The influence of stability of fixation and soft-tissue preservation. *Clin Orthop Relat Res* 1989(238):249-281.

28. Ilizarov GA: The tension-stress effect on the genesis and growth of tissues: Part II. The influence of the rate and frequency of distraction. *Clin Orthop Relat Res* 1989(239):263-285.

29. Ilizarov GA, Ledyaev VI: The replacement of long tubular bone defects by lengthening distraction osteotomy of one of the fragments: 1969. *Clin Orthop Relat Res* 1992(280):7-10.

30. Kocaoglu M, Eralp L, Rashid H, Sen C, Bilsel K: Reconstruction of segmental bone defects due to chronic osteomyelitis with use of an external fixator and an intramedullary nail. *J Bone Joint Surg Am* 2006;88(10):2137-2145.

31. Clasper JC, Parker SJ, Simpson AH, Watkins PE: Contamination of the medullary canal following pin-tract infection. *J Orthop Res* 1999;17(6):947-952.

32. Paley D, Herzenberg JE: Intramedullary infections treated with antibiotic cement rods: Preliminary results in nine cases. *J Orthop Trauma* 2002;16(10):723-729.

33. Sen C, Kocaoglu M, Eralp L, Gulsen M, Cinar M: Bifocal compression-distraction in the acute treatment of grade III open tibia fractures with bone and soft-tissue loss: A report of 24 cases. *J Orthop Trauma* 2004;18(3):150-157.

34. Sen C, Eralp L, Gunes T, Erdem M, Ozden VE, Kocaoglu M: An alternative method for the treatment of nonunion of the tibia with bone loss. *J Bone Joint Surg Br* 2006;88(6):783-789.

35. Meffert RH, Inoue N, Tis JE, Brug E, Chao EY: Distraction osteogenesis after acute limb-shortening for segmental tibial defects: Comparison of a monofocal and a bifocal technique in rabbits. *J Bone Joint Surg Am* 2000;82(6):799-808.

CHAPTER 20

TREATMENT OF SEGMENTAL BONE LOSS DUE TO TUMORS

HIROYUKI TSUCHIYA, MD, PhD

INTRODUCTION

Distraction osteogenesis performed with the ring fixator invented by Ilizarov and callotasis performed with the unilateral fixator developed by de Bastiani have been widely adopted to treat several orthopaedic problems such as limb-length discrepancy, deformity, nonunion, osteomyelitis, and congenital or acquired skeletal defects.[1-4] Skeletal defects related to bone tumor, trauma, and infection have been treated with free autografts, vascularized bone transfers, allografts, heat-treated autografts, artificial bone substitutes, spacers, and prostheses. In the case of skeletal reconstruction, however, bone defects ideally should be repaired using living bone. The main advantage of distraction osteogenesis is that it can achieve regeneration of living bone that has the same strength and width as the native bone. Peripheral nerves, vessels, muscles, tendons, ligaments, and skin also are gradually lengthened in proportion to the lengthening of the bone. This chapter reviews applications of distraction osteogenesis for tumor surgery.

RECONSTRUCTION AFTER MALIGNANT TUMOR EXCISION

Patient Selection

Patient selection is of paramount importance. Patients with low-grade tumors can safely undergo distraction osteogenesis because they have no chemotherapy-related risk factors and they have healthy, well-preserved soft tissues; both of these factors lead to good bone regeneration. Patients with diaphyseal or metaphyseal defects are very good candidates for reconstruction with distraction osteogenesis because the joint is preserved and reconstruction provides excellent limb function. Patients with tumors that respond favorably to chemotherapy also are good candidates for this treatment because their prognosis is good. Distraction osteogenesis also is indicated in patients with defects smaller than 15 cm, a great deal of preserved healthy tissue, and a good prognosis. By combining the use of an intramedullary nail with distraction osteogenesis, even defects larger than 15 cm can be treated.

Distraction Osteogenesis Technique

Ilizarov initially generated bone with distraction physiolysis, in which the growth plate is mechanically distracted without performing an osteotomy and bone forms as a result. Subsequently, Ilizarov developed distraction osteogenesis, which features de novo bone formation between vascular bone surfaces created by osteotomy and gradual distraction.[2-4] I prefer to use four basic methods: simple lengthening, bone transport, shortening-distraction, and lengthening combined with

---

Neither Dr. Tsuchiya nor any immediate family member has received anything of value from or owns stock in a commercial company or institution related directly or indirectly to the subject of this chapter.

intramedullary nailing. Intramedullary nailing helps reduce external fixation time. Lengthening is performed over an intramedullary nail with either proximal or distal locking screws when primary intramedullary nailing is feasible before distraction (primary nailing). Screws are placed on the unlocked side after distraction is complete, and the external fixator maintains the length of distraction. When primary nailing is difficult to perform, intramedullary nailing is performed after distraction is complete (delayed nailing).[5,6]

Principles of Reconstruction

A recent subject of interest in limb-saving surgery in the tumor patient is the improvement of limb function without negatively affecting survival rates.[7] Several modalities are available for the treatment of bone loss, including autografts, heat-treated bone, allografts, biomaterials, prostheses, and distraction osteogenesis. To refine limb-saving surgery and provide natural limb function, the linkage between distraction osteogenesis and primary reconstruction after massive tumor resection was established at my institution in 1989. Recently, several authors reported on the advantages[5,6,8-16] and disadvantages[15] of distraction osteogenesis performed after tumor surgery.

Ideal bone reconstruction should feature resistance to infection, durability, long-lasting stability and biologic affinity, and, eventually, good limb function.[8] A characteristic of distraction osteogenesis is the regeneration of living bone together with muscles, tendons, nerves, and skin. Tumor reconstruction by means of distraction osteogenesis consists of several steps: preconstruction of a frame, adequate tumor excision, osteotomy, and distraction performed with or without chemotherapy. The distraction procedure is the same as that used for trauma or congenital cases. My classification of reconstruction based on the location of the bone defect after tumor excision includes five types: diaphyseal reconstruction, metaphyseal reconstruction, epiphyseal reconstruction, subarticular reconstruction, and arthrodesis.[5] After adequate tumor excision, a preconstructed Ilizarov frame or unilateral fixator is used. Patients with high-grade tumors usually undergo a regular course of postoperative chemotherapy. Postoperative rehabilitation entails weight bearing while using crutches and range-of-motion exercises for the knee, initiated after subsidence

of bleeding and wound pain or 3 weeks after surgery, when the patellar tendon is reattached.

Low-grade malignant tumors such as parosteal osteosarcoma, low-grade central osteosarcoma, chondrosarcoma, and adamantinoma are usually treated with wide or marginal excision. Healthy soft tissue sometimes has to be sacrificed for tumor excision, and this loss may lead to poor blood supply, affecting regeneration. After adequate tumor excision, distraction osteogenesis can be applied safely and successfully. A diaphyseal defect is treated simply with bone transport or a shortening-distraction procedure with or without an intramedullary nail (**Figure 1**). I usually use a shortening-distraction procedure with a femoral defect smaller than 10 cm or a tibial defect smaller than 5 cm. Careful attention should be paid to the possibility of nerve injury and circulatory disturbance. Difficulty with wound closure and invagination of muscle also are limiting factors when shortening the defect.

High-grade malignant tumors such as osteosarcoma, Ewing sarcoma, and malignant fibrous histiocytoma usually are treated with wide or radical resection and are accompanied by loss of healthy soft tissue. In most cases, chemotherapy is performed pre- and postoperatively, sometimes in conjunction with radiation therapy. The clinical effects of chemotherapy and radiation on bone formation are still unclear, but they may be negative.[16,17] My colleagues and I found that most healthy soft tissue can be preserved for good bone formation by means of an intentional marginal procedure with the support of caffeine-assisted chemotherapy. In addition, important structures such as the epiphysis and the ligaments that contribute to joint stability can be preserved.[7] Epiphyseal sparing and reconstruction with distraction osteogenesis are the only chance for restoration of the affected limb to as close to normal as possible (**Figure 2**). Epiphyseal preservation is indicated by tumor extension seen on MRI and the response to preoperative chemotherapy; that is, the epiphysis can be preserved when little or no involvement of tumor is seen on MRI and a remarkable response to preoperative chemotherapy is observed.

Pitfalls and Common Errors

Delayed consolidation, fracture, deep infection, pes equinus, skin invagination, nerve palsy, skin necrosis, defor-

FIGURE 1

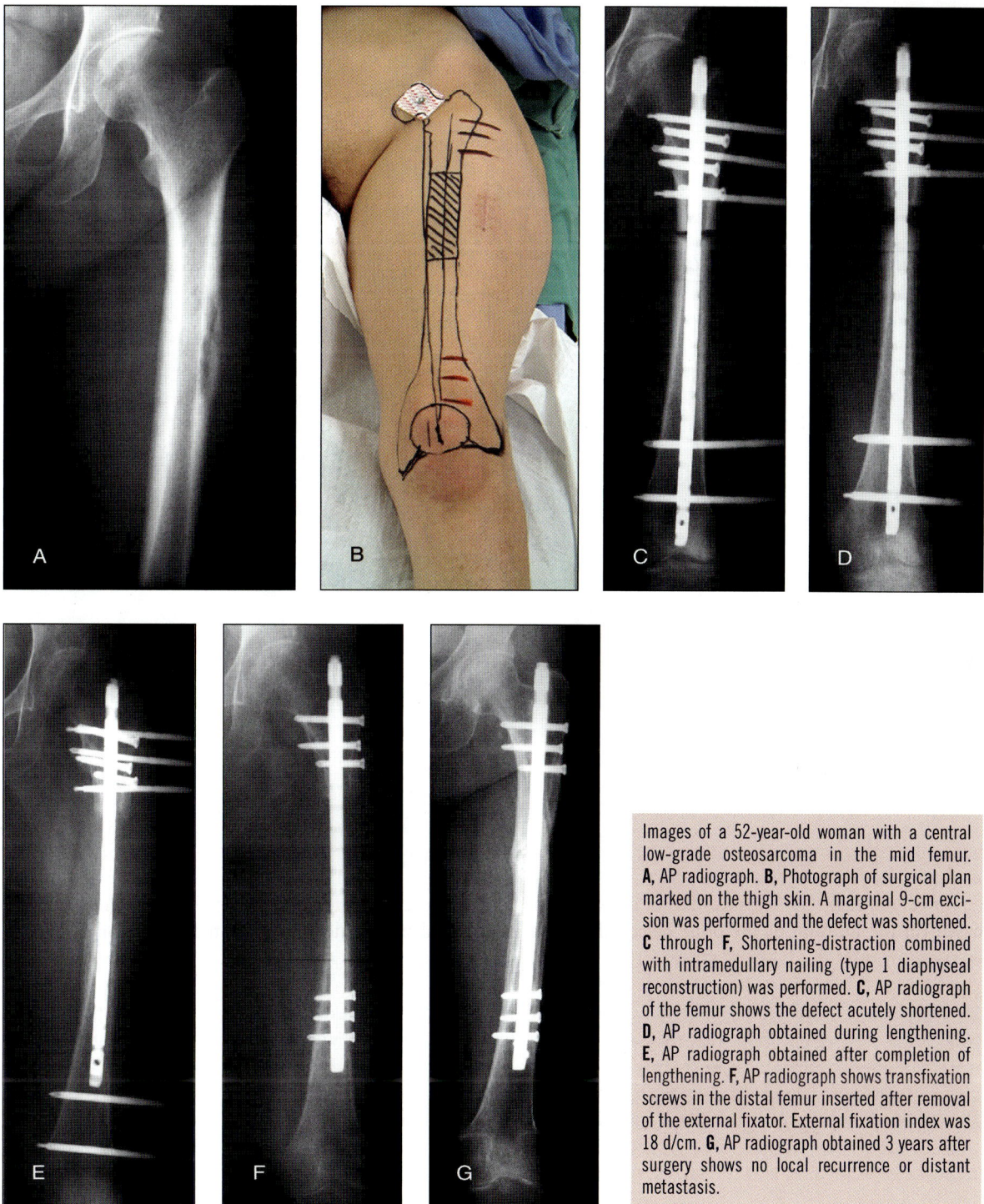

Images of a 52-year-old woman with a central low-grade osteosarcoma in the mid femur. **A,** AP radiograph. **B,** Photograph of surgical plan marked on the thigh skin. A marginal 9-cm excision was performed and the defect was shortened. **C** through **F,** Shortening-distraction combined with intramedullary nailing (type 1 diaphyseal reconstruction) was performed. **C,** AP radiograph of the femur shows the defect acutely shortened. **D,** AP radiograph obtained during lengthening. **E,** AP radiograph obtained after completion of lengthening. **F,** AP radiograph shows transfixation screws in the distal femur inserted after removal of the external fixator. External fixation index was 18 d/cm. **G,** AP radiograph obtained 3 years after surgery shows no local recurrence or distant metastasis.

FIGURE 2

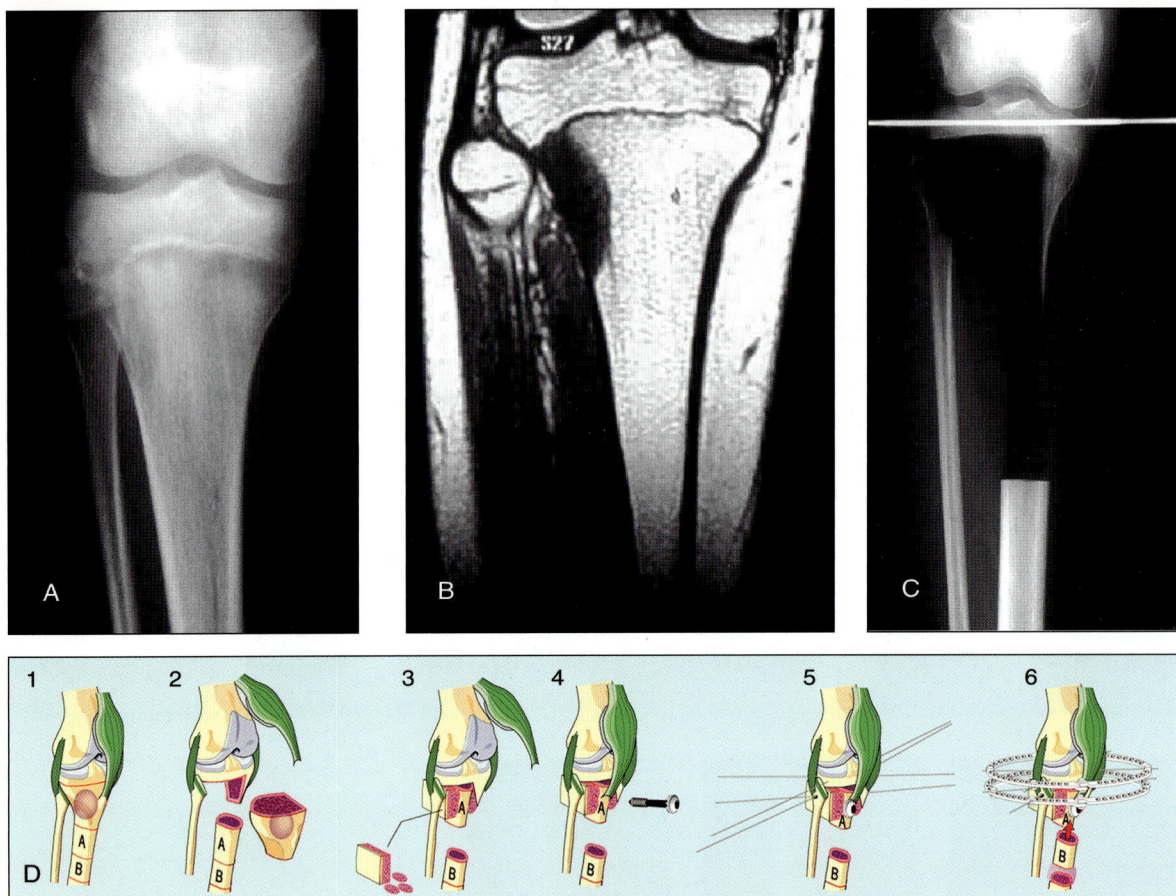

Images of a 13-year-old girl with a high-grade osteosarcoma in the proximal tibia who underwent epiphyseal preservation and type 2 metaphyseal reconstruction. Preoperative AP radiograph (**A**) and coronal T1-weighted MRI (**B**). **C,** AP radiograph after tumor resection. The surgeon decided to preserve the epiphysis because preoperative chemotherapy was judged very effective and the lesion was localized. **D,** Diagram shows steps in type 2 metaphyseal reconstruction; wires are inserted into the preserved epiphysis: (1) planned osteotomy lines, (2) tumor excision, (3) periarticular reconstruction using bone cylinder A, (4) reattachment of patellar tendon, (5) wire fixation, and (6) ring fixation.

(continued)

mity, premature consolidation, and joint subluxation or dislocation are complications that may be encountered during or after treatment. These complications are successfully solved by surgical or nonsurgical treatment. At present, it is not possible to completely avoid complications in limb-saving tumor surgery, regardless of what reconstructive method is used. Reconstruction is more likely to be successful with distraction osteogenesis even when complications occur because living bone is easier to handle than dead bone or a prosthesis.

Postoperative Care

The steps involved in distraction osteogenesis include stable fixation of the fragments, treatment (latency, dis-

FIGURE 2 (*continued*)

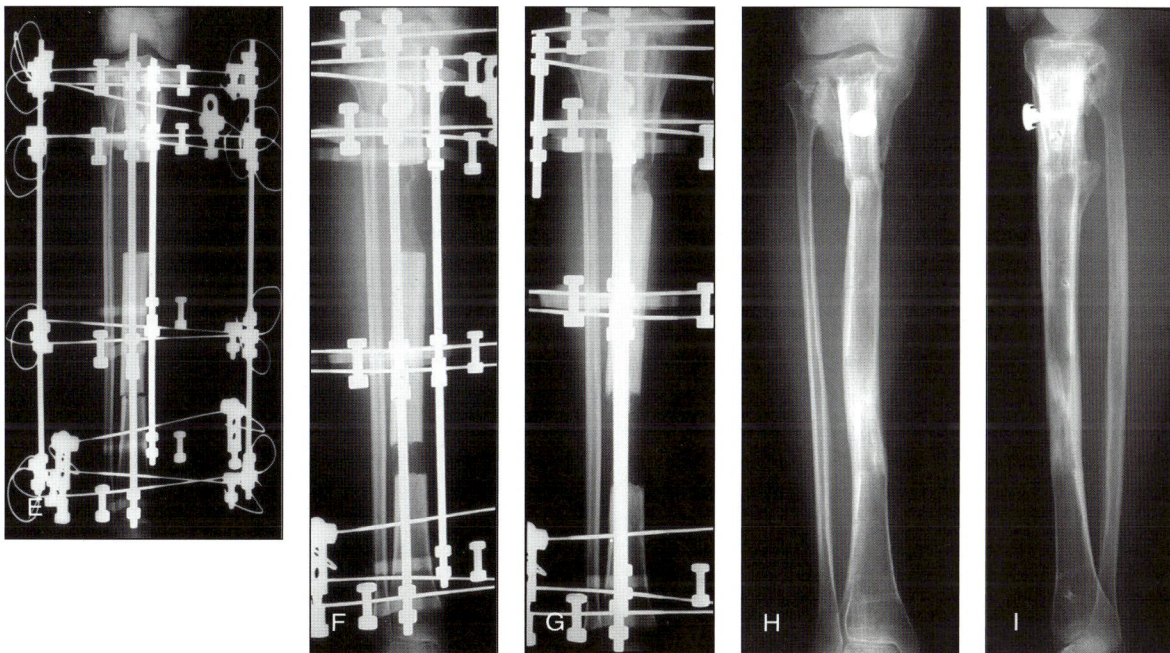

AP radiographs show tibia before (**E**), during (**F**), and after (**G**) transport. A cylinder of bone was taken from the diaphysis and the periartic-ular structure was stabilized first. The patellar tendon was reattached to the cylinder bone with a spike washer and screw. Bone transport was then conducted to reconstruct the newly created diaphyseal defect. The external fixation index was 56 d/cm. AP (**H**) and lateral (**I**) radiographs obtained 4 years postoperatively show no recurrence and no metastasis. The patient was using the limb normally and enjoying athletic activities.

traction, and consolidation phases), regenerate assessment, and removal of the frame. Distraction is started 7 to 14 days after osteotomy at a rate of 0.5 mm twice daily or 0.25 mm four times daily. This rate is later either reduced to zero if the callus formation is delayed or impaired, or increased to 1.5 mm/d if the callus formation is likely to consolidate prematurely. The external fixator is removed when sufficient consolidation is attained. Usually, consolidation takes 1.5 to 2 times as long as distraction. After removal of the external fixator, a cast or an orthosis is applied for approximately 4 weeks. In the case of very poor callus formation, distraction is delayed, or compression and distraction of a moving segment (accordion maneuver) is performed. If these procedures fail, an iliac bone graft should be applied to the lengthened site.

Distraction osteogenesis is safe and useful for biologic bone reconstruction after tumor resection. The main advantage of distraction osteogenesis is regeneration of living bone, and the disadvantage is the psychosocial burden and complications resulting from long-term external fixation. The Ilizarov fixator is used mainly for juxta-articular reconstruction, and a unilateral fixator for diaphyseal reconstruction or arthrodesis. Epiphyseal preservation and reconstruction by means of distraction osteogenesis can provide excellent outcomes in selected cases, resulting in sturdy reconstruction and reproduction of the native limb. Tumor surgery has progressed from amputation to limb-saving surgery to joint-saving surgery.[10]

Reconstruction of bone loss due to tumor involves some difficulties, such as an extensive defect, loss of healthy soft tissue, and the need for chemotherapy. In the case of high-grade tumors, accurate timing of antibiotics administration, change of dressing, and adjustment of the lengthening rate are essential to achieve reconstruction. Joint preservation and bone regeneration by means of distraction osteogenesis constitute a highly conservative limb-saving surgery.

REFERENCES

1. De Bastiani G, Aldegheri R, Renzi-Brivio L, Trivella G: Limb lengthening by callus distraction (callotasis). *J Pediatr Orthop* 1987;7(2):129-134.

2. Ilizarov GA: The tension-stress effect on the genesis and growth of tissues: Part I. The influence of stability of fixation and soft-tissue preservation. *Clin Orthop Relat Res* 1989(238):249-281.

3. Ilizarov GA: The tension-stress effect on the genesis and growth of tissues: Part II. The influence of the rate and frequency of distraction. *Clin Orthop Relat Res* 1989(239):263-285.

4. Ilizarov GA: *The Transosseous Osteosynthesis: Theoretical and Clinical Aspects of the Regeneration and Growth of Tissue.* New York, NY, Springer, 1992.

5. Tsuchiya H, Tomita K, Minematsu K, Mori Y, Asada N, Kitano S: Limb salvage using distraction osteogenesis: A classification of the technique. *J Bone Joint Surg Br* 1997;79(3):403-411.

6. Tsuchiya H, Kitano S, Tomita K: Periarticular reconstruction using distraction osteogenesis after en bloc tumor resection. *Arch Am Acad Orthop Surg* 1999;2: 68-75.

7. Tsuchiya H, Tomita K, Mori Y, Asada N, Yamamoto N: Marginal excision for osteosarcoma with caffeine assisted chemotherapy. *Clin Orthop Relat Res* 1999(358):27-35.

8. Cara JA, Forriol F, Canadell J: Bone lengthening after conservative oncologic surgery. *J Pediatr Orthop B* 1993;2(1):57-61.

9. González-Herranz P, Burgos-Flores J, Ocete-Guzmán JG, López-Mondejar JA, Amaya S: The management of limb-length discrepancies in children after treatment of osteosarcoma and Ewing's sarcoma. *J Pediatr Orthop* 1995;15(5):561-565.

10. Kapukaya A, Subaşi M, Kandiya E, Ozateş M, Yilmaz F: Limb reconstruction with the callus distraction method after bone tumor resection. *Arch Orthop Trauma Surg* 2000;120(3-4):215-218.

11. Millett PJ, Lane JM, Paletta GA Jr: Limb salvage using distraction osteogenesis. *Am J Orthop (Belle Mead NJ)* 2000;29(8):628-632.

12. Said GZ, el-Sherif EK: Resection-shortening-distraction for malignant bone tumours: A report of two cases. *J Bone Joint Surg Br* 1995;77(2):185-188.

13. Stoffelen D, Lammens J, Fabry G: Resection of a periosteal osteosarcoma and reconstruction using the Ilizarov technique of segmental transport. *J Hand Surg Br* 1993;18(2):144-146.

14. Tsuchiya H, Tomita K, Shinokawa Y, Minematsu K, Katsuo S, Taki J: The Ilizarov method in the management of giant-cell tumours of the proximal tibia. *J Bone Joint Surg Br* 1996;78(2):264-269.

15. Ozaki T, Nakatsuka Y, Kunisada T, et al: High complication rate of reconstruction using Ilizarov bone transport method in patients with bone sarcomas. *Arch Orthop Trauma Surg* 1998;118(3):136-139.

16. Tsuchiya H, Tomita K: Distraction osteogenesis for treatment of bone loss in the lower extremity. *J Orthop Sci* 2003;8(1):116-124.

17. Subasi M, Kapukaya A: Distraction osteogenesis for treatment of bone loss in the lower extremity. *J Orthop Sci* 2003;8(6):882-884.

LIMB LENGTHENING IN SKELETALLY MATURE PATIENTS

S. ROBERT ROZBRUCH, MD

INTRODUCTION

Distraction osteogenesis using the Ilizarov method is a widely used technique for leg lengthening,[1-3] deformity correction,[4-7] and the reconstruction of nonunions and bone defects.[5,8-11] The process has two successive stages: distraction and consolidation.[3,12] External fixation generally has been considered necessary for both stages.

Different issues occur in limb lengthening in skeletally mature patients than in growing children. Adult patients have closed growth plates and longer and wider bones, and typically bony union takes longer to achieve in adults than in children. The consolidation phase can be prolonged in adults; 1 cm of lengthening often is estimated to take 2 months.[1] This prolonged time in an external fixation frame confers several disadvantages. First, a greater chance exists of health-related complications, including pin-tract infection and decreased range of motion in the surrounding joints. Second, the process can affect the patient psychologically, increasing frustration and decreasing compliance. Finally, when the frame is removed, the regenerate bone is at risk for fracture because of the lack of any internal stabilization. O'Carrigan et al[13] reported an 8% fracture rate after frame removal in a review of 650 patients with 986 lengthening segments. Simpson and Kenwright[14] reported a frac-

ture rate of 9.4% in a series of 180 lengthening segments.

Closed growth plates and larger bones found in adults allow the use of hybrid techniques that include both internal (eg, intramedullary rods and plates) and external fixation. Methods of lengthening that minimize or eliminate time in external fixation and protect against refracture include lengthening and then nailing (LATN),[15] lengthening over a nail (LON),[12,16-18] lengthening and then plating (LAP), lengthening over a plate,[19] and the use of a fully implantable limb-lengthening nail,[20] which is discussed in a separate chapter.

To address the prolonged consolidation phase in adults, we often implement adjuvant treatments that have been shown to enhance bone formation. These include ultrasound,[21-24] electric bone stimulation,[25,26] and injection of bone marrow aspirate concentrate into the unhealed regenerate bone.[4,27,28] To enhance regenerate bone healing, we occasionally have used pharmacologic agents such as parathyroid hormone[29-31] and bisphosphonates.[32-34]

LENGTHENING AND THEN NAILING

LATN (**Figure 1**) is a new technique my colleagues and I developed that uses external fixation for lengthening

Dr. Rozbruch or an immediate family member has received royalties from EBI and SBI, is a member of a speakers' bureau or has made paid presentations on behalf of Smith & Nephew, serves as a paid consultant to or is an employee of EBI and SBI, has received research or institutional support from Smith & Nephew, and has received nonincome support (such as equipment or services), commercially derived honoraria, or other non–research-related funding (such as paid travel) from SBI and EBI.

FIGURE 1

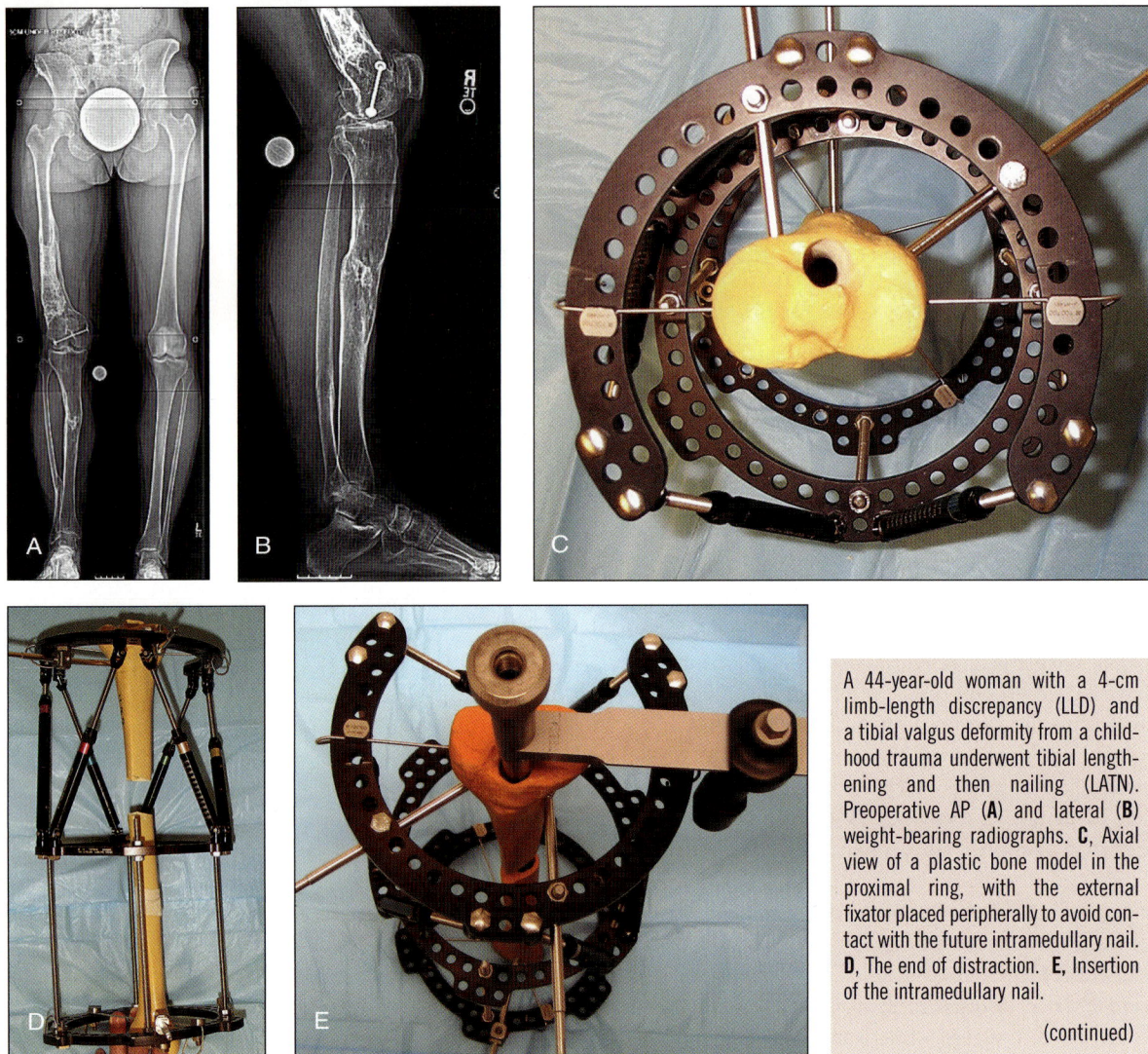

A 44-year-old woman with a 4-cm limb-length discrepancy (LLD) and a tibial valgus deformity from a childhood trauma underwent tibial lengthening and then nailing (LATN). Preoperative AP (**A**) and lateral (**B**) weight-bearing radiographs. **C**, Axial view of a plastic bone model in the proximal ring, with the external fixator placed peripherally to avoid contact with the future intramedullary nail. **D**, The end of distraction. **E**, Insertion of the intramedullary nail.

(continued)

during the distraction phase. The external fixator is applied so that an intramedullary nail can be inserted while the frame is in place, without contact between the internal and external fixation pins and wires. Once the final length has been achieved, a reamed, locked intramedullary nail is inserted across the regenerate bone and the frame is removed. The intramedullary nail supports the bone during the consolidation phase, allowing removal of the external fixator after the distrac-

tion phase of lengthening. The goal is to decrease the time needed for external fixation and to protect the bone from deformation and refracture.

Surgical Technique

For LATN in the tibia, a fibular osteotomy is performed under tourniquet control. A 3-cm incision is made on the lateral aspect of the middle leg and the fibula is approached in the interval between the lateral and pos-

FIGURE 1 (*continued*)

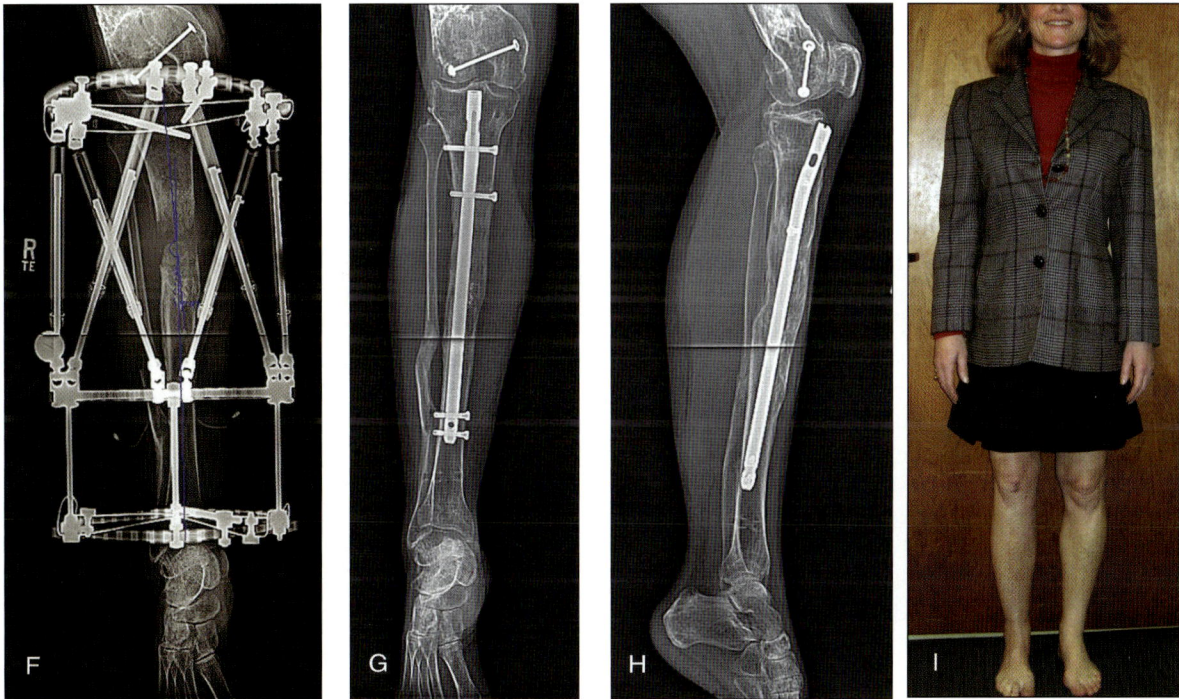

F, AP radiograph obtained at the end of distraction shows 4-cm lengthening and deformity correction. AP (**G**) and lateral (**H**) radiographs and clinical photograph (**I**) obtained 3.5 months following insertion of intramedullary nail and removal of frame. Note bony union on the radiographs. (Parts C through F reproduced with permission from Rozbruch SR, Kleinman D, Fragomen AT, Ilizarov I: Limb lengthening and then insertion of an intramedullary nail. *Clin Orthop Relat Res* 2008;466:2923-2932.)

terior compartments. The fibular osteotomy is then performed using a multiple–drill-hole technique with a 1.8-mm wire and completed with an osteotome. The tourniquet is not used for the remainder of the surgery. A three-ring Taylor spatial frame (TSF) (Smith & Nephew, Memphis, TN) is applied using a rings-first method.[7,35] The proximal ring is stabilized with a 1.8-mm tensioned transverse wire, a 1.8-mm tibiofibular wire, an anteromedial half pin, and an anterolateral half pin. The configuration of this proximal ring fixation is unique in that the bone fixation is placed peripherally within the proximal tibia to allow future insertion of an intramedullary nail, avoiding any contact with the external fixation pins (**Figure 1, *C***). The 1.8-mm wires are placed more posteriorly in the tibia than is typical. The half pins are placed using a cannulated wire tech-

nique for precision. The anteromedial half pin is at the periphery of the tibia and is placed in an anterior-to-posterior direction. The anterolateral half pin also is at the periphery of the tibia and is placed in an antero-lateral-to-posterior central direction. The proximal ring is the reference ring, and the TSF mounting parameters[35] are measured in relation to this ring. The origin[35] is placed at the level of deformity within the diaphysis. When no deformity exists, the origin is assigned to the center of the bone at the osteotomy level 10 to 12 cm distal to the knee joint. Next, a ring block consisting of two rings connected with four rods is applied to the mid distal tibia orthogonal to the tibial diaphysis. The distal ring is stabilized with a 1.8-mm transverse wire 1.5 cm proximal to the ankle joint, a 1.8-mm tibiofibular wire 2 cm proximal to the ankle joint, and a 6-mm half pin placed in an anteromedial-to-posterolateral direction. The middle ring has no fixation. The proximal and middle rings are then connected with six TSF struts and the lengths are recorded. The struts then are removed for the tibial osteotomy.

The tibial osteotomy is performed in a percutaneous fashion using a multiple–drill-hole technique. The osteotomy is then stabilized in a nondisplaced position by reattaching the struts. Distraction is started 7 to 10 days postoperatively. The distraction schedule is planned using the TSF internet-based software (Smith & Nephew, Memphis, TN), which implements the total residual method. The entire deformity is carefully corrected at the osteotomy site before nail insertion.

After final length and deformity correction are achieved, the second-stage surgery is scheduled with minimal delay. We do not operate if the patient has an active pin-tract infection. No tourniquet is used for surgery. The external fixator is sprayed with an antiseptic solution and prepared into the surgical field. Antiseptic-soaked sponges are placed around all pin sites. The frame is covered with sterile towels to avoid contact as much as possible. A 4.5-mm solid syndesmosis screw is inserted 1 cm proximal to the distal tibial pin fixation to prevent proximal fibular migration. The screw is placed in an oblique fashion, engaging two fibular cortices and two tibial cortices. The nail diameter and length were templated before surgery and a custom interlocking hole was made so that two interlocking screws can be inserted into the proximal segment without using the standard proximal interlocking screw hole. The standard proximal hole typically is located at the same level as the previously placed external fixation pins, and this would lead to contamination. A minimal incision technique is used for intramedullary nail insertion. With the knee flexed, a percutaneous Steinmann pin is placed at the optimal location for nail entry in the proximal tibia. This pin is placed using biplanar fluoroscopy, carefully avoiding contact with previously placed external fixator pins. A 2-cm incision is made, and the patellar tendon is incised longitudinally. A 10-mm cannulated drill is used to open the intramedullary canal. The guidewire is passed across the regenerate bone and into the distal fragment, ending at the syndesmosis screw. Serial reaming is performed until cortical chatter is achieved, and a nail 1 mm smaller than the last reamer used is inserted. The maximum amount of reaming particles are retained within the tibia. The regenerate site is not opened, and no reaming particles are removed. One proximal interlocking screw is inserted using a special jig that allows clearance of the proximal ring. The second proximal interlocking screw and the two distal interlocking screws are placed using a freehand technique. The surgical wounds are irrigated, closed, and covered with antiseptic sponges. The external fixator is then removed without risk of tibial displacement or shortening. The pin sites are irrigated, but not curettaged or closed. The surgical wounds and pin sites are covered with a dry, sterile dressing. If gastrocnemius recession is performed, it is done after frame removal.

No cast or splint is used postoperatively. Twenty-pound partial weight bearing is allowed after surgery in unilateral cases. In bilateral cases, protected weight bearing with crutches is allowed for transfers and walking fewer than 10 steps at a time, for a maximum of 50 steps per day. Prophylactic intravenous antibiotics are administered for 48 hours after surgery.

Clinical Results

My colleagues and I reported our experience in a retrospective case-matched comparison study of 39 limbs (in 27 patients) lengthened with LATN versus lengthening using classic techniques.[15] The LATN group wore the external fixator for less time than the classic group (12 versus 29 weeks). The LATN group had a lower external fixation index (0.5 versus 1.9) and a lower bone healing index (0.8 versus 1.9) than the classic group. LATN confers advantages over the classic method, including shorter times needed in external fixation, quicker bone healing, and protection against refracture.

LENGTHENING AND THEN PLATING

The LAP technique (**Figure 2**) was developed to decrease the time spent in the frame when the osteotomy is in close proximity to a joint. External fixation is used for lengthening during the distraction phase. The external fixator is applied so that a plate can be inserted while the frame is in place; however, this must be done without contact between the internal and external fixation pins and wires. Once final length and deformity correc-

FIGURE 2

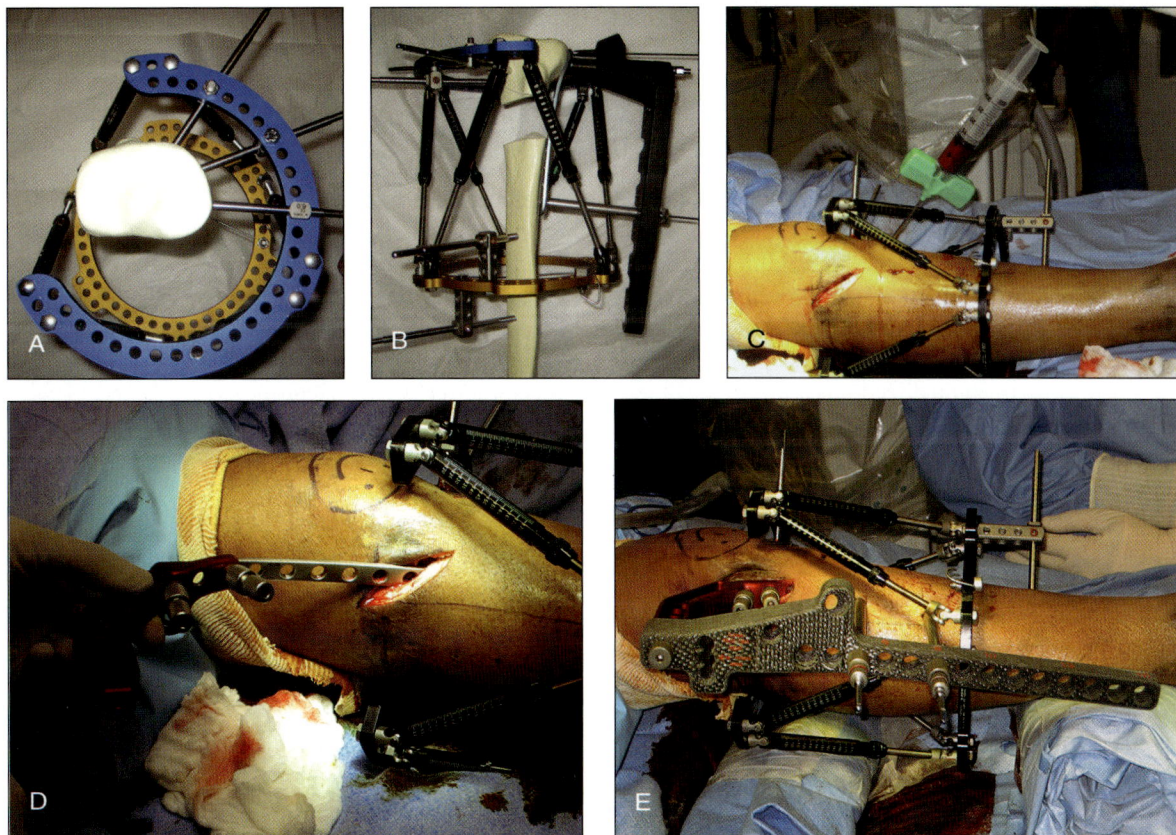

Images of tibial lengthening and then plating (LAP). **A,** Axial view of a plastic bone model in an external fixator shows the proximal ⅔ ring positioned with the opening on the lateral side and the half pin configuration on the medial side. **B,** Insertion of the plate from the lateral side at the end of lengthening. Note the targeting jig location in relation to the distal ring. Intraoperative photographs show the proximal lateral tibial incision and injection of bone marrow aspirate concentrate into the regenerate bone (**C**), plate insertion (**D**), and the jig applied for percutaneous screw insertion (**E**).

tion have been achieved, a locked plate is inserted across the regenerate bone and the frame is removed. The plate supports the bone during the consolidation phase, allowing removal of the external fixator after the distraction phase of lengthening. The goal is to decrease the time required in external fixation and protect the bone from deformation and refracture. This technique was introduced as an alternative to LATN when the osteotomy must be performed in the proximal tibia or distal femur. A proximal tibial osteotomy may be necessary if the apex of the deformity is located there, as

with genu varum and shortening. Alternatively, the treatment may be bifocal, with nonunion repair or ankle fusion occurring in the distal tibia while lengthening takes place in the proximal tibia. Of note, I also have used LAP in the distal tibial.

Surgical Technique

For LAP in the tibia, a fibular osteotomy is performed in the same manner as described for LATN. A ⅔ three-ring TSF is applied using a rings-first method. A ring is used at the proximal tibia, with the opening of the ring facing laterally. The pin fixation is placed from the medial side, leaving the lateral approach undisturbed. The reference pin is placed in a medial-to-lateral direction perpendicular to the proximal mechanical axis using a cannulated wire technique. The second pin is placed in an anteromedial-to-posterolateral direction to set the ring in both the coronal and sagittal planes. The third pin is placed in an anteromedial-to-posterolateral direction using a cannulated wire technique and captures the fibular head. First, the 1.8-mm wire is directed from the proximal fibula in an anteromedial direction. Then, a cube is placed on the ring at the location of the wire. A cannulated 4.8-mm drill is used in an anteromedial-to-posterolateral direction, ending at the fibular head, and a 6-mm pin is inserted. The distal ring is applied so that the pin fixation will be distal to the future plating. Placing three to four locking screws into the distal fragment at plate insertion is desirable.

The proximal ring is the reference ring, and the TSF mounting parameters are measured in relation to this ring. The ring orientation requires the input of rotatory frame offset into the TSF program because the master tab of the reference ring is rotated. The origin is placed at the level of deformity within the metaphysis. When no deformity exists, the origin is assigned to the center of the bone at the osteotomy level 5 cm distal to the knee joint just beyond the tibial tubercle.

After lengthening is completed, a second surgery is performed to insert the plate. The plate is inserted with the TSF in place. Pin sites are covered with antiseptic-soaked sponges and the frame is prepared into the field. The frame is maximally covered with towels to minimize contact and contamination. A 5-cm incision is made at the proximal lateral tibia. The iliotibial band insertion on the Gerdy tubercle is released, and the split in the anterior fascia is used as a portal for the plate. A locked plate is inserted along the lateral aspect of the tibia in an anterograde direction using biplanar fluoroscopy for optimal positioning. The plate targeting device is attached to the plate and used for screw insertion. The first screw is nonlocking and placed at the proximal plate to pull the plate to the bone. All subsequent screws are locking screws. Care is taken to avoid deforming the plate. Often, the distal plate is translated off the bone. Typically, four screws are inserted in both the proximal and distal segments. The frame is then removed, carefully avoiding contact between the internal and external fixation.

Clinical Results

LAP was used to treat 18 limbs (7 femora and 11 tibias) in 16 patients (unpublished presentation, Rozbruch et al, Limb Lengthening and Reconstruction Society annual meeting, July 11-13, 2008, Albuquerque, NM). An external fixator was applied to accomplish lengthening and/or deformity correction in the distraction phase. Subsequently, during a single surgery, a locked plate and screws were inserted in a minimally invasive fashion to support consolidation of the regenerate bone, after which the external fixation was removed. Initial pin/wire/ring placement was planned carefully to avoid contact with and to facilitate insertion of the internal fixation (**Figure 3**).

The mean patient age was 37 years; mean follow-up was 9.7 months. Mean limb-length discrepancy improvement was from 3.0 cm to 2 mm, and the average lengthening accomplished was 4.5 cm in the femur and 3.3 cm in the tibia. Mean time spent in the external fixation frame after osteotomy for lengthening was 2.7 months in the femur and 3.2 months in the tibia. The mean external fixation index for lengthening was 0.67 mo/cm in the femur and 1.05 mo/cm in the tibia (combined femoral and tibial range, 0.4 to 1.8 months). Full weight bearing was tolerated 5.41 months after osteotomy and was considered the time of bony healing. The average bone healing index was 1.65 mo/cm. In the tibial group, complications included one plate breakage that required removal of the hardware and reapplication of external fixation, and a plate bend with a mild change of alignment.

My colleagues and I concluded that LAP can be a safe and effective procedure for limb lengthening and deformity correction. LAP reduces the patient's time spent in external fixation by substituting a plate during all or part of the consolidation phase. This technique also helps protect against refracture after frame removal. The distal femoral plates are quite strong, which allows plate insertion soon after the end of distraction. The tibial plates are less strong and require more advanced bony healing before plate insertion. Currently, my colleagues and I use tibial LAP to moderately decrease the time spent in external fixation and to prevent refracture. We do not substitute the plate immediately at the end of the

FIGURE 3

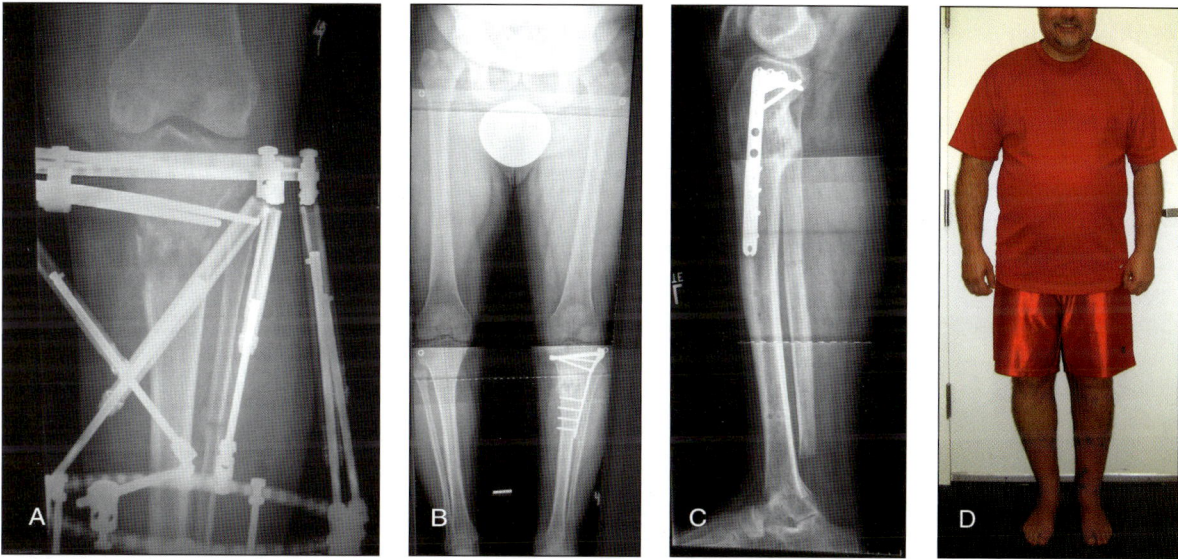

Images of a 46-year-old man with an infected pilon fracture who underwent ankle fusion with a circular frame and proximal tibial lengthening using the LAP technique. Total external fixation time was 6 months. **A,** AP radiograph obtained at the end of distraction shows 3.5-cm lengthening. AP (**B**) and lateral (**C**) weight-bearing radiographs and clinical photograph (**D**) obtained 3 months after plating.

distraction phase; rather, we wait until the regenerate bone healing has progressed to a reasonable degree. Most recently, we have used a custom-made tibial plate that is 2 mm wider and thicker than the standard plate. We also have removed the plate holes adjacent to the regenerate bone.

LENGTHENING OVER A NAIL

LON has been used in both the femur and the tibia to decrease the time spent in external fixation and to prevent refracture. At the initial surgery, an osteotomy is performed and the intramedullary nail is inserted and locked proximally. Then, the external fixator is applied so there is no contact between the internal and external fixation devices (**Figure 4**). The external fixator lengthens the bone over the intramedullary nail. Once distraction is complete, the intramedullary nail is locked distally and the frame is removed.

Surgical Technique
In preparation for LON in the femur, a custom-made intramedullary nail is ordered. The length and diame-ter are determined by the preoperative radiographs. The intramedullary canal is measured at its smallest point, which becomes the intramedullary nail diameter, typically 9, 10, or 11 mm in diameter. The intramedullary nail is straight, with no sagittal bow, and has a uniform diameter throughout (including the proximal part). The intramedullary nail should fill the canal but not be too tight.

The patient is positioned on a radiolucent table with fluoroscopic access to the entire femur. A bump is placed under the buttock to tilt the pelvis 15°, which facilitates AP and lateral views of the hip. The osteotomy site is chosen. If a femoral deformity exists, the osteotomy is performed at the apex of the anterior bow as seen on a lateral view. In addition, the migration of the distal nail that will occur with lengthening must be calculated to ensure that adequate intramedullary nail remains in the distal fragment. The osteotomy site is approached in a percutaneous fashion through a 1-cm stab incision. Multiple holes are drilled at varying angles in the axial plane in a transverse fashion. This first step of the osteotomy also serves to vent the femoral canal during

FIGURE 4

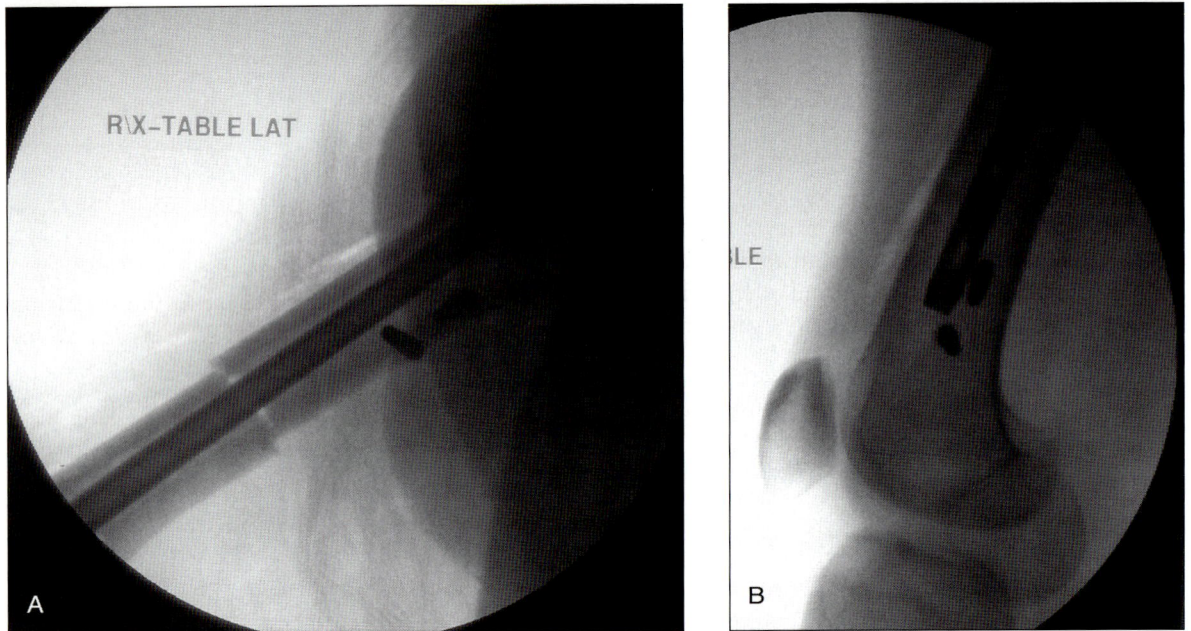

Lateral fluoroscopic views obtained during a lengthening over a nail (LON) procedure show the two proximal (**A**) and the two distal (**B**) femoral pins placed posterior to the intramedullary nail. Note that the pins make no contact with the nail.

reaming. In addition, the reamings exude through these holes and serve as bone graft. Next, the entry site at the piriformis fossa is approached in a percutaneous fashion using a Steinmann pin; the hip is adducted with the patella facing upward. The pin is inserted into the femoral intramedullary canal. A 3-cm incision is made over the pin, and a 10-mm cannulated drill is used to open the entry site into the canal. Next, the beaded guidewire is inserted into the canal and flexible reamers are used sequentially to prepare the canal. The canal is reamed 2 mm larger than the intramedullary nail to be inserted so that the nail will slide through the distal segment.

The intramedullary nail is then inserted up to the osteotomy location and the guidewire is pulled back to this point. The osteotomy is completed with an osteotome, and the guidewire and then the intramedullary nail are passed into the distal segment. Femoral rotation is carefully monitored; correction can

be performed at this time if a deformity exists. A jig is used to insert the proximal locking screw, and the jig is then removed.

A rail frame is then applied to the thigh parallel to the intramedullary nail in both the coronal and sagittal planes. External fixation pins are placed posterior to the intramedullary nail using cannulated wire technique (**Figure 4**). The first external fixator pin is inserted both perpendicular and posterior to the intramedullary nail at the level of the lesser trochanter, carefully avoiding contact between the internal and external fixation devices. The rail frame is applied to the pin and is used as a guide for inserting the most distal pin. One additional pin is inserted into the proximal and distal pin clamps. Usually, two 6-mm hydroxyapatite-coated half pins are used in both the proximal and distal segments. The pins and the bone around the intramedullary nail are rotated to confirm that the osteotomy is complete, and the rail frame is reapplied. Distraction is started on postoperative day 5, at a rate of 1 mm/d. Radiographs obtained after about 1 week of distraction are evaluated to confirm separation of the osteotomy site. The rate of distraction can be increased if necessary.

At the end of distraction, the patient is returned to the operating room for insertion of locking screws into the distal aspect of the intramedullary nail and frame removal. The frame is prepared into the surgical field and the pin sites are covered with antiseptic-soaked sponges. The frame is covered with towels, carefully avoiding contact between internal and external fixation. Using a freehand technique, two interlocking screws are inserted into the distal aspect of the intramedullary nail under fluoroscopic guidance. The external fixator is removed (**Figure 5**).

Clinical Results

Paley et al[12] reported on 29 patients (32 femora) who had undergone femoral LON, with the nail and the external fixator applied concomitantly at the time of the femoral osteotomy. After gradual distraction at a rate of 1 mm/d, the nail was locked and the fixator was removed. The mean patient age was 26 years (range, 10 to 53 years), and the mean lengthening was 5.8 cm (range, 2 to 13 cm). For comparison, 31 patients (32 limbs) who had undergone standard Ilizarov femoral lengthening were matched with the group that had undergone LON. The matching was based on the amount of lengthening, the age of the patient, the etiology of the deficiency, and the difficulty level of the procedure. LON reduced the average duration of external fixation by almost one half. The radiographic consolidation index (the number of months needed for radiographic consolidation for each centimeter of lengthening) for the limbs that had undergone LON was reduced significantly ($P < 0.001$) compared with that for the matched-case group. Knee range of motion returned to normal at a mean rate of 2.2 times faster in the group that had undergone LON. Six refractures of the distracted bone occurred in the matched-case group. In the group that had undergone LON, one nail and one proximal locking screw failed. Paley et al concluded that the advantages of LON include a decrease in the duration of external fixation, protection against refracture, and earlier rehabilitation.

Kocaoglu et al[17] reported on a combined technique of fixator-assisted nailing and LON for the treatment of femoral deformities associated with shortening. They reported on 28 femora in 25 patients with a median age of 27 years underwent reconstruction with an intramedullary nail and a unilateral fixator. The mean shortening was 6.33 cm, and the mean preoperative mechanical axis deviation was 33.86 mm. Deformity correction was performed acutely and secured by the intramedullary nail, which was locked distally. The same external fixator was used for both the deformity correction and the lengthening. At the end of the distraction period, proximal locking screws were placed in the intramedullary nail and the external fixator was removed. The mean duration of external fixation was 83.29 days, the mean external fixation index was 14.98 d/cm, the mean lengthening was 6.02 cm, the mean mechanical axis deviation at the end of the treatment was 11.29 mm, and the mean bone healing index was 36.66 d/cm. Kocaoglu et al concluded that femoral lengthening and deformity correction can be achieved with classic methods for application of an external fixator, but the long period of external fixation, patient discomfort, and plastic deformation of the regenerate bone after fixator removal are major disadvantages. With the combined techniques, the external fixation duration was reduced compared with that required for classic treatment with an external fixator and patient comfort was increased. In addition, the intramedullary nail prevented fracture and deformation of the regenerate bone.

The LON technique does have certain inherent limitations, mainly in the concurrent use of internal and external fixation.[16,18] Song et al[18] reported a 14% rate of deep infection after LON. Kocaoglu et al[16] reported on 42 segments (35 femora and 7 tibias) lengthened in 35 patients with a mean patient age of 26.6 years, a mean lengthening of 6.3 cm (range, 2.5 to 11.5 cm), a mean external fixation index of 18.7 d/cm, and a mean lengthening index of 31.2 d/cm. Eighteen complications occurred in 16 (38%) of the 42 segments, for a complication rate of 0.43 per segment. Sixteen of the complications required additional surgical intervention. Kocaoglu et al concluded that LON provides increased patient comfort and reduces the external fixation period. If the problems encountered are treated aggressively, treatment results can be quite satisfactory.

FIGURE 5

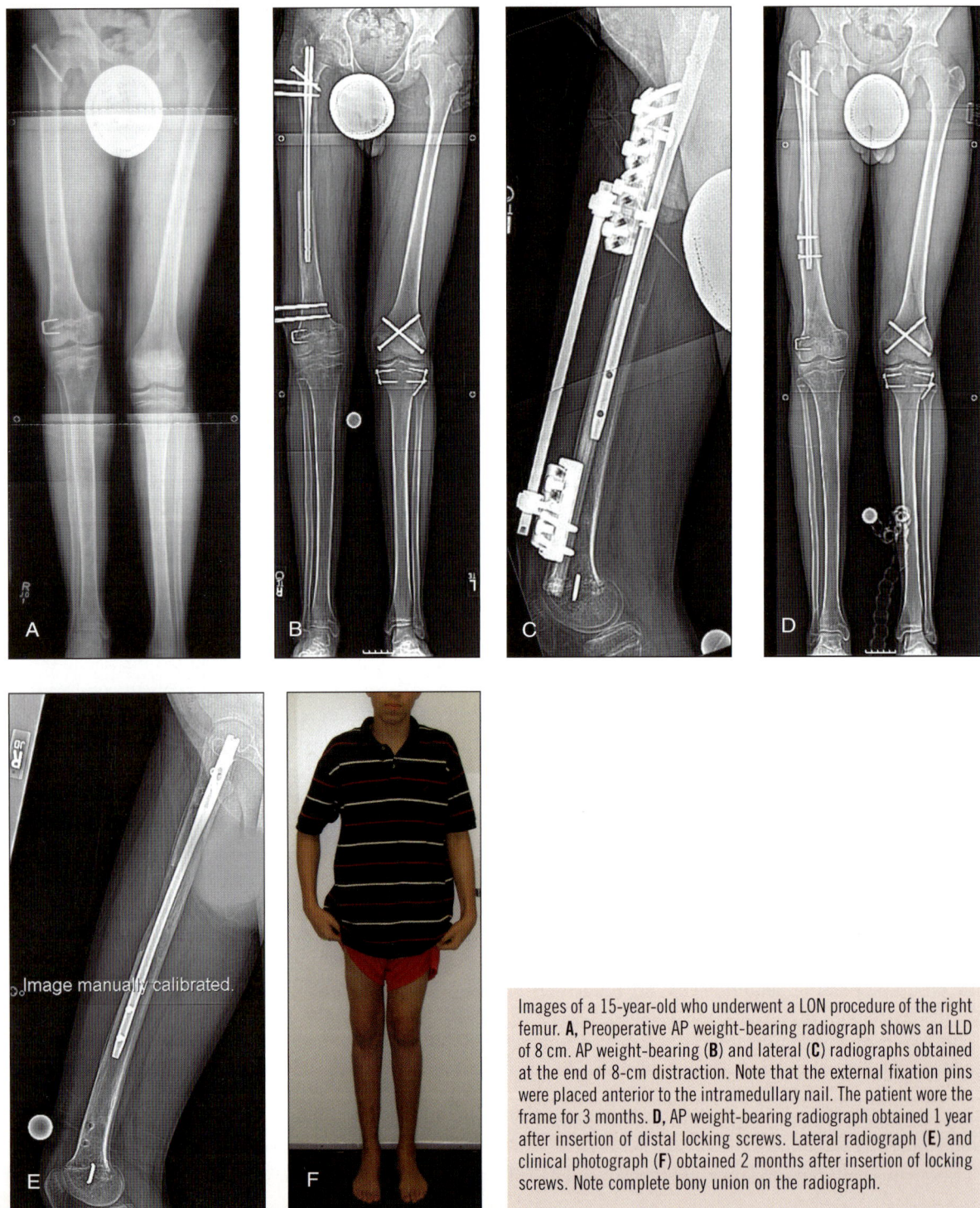

Images of a 15-year-old who underwent a LON procedure of the right femur. **A,** Preoperative AP weight-bearing radiograph shows an LLD of 8 cm. AP weight-bearing (**B**) and lateral (**C**) radiographs obtained at the end of 8-cm distraction. Note that the external fixation pins were placed anterior to the intramedullary nail. The patient wore the frame for 3 months. **D,** AP weight-bearing radiograph obtained 1 year after insertion of distal locking screws. Lateral radiograph (**E**) and clinical photograph (**F**) obtained 2 months after insertion of locking screws. Note complete bony union on the radiograph.

REFERENCES

1. Fischgrund J, Paley D, Suter C: Variables affecting time to bone healing during limb lengthening. *Clin Orthop Relat Res* 1994(301):31-37.

2. Ilizarov GA: *Transosseous Osteosynthesis.* Berlin, Germany, Springer-Verlag, 1992.

3. Ilizarov GA: Clinical application of the tension-stress effect for limb lengthening. *Clin Orthop Relat Res* 1990(250):8-26.

4. Pinzur MS: Use of platelet-rich concentrate and bone marrow aspirate in high-risk patients with Charcot arthropathy of the foot. *Foot Ankle Int* 2009;30(2):124-127.

5. Pugh K, Rozbruch SR: Nonunions and malunions, in Baumgaertner MR, Tornetta P, eds: *Orthopaedic Knowledge Update: Trauma,* ed 3. Rosemont, IL, American Academy of Orthopaedic Surgeons, 2005, pp 115-130.

6. Rozbruch SR, Paley D, Bhave A, Herzenberg JE: Ilizarov hip reconstruction for the late sequelae of infantile hip infection. *J Bone Joint Surg Am* 2005;87(5):1007-1018.

7. Rozbruch SR, Fragomen AT, Ilizarov S: Correction of tibial deformity with use of the Ilizarov-Taylor spatial frame. *J Bone Joint Surg Am* 2006;88(Suppl 4):156-174.

8. Nho SJ, Helfet DL, Rozbruch SR: Temporary intentional leg shortening and deformation to facilitate wound closure using the Ilizarov/Taylor spatial frame. *J Orthop Trauma* 2006;20(6):419-424.

9. Rozbruch SR, Ilizarov S, Blyakher A: Knee arthrodesis with simultaneous lengthening using the Ilizarov method. *J Orthop Trauma* 2005;19(3):171-179.

10. Rozbruch SR, Weitzman AM, Watson JT, Freudigman P, Katz HV, Ilizarov S: Simultaneous treatment of tibial bone and soft-tissue defects with the Ilizarov method. *J Orthop Trauma* 2006;20(3):197-205.

11. Rozbruch SR, Pugsley JS, Fragomen AT, Ilizarov S: Repair of tibial nonunions and bone defects with the Taylor Spatial Frame. *J Orthop Trauma* 2008;22(2):88-95.

12. Paley D, Herzenberg JE, Paremain G, Bhave A: Femoral lengthening over an intramedullary nail: A matched-case comparison with Ilizarov femoral lengthening. *J Bone Joint Surg Am* 1997;79(10):1464-1480.

13. O'Carrigan T, Paley D, Herzenberg JE: Obstacles in limb lengthening: Fractures, in Rozbruch SR, Ilizarov S, eds: *Limb Lengthening and Reconstruction Surgery.* New York, NY, Informa Healthcare, 2007, pp 675-679.

14. Simpson AH, Kenwright J: Fracture after distraction osteogenesis. *J Bone Joint Surg Br* 2000;82(5):659-665.

15. Rozbruch SR, Kleinman D, Fragomen AT, Ilizarov S: Limb lengthening and then insertion of an intramedullary nail: A case-matched comparison. *Clin Orthop Relat Res* 2008;466(12):2923-2932.

16. Kocaoglu M, Eralp L, Kilicoglu O, Burc H, Cakmak M: Complications encountered during lengthening over an intramedullary nail. *J Bone Joint Surg Am* 2004;86-A(11):2406-2411.

17. Kocaoglu M, Eralp L, Bilen FE, Balci HI: Fixator-assisted acute femoral deformity correction and consecutive lengthening over an intramedullary nail. *J Bone Joint Surg Am* 2009;91(1):152-159.

18. Song HR, Oh CW, Mattoo R, et al: Femoral lengthening over an intramedullary nail using the external fixator: Risk of infection and knee problems in 22 patients with a follow-up of 2 years or more. *Acta Orthop* 2005;76(2):245-252.

19. Iobst CA, Dahl MT: Limb lengthening with submuscular plate stabilization: A case series and description of the technique. *J Pediatr Orthop* 2007;27(5):504-509.

20. Cole JD, Justin D, Kasparis T, DeVlught D, Knobloch C: The intramedullary skeletal kinetic distractor (ISKD): First clinical results of a new intramedullary nail for lengthening of the femur and tibia. *Injury* 2001;32(Suppl 4):129-139.

21. Claes L, Willie B: The enhancement of bone regeneration by ultrasound. *Prog Biophys Mol Biol* 2007;93(1-3):384-398.

22. El-Mowafi H, Mohsen M: The effect of low-intensity pulsed ultrasound on callus maturation in tibial distraction osteogenesis. *Int Orthop* 2005;29(2):121-124.

23. Malizos KN, Hantes ME, Protopappas V, Papachristos A: Low-intensity pulsed ultrasound for bone healing: An overview. *Injury* 2006;37(Suppl 1):S56-S62.

24. Tsumaki N, Kakiuchi M, Sasaki J, Ochi T, Yoshikawa H: Low-intensity pulsed ultrasound accelerates maturation of callus in patients treated with opening-wedge high tibial osteotomy by hemicallotasis. *J Bone Joint Surg Am* 2004;86-A(11):2399-2405.

25. Ceballos A, Pereda O, Ortega R, Balmaseda R: Electrically-induced osteogenesis in external fixation treatment. *Acta Orthop Belg* 1991;57(2):102-108.

26. Kawamoto K, Kim WC, Tsuchida Y, et al: Effects of alternating current electrical stimulation on lengthening callus. *J Pediatr Orthop B* 2005;14(4):299-302.

27. Nishimoto S, Oyama T, Matsuda K: Simultaneous concentration of platelets and marrow cells: A simple and useful technique to obtain source cells and growth factors for regenerative medicine. *Wound Repair Regen* 2007;15(1):156-162.

28. Jäger M, Jelinek EM, Wess KM, et al: Bone marrow concentrate: A novel strategy for bone defect treatment. *Curr Stem Cell Res Ther* 2009;4(1):34-43.

29. Aleksyniene R, Eckardt H, Bundgaard K, Lind M, Hvid I: Effects of parathyroid hormone on newly regenerated bone during distraction osteogenesis in a rabbit tibial lengthening model: A pilot study. *Medicina (Kaunas)* 2006;42(1):38-48.

30. Black MT, Munn JG, Allsop AE: On the catalytic mechanism of prokaryotic leader peptidase 1. *Biochem J* 1992;282(Pt 2):539-543.

31. Chalidis B, Tzioupis C, Tsiridis E, Giannoudis PV: Enhancement of fracture healing with parathyroid hormone: Preclinical studies and potential clinical applications. *Expert Opin Investig Drugs* 2007;16(4):441-449.

32. Kiely P, Ward K, Bellemore CM, Briody J, Cowell CT, Little DG: Bisphosphonate rescue in distraction osteogenesis: A case series. *J Pediatr Orthop* 2007;27(4):467-471.

33. Little DG, Smith NC, Williams PR, et al: Zoledronic acid prevents osteopenia and increases bone strength in a rabbit model of distraction osteogenesis. *J Bone Miner Res* 2003;18(7):1300-1307.

34. Little DG, Kiely P: Enhancements of regenerate bone healing, in Rozbruch S, Ilizarov S, eds: *Limb Lengthening and Reconstruction Surgery.* New York, NY, Informa Healthcare, 2007, pp 53-67.

35. Taylor JC: Taylor spatial frame, in Rozbruch S, Ilizarov S, eds: *Limb Lengthening and Reconstruction Surgery.* New York, NY, Informa Healthcare, 2007, pp 613-637.

MONITORING OF REGENERATE BONE

INTRODUCTION

One of the most elusive components of limb lengthening using external fixators is the timing of fixator removal. Although prolonged fixator time may allow the regenerate bone to mature, this is associated with a psychologic burden for the patient,[1] adjacent-bone osteopenia,[2] persistent pain,[3] and pin-tract infections;[4] thus, surgeons are motivated to decrease the time a patient spends in the fixator. The danger is that the fixator may be removed prematurely, which may result in the dreaded complication of bending or fracture. The formation of good regenerate bone to allow fixator removal is directly linked to the rate of lengthening.[5] Monitoring the regenerate bone during the lengthening procedure is as vital as assessing the regenerate bone before fixator removal.

MONITORING DURING DISTRACTION

Ilizarov's[5] seminal paper on the tension-stress effect on the rate and frequency of distraction revealed that regenerate bone formation requires an optimal rate of distraction. He found that slower rates are associated with premature consolidation and faster rates are associated with poor regenerate bone formation. The frequency of distraction usually is four times per day, and typically, the optimal distraction rate is 1 mm/d; however, this distraction rate can be altered depending on the quality of the newly formed regenerate.

Assessment of the newly formed regenerate is difficult during the early stages of lengthening because the calcification of the osteoid that forms in the distraction gap usually is not evident for a couple of weeks. Ultrasonography has been advocated for early detection of callus formation and/or defects,[6,7] but it is useful only during the first few weeks of lengthening.[6] After this early period, standard radiography is the primary method of regenerate bone assessment. Donnan et al[8] described a classification of regenerate bone based on the shape, polarity, and consistency of the regenerate; unfortunately, clear outcome predictions could not be discerned, perhaps partly because of the small sample size ($n = 30$) in their study. Li et al[9] described a regenerate classification based on callus shape and radiographic features (pattern and density). They demonstrated fair to moderate interobserver and intraobserver agreement for identifying the various callus shapes and types. Although the callus types described by Li et al provide insight into osteogenesis, the classification is not widely used, likely because of its complexity. Nonetheless, a simplified version of this classification can be used to guide distraction rates to optimize regenerate bone formation. Our modified Li classifica-

Dr. Saran or an immediate family member has received research or institutional support from Stryker. Neither Dr. Hamdy nor any member of his immediate family has received anything of value from or owns stock in a commercial company or institution related directly or indirectly to the subject of this chapter.

FIGURE 1

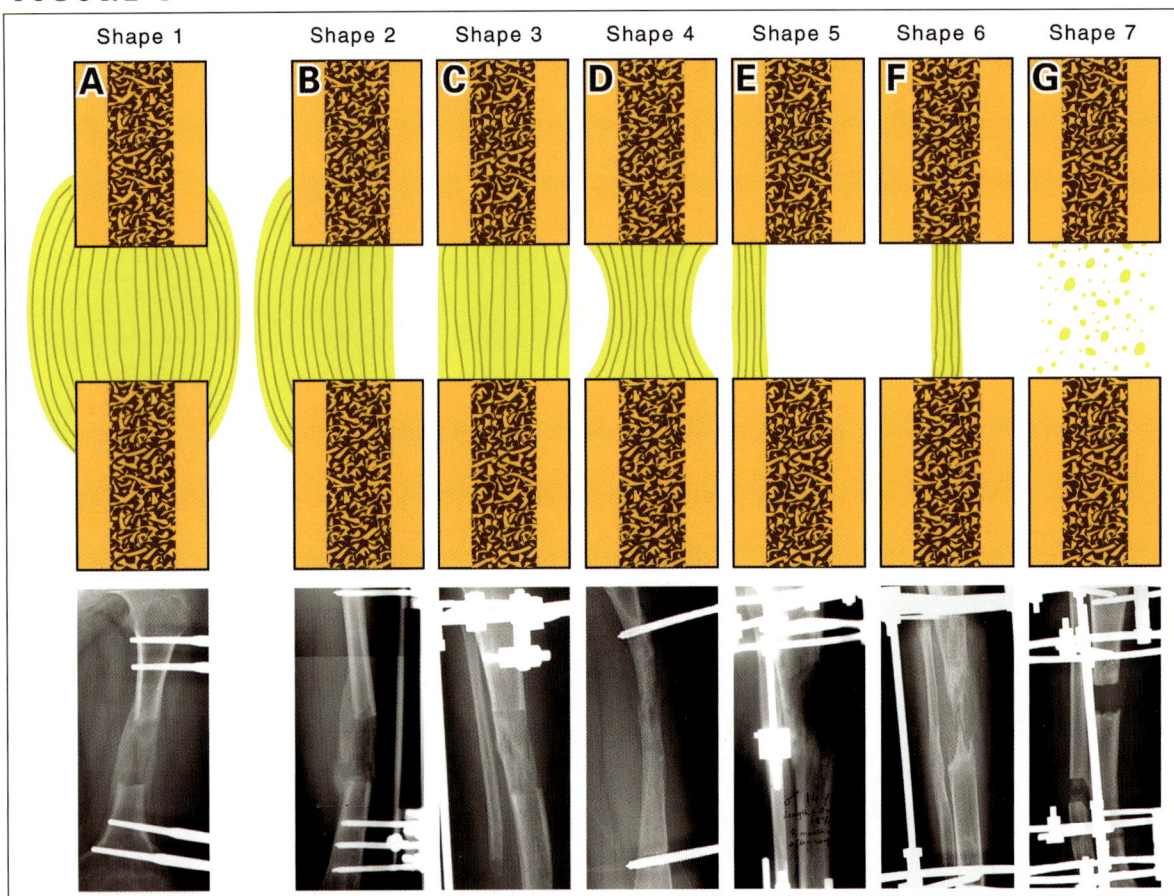

Illustrations and radiographs demonstrate the modified Li classification of callus shape in healing regenerate bone. **A,** Shape 1 regenerate: New bone is seen throughout the distraction gap and extends beyond the outer borders of the adjacent cortical bone. **B,** Shape 2 regenerate: New bone is seen toward one side of the distraction gap with extension beyond the outer borders of the adjacent cortical bone. **C,** Shape 3 regenerate: Fusiform new bone formation is seen throughout the distraction gap with margins parallel to the adjacent cortical bone. **D,** Shape 4 regenerate: A spindle- or biconcave-shaped regenerate is seen. **E,** Shape 5 regenerate: One-sided bone formation is seen without extension beyond the outer borders of the adjacent cortical bone. **F,** Shape 6 regenerate: A central regenerate has formed, with limited new bone formation in the lateral portions of the distraction gap, representing a severe spindle-shaped regenerate. **G,** Shape 7 regenerate: Only speckled bone formation is present.

tion includes seven callus shapes (**Figure 1**). Shapes 1 through 3 show satisfactory regenerate bone that should heal without sequelae. Shape 4 suggests that the rate of distraction is too fast. Shapes 5 through 7 are examples of poorly formed regenerate that may require bone enhancement before fixator removal to minimize complications such as bending or fracture of the regenerate after fixator removal.

MONITORING FOR FIXATOR REMOVAL
Mechanical Testing

The ideal method to determine when to remove the fixator would be a quick and easy biomechanical test that would indicate when a threshold level of regenerate bone stiffness has been achieved such that bending or fracture will not occur after fixator removal. Richardson et al[10] assessed sagittal plane stiffness in patients with tibial fractures treated with external fixation. They found that no patients with stiffness greater than 10 Nm/degree at the time of fixator removal experienced refracture. Using a safety margin of 50%, they suggested a stiffness of 15 Nm/degree as a safe cutoff for fixator removal in adults with tibial fractures treated by external fixation. In a follow-up study using this criterion, Richardson et al[11] reported no refractures in 95 patients. Wade et al[12] reported four malunions in 76 patients aged 13 to 87 years when using the same guidelines. Dwyer et al[13] reported on 15 femoral and 15 tibial lengthenings in patients aged 13 to 29 years. They reported two tibial failures (both at 1 Nm/degree) and one femoral failure (19.2 Nm/degree); however, no regenerate fractures occurred in patients with sagittal tibial stiffness of at least 15 Nm/degree and sagittal femoral stiffness of at least 20 Nm/degree, and suggested these as the safe threshold levels for frame removal. Chotel et al[14] studied stiffness in 11 patients aged 5.5 to 16.7 years who had undergone limb lengthening before an osteotomy. Chotel et al showed that the normal stiffness of tibias and femora was quite variable, and they recommended that adult threshold levels were inappropriate for children undergoing lengthenings. Because of the variability of stiffness seen in children, guidelines that have been evaluated and validated are required before in vivo mechanical testing can be recommended as a safe method for determining when to remove the fixator in limb lengthening.

Standard Radiography

Fischgrund et al[15] described a method using standard radiography to determine when to remove the fixator in patients undergoing distraction osteogenesis. The authors maintained a low fracture rate of 3% after fixator removal using this method, which requires at least three uninterrupted 2-mm-thick cortices to have formed across the distraction gap before fixator removal is allowed (**Figure 2**). Although this remains the primary method of regenerate bone assessment for fixator removal, a reliability study by Starr et al[16] showed that this technique is highly subjective. Starr et al reported that interobserver (0.127) and intraobserver (0.290) coefficients for the number of cortices were only slightly better than chance, and interobserver (0.352) and intraobserver (0.461) coefficients for whether to remove

FIGURE 2

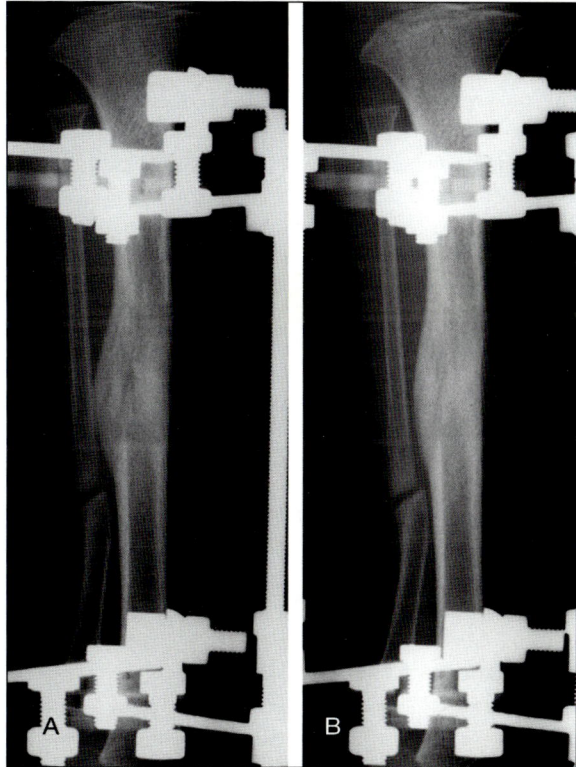

AP radiographs of a lengthened tibia show healing of the regenerate bone 1 month before (**A**) and immediately before (**B**) frame removal. The current standard is to remove the fixator when at least three 2-mm-thick cortices are seen on orthogonal views. Unfortunately, determination of neocorticalization of the regenerate is highly variable. Although the regenerate bone was developing nicely 1 month before frame removal and may have been adequate for frame removal, we were reluctant to define the medial and lateral new bone as cortices at this time.

the fixator based on the number of cortices were only fair to moderately better than chance. Several other methods, including dual-energy x-ray absorptiometry (DEXA), quantitative CT, and pixel value ratios (PVRs), have been proposed to provide more objective measures of this subjective determination.

Dual-Energy X-ray Absorptiometry

DEXA scanning is a method used to determine bone mineral content (BMC) and bone mineral density

(BMD). In a sheep study by Reichel et al,[17] the biomechanical strength of lengthened tibias was correlated with BMD, suggesting that BMD could be used as a surrogate for biomechanical strength. Similarly, clinical studies have shown that stiffness of regenerate correlates with BMC.[18,19] Saran and Hamdy[20] evaluated 26 patients who underwent 28 lengthenings using DEXA to determine appropriate removal of the fixator. In this study,[20] the fixator was removed when the BMD, as measured on monthly DEXA scans, had plateaued to an increase of less than 10% and the plain radiographs did not reveal any major defects or transverse lucencies in the regenerate bone. Using these criteria, the fracture rate after fixator removal (3.6%) and the average bone healing index (47 days/cm) were maintained at acceptable rates. Our opinion is that although DEXA may provide an objective measure to help determine timing for fixator removal, it can be used only as an adjunct to plain radiography because DEXA currently does not account for bone defects that may predispose regenerate bone to bending or fracture.

Quantitative CT

Quantitative CT provides densitometric data for cortical and trabecular bone by comparing tissue densities with standardized reference data through linear attenuation coefficients.[21] Multiple studies have shown that quantitative CT measurements correlate with biomechanical regenerate stiffness as seen in the BMD and BMC measurements obtained from DEXA scans.[22-25] An animal model comparison study by Markel and Chao[23] revealed that although quantitative CT had a stronger correlation with torsional stiffness and torque than DEXA, the difference between the two techniques was not significant. Aronson and Shin[25] compared multiple imaging modalities, including quantitative CT, with histologic and mechanical properties in a series of 65 unilateral canine tibial lengthenings and found that quantitative CT correlated with mechanical strength of newly formed bone. Quantitative CT provides the user with a high-resolution assessment of regenerate structure as well as densitometric data, which, when used together, may help derive an objective criterion for fixator removal. Although quantitative CT has great potential, it is used infrequently in clinical practice because objective criteria for fixator removal using this technique are not yet defined and evaluated. Additionally, higher costs, limited availability, and higher relative radiation doses further preclude its widespread use.

Pixel Value Ratio

Shim et al[26] described a technique using the pixel value from digital radiographs that were obtained during usual monitoring of the regenerate bone to provide valuable information about bone density changes (**Figure 3**). They noted that the pixel value changed in a sigmoid curve pattern while the patient was in the fixator and that the relative pixel value was greater than 95% in three of four cortices at the time of fixator removal. Hazra et al[27] found that PVR correlated well with BMD ratio (Pearson correlation coefficient = 0.79) in patients undergoing tibial lengthening. Zhao et al[28] evaluated a PVR guideline for fixator removal in patients undergoing lengthening over an intramedullary nail and reported no nail or screw breakage and no refractures. Pixel values were determined on AP and lateral views of the anterior, posterior, medial, and lateral areas of each tibia. Each of the four areas was represented as an average pixel value by calculating the mean value of the proximal and distal segments. These values were then compared with the pixel value of the adjacent bone, and the resultant value was called the PVR. When the PVR was equal to 1, the corticalization of the regenerate area was considered similar to that of the adjacent bone. Values less than 1 represent less-mature regenerate bone. Partial weight bearing with crutches was allowed when two cortices had a PVR of 1, and full weight bearing without crutches was permitted when three cortices had a PVR of 1. The utility of these guidelines for standard distraction osteogenesis is unknown because of the use of intramedullary nails. Furthermore, whereas the correlation of biomechanical stiffness with BMD and BMC has been scientifically shown,[17-19] no direct correlation has been determined; therefore, the correlation between PVR and strength of regenerate bone remains somewhat hypothetical. Nonetheless, PVR seems to be a promising new noninvasive assessment tool that is readily available through most picture archiving and communication systems. With further work and guideline testing, the PVR method potentially can be used as widely as standard radiography for determining the timing of fixator removal.

FIGURE 3

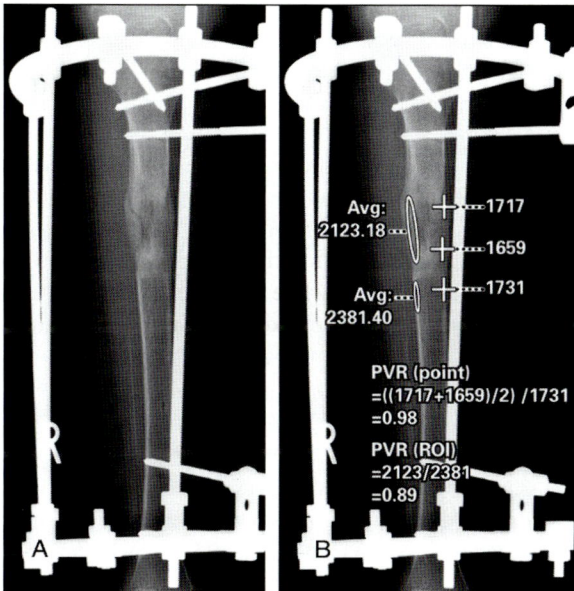

Digital AP radiographs of a lengthened tibia obtained before frame removal before (**A**) and after (**B**) pixel values of the neocortical regions of the distraction gap were added. Point pixel values (+) or average (Avg) pixel values in a region of interest (ROI), represented by the ellipses (...), can be determined using most picture archiving and communication systems used for digital radiography. These values then can be used to create a pixel value ratio (PVR). The point PVR was calculated by comparing the pixel values of the neocortical bone with the adjacent cortical bone using pixel values, and the PVR of the ROI was calculated using the average pixel value of the ROI. As the PVR of regenerate bone to adjacent cortex nears 1, the bone mineral density and biomechanical strength of the regenerate bone is thought to approximate that of the adjacent bone. The exact methods used to determine PVRs and criteria for frame removal based on these values are not yet determined.

CONCLUSION

Appropriate timing for fixator removal after distraction osteogenesis continues to be a challenging component of limb lengthening. Current standard practice dictates that the fixator be removed when three of four cortices have formed on AP and lateral radiographs. In vivo mechanical testing, DEXA, quantitative CT, and PVR all have been suggested as possible adjuncts to help in this decision-making process, but standard radiography remains the primary method. As guidelines for its use are better defined, the PVR method may become more widely used.

REFERENCES

1. Eldridge JC, Bell DF: Problems with substantial limb lengthening. *Orthop Clin North Am* 1991;22(4): 625-631.

2. Cattermole HC, Cook JE, Fordham JN, Muckle DS, Cunningham JL: Bone mineral changes during tibial fracture healing. *Clin Orthop Relat Res* 1997(339): 190-196.

3. García-Cimbrelo E, Olsen B, Ruiz-Yagüe M, Fernandez-Baíllo N, Munuera-Martínez L: Ilizarov technique: Results and difficulties. *Clin Orthop Relat Res* 1992(283):116-123.

4. Velazquez RJ, Bell DF, Armstrong PF, Babyn P, Tibshirani R: Complications of use of the Ilizarov technique in the correction of limb deformities in children. *J Bone Joint Surg Am* 1993;75(8):1148-1156.

5. Ilizarov GA: The tension-stress effect on the genesis and growth of tissues: Part II. The influence of the rate and frequency of distraction. *Clin Orthop Relat Res* 1989(239):263-285.

6. Hamdy RC, Walsh W, Olmedo M, Wallach M, Ehrlich MG: Correlation between ultrasound imaging and mechanical and physical properties of lengthened bone: An experimental study in a canine model. *J Pediatr Orthop* 1995;15(2):206-211.

7. Hughes TH, Maffulli N, Green V, Fixsen JA: Imaging in bone lengthening: A review. *Clin Orthop Relat Res* 1994(308):50-53.

8. Donnan LT, Saleh M, Rigby AS, McAndrew A: Radiographic assessment of bone formation in tibia during distraction osteogenesis. *J Pediatr Orthop* 2002;22(5): 645-651.

9. Li R, Saleh M, Yang L, Coulton L: Radiographic classification of osteogenesis during bone distraction. *J Orthop Res* 2006;24(3):339-347.

10. Richardson JB, Kenwright J, Cunningham JL: Fracture stiffness measurement in the assessment and management of tibial fractures. *Clin Biomech (Bristol, Avon)* 1992;7(2):75-79.

11. Richardson JB, Cunningham JL, Goodship AE, O'Connor BT, Kenwright J: Measuring stiffness can define healing of tibial fractures. *J Bone Joint Surg Br* 1994;76(3):389-394.

12. Wade RH, Moorcroft CI, Thomas PB: Fracture stiffness as a guide to the management of tibial fractures. *J Bone Joint Surg Br* 2001;83(4):533-535.

13. Dwyer JS, Owen PJ, Evans GA, Kuiper JH, Richardson JB: Stiffness measurements to assess healing during leg lengthening: A preliminary report. *J Bone Joint Surg Br* 1996;78(2):286-289.

14. Chotel F, Braillon P, Sailhan F, et al: Bone stiffness in children: Part I. In vivo assessment of the stiffness of femur and tibia in children. *J Pediatr Orthop* 2008; 28(5):534-537.

15. Fischgrund J, Paley D, Suter C: Variables affecting time to bone healing during limb lengthening. *Clin Orthop Relat Res* 1994(301):31-37.

16. Starr KA, Fillman R, Raney EM: Reliability of radiographic assessment of distraction osteogenesis site. *J Pediatr Orthop* 2004;24(1):26-29.

17. Reichel H, Lebek S, Alter C, Hein W: Biomechanical and densitometric bone properties after callus distraction in sheep. *Clin Orthop Relat Res* 1998(357):237-246.

18. Tselentakis G, Owen PJ, Richardson JB, et al: Fracture stiffness in callotasis determined by dual-energy X-ray absorptiometry scanning. *J Pediatr Orthop B* 2001; 10(3):248-254.

19. Chotel F, Braillon P, Sailhan F, et al: Bone stiffness in children: Part II. Objectives criteria for children to assess healing during leg lengthening. *J Pediatr Orthop* 2008;28(5):538-543.

20. Saran N, Hamdy RC: DEXA as a predictor of fixator removal in distraction osteogenesis. *Clin Orthop Relat Res* 2008;466(12):2955-2961.

21. Lang TF: Quantitative computed tomography. *Radiol Clin North Am* 2010;48(3):589-600.

22. Harp JH, Aronson J, Hollis M: Noninvasive determination of bone stiffness for distraction osteogenesis by quantitative computed tomography scans. *Clin Orthop Relat Res* 1994(301):42-48.

23. Markel MD, Chao EY: Noninvasive monitoring techniques for quantitative description of callus mineral content and mechanical properties. *Clin Orthop Relat Res* 1993(293):37-45.

24. Markel MD, Morin RL, Wikenheiser MA, Lewallen DG, Chao EY: Quantitative CT for the evaluation of bone healing. *Calcif Tissue Int* 1991;49(6):427-432.

25. Aronson J, Shin HD: Imaging techniques for bone regenerate analysis during distraction osteogenesis. *J Pediatr Orthop* 2003;23(4):550-560.

26. Shim JS, Chung KH, Ahn JM: Value of measuring bone density serial changes on a picture archiving and communication systems (PACS) monitor in distraction osteogenesis. *Orthopedics* 2002;25(11):1269-1272.

27. Hazra S, Song HR, Biswal S, et al: Quantitative assessment of mineralization in distraction osteogenesis. *Skeletal Radiol* 2008;37(9):843-847.

28. Zhao L, Fan Q, Venkatesh KP, Park MS, Song HR: Objective guidelines for removing an external fixator after tibial lengthening using pixel value ratio: A pilot study. *Clin Orthop Relat Res* 2009;467(12):3321-3326.

INDEX